ADVANCES IN

Pharmacology and Chemotherapy

VOLUME 15

ADVISORY BOARD

ADVANCES IN

Pharmacology and Chemotherapy

EDITED BY

Silvio Garattini

Istituto di Ricerche Farmacologiche "Mario Negri"
Milano, Italy

A. Goldin

National Cancer Institute
Bethesda, Maryland

F. Hawking

Commonwealth Institute of Helminthology
St. Albans, Herts., England

I. J. Kopin

National Institute of Mental Health
Bethesda, Maryland

Consulting Editor

R. J. Schnitzer

Mount Sinai School of Medicine
New York, New York

VOLUME 15—1978

ACADEMIC PRESS New York San Francisco London

A Subsidiary of Harcourt Brace Jovanovich, Publishers

ACADEMIC PRESS, INC.
111 Fifth Avenue, New York, New York 10003

United Kingdom Edition published by
ACADEMIC PRESS, INC. (LONDON) LTD.
24/28 Oval Road, London NW1 7DX

LIBRARY OF CONGRESS CATALOG CARD NUMBER: 61–18298

ISBN 0–12–032915–8

PRINTED IN THE UNITED STATES OF AMERICA

CONTENTS

Daunomycin: An Anthracycline Antibiotic Effective in Acute Leukemia

DANIEL D. VON HOFF, MARCEL ROZENCWEIG, AND MILAN SLAVIK

Drug Information Services

CONSTANTINE J. GILLESPIE

Pharmacology and Neurochemistry of Apomorphine

GAETANO DI CHIARA AND GIAN LUIGI GESSA

Structural Requirements for Tetracycline Activity

J. R. BROWN AND D. S. IRELAND

Neurotransmitter Mechanisms during Mental Illness Induced by Alterations in Thyroid Function

RADHEY L. SINGHAL AND RAM B. RASTOGI

Immune Modulation and Cancer Control

STANISLAW M. MIKULSKI, MICHAEL A. CHIRIGOS, AND FRANCO M. MUGGIA

Suramin: With Special Reference to Onchocerciasis

F. HAWKING

CONTRIBUTORS TO THIS VOLUME

Numbers in parentheses indicate the pages on which the authors' contributions begin.

J. R. BROWN (161), *Department of Pharmacy, University of Manchester, Manchester, England*

GAETANO DI CHIARA (87), *Institute of Pharmacology, University of Cagliari, Cagliari, Italy*

MICHAEL A. CHIRIGOS (263), *Viral Oncology Program, National Cancer Institute, National Institutes of Health, Bethesda, Maryland*

GIAN LUIGI GESSA (87), *Institute of Pharmacology, University of Cagliari, Cagliari, Italy*

CONSTANTINE J. GILLESPIE (51), *Library, National Institutes of Health, Bethesda, Maryland*

F. HAWKING (289), *The Commonwealth Institute of Helminthology, St. Albans, England*

D. S. IRELAND* (161), *Department of Pharmacy, University of Manchester, Manchester, England*

STANISLAW M. MIKULSKI (263), *Cancer Therapy Evaluation Program, National Cancer Institute, National Institutes of Health, Bethesda, Maryland*

FRANCO M. MUGGIA (263), *Cancer Therapy Evaluation Program, National Cancer Institute, National Institutes of Health, Bethesda, Maryland*

RAM B. RASTOGI† (203), *Department of Pharmacology, Faculty of Medicine, University of Ottawa, Ottawa, Ontario, Canada*

MARCEL ROZENCWEIG (1), *Investigational Drug Branch, Division of Cancer Treatment, National Cancer Institute, National Institutes of Health, Bethesda, Maryland*

* Present address: Fazakerley Hospital, Liverpool, England.

† Present address: Nordic Research Laboratories, Connlab Holdings Limited, Montreal, Quebec, Canada.

RADHEY L. SINGHAL (203), *Department of Pharmacology, Faculty of Medicine, University of Ottawa, Ottawa, Ontario, Canada*

MILAN SLAVIK (1), *Investigational Drug Branch, Division of Cancer Treatment, National Cancer Institute, National Institutes of Health, Bethesda, Maryland*

DANIEL D. VON HOFF (1), *Investigational Drug Branch, Division of Cancer Treatment, National Cancer Institute, National Institutes of Health, Bethesda, Maryland*

Daunomycin: An Anthracycline Antibiotic Effective in Acute Leukemia

DANIEL D. VON HOFF, MARCEL ROZENCWEIG, AND MILAN SLAVIK

Investigational Drug Branch, Division of Cancer Treatment
National Cancer Institute
National Institutes of Health, Bethesda, Maryland

I. Introduction

The Division of Cancer Treatment (DCT) of the National Cancer Institute (NCI) in its drug development function sponsors clinical trials with investigational anticancer drugs. These drugs are gathered from various sources, with about two-thirds coming from the DCT drug-screening program and about one-third from a cooperative drug exchange program conducted throughout the world. Among the interesting anticancer drugs developed abroad is daunomycin, an antitumor antibiotic of the anthracycline group. The drug was isolated in 1963, and in the last 13 years a large amount of preclinical and clinical data has accumulated. This information requires an updated analysis, particularly in light of the fact the drug has shown a substantial amount of activity in acute leukemia refractory to other antileukemic drugs.

II. Chemical and Pharmaceutical Aspects

A. Description

In 1961, Arcamone and his colleagues studied substances isolated from *Streptomyces* cultures that had been obtained from a soil sample from India. These substances had a marked influence on Ehrlich ascites tumors and Sarcoma 180 tumors in mice (Arcamone *et al.,* 1961).

Daunomycin is an antitumor antibiotic of the anthracycline group, which was isolated in the Farmitalia Research Laboratories in Milan, Italy, from cultures of *Streptomyces peucetius* by Grein *et al.* in 1963. The major part of the drug was found in the culture media of the mycelium and was isolated by means of solvent extraction, cation resins, and paper or column chromatography. The yield was 5–15 mg of product per liter of culture media. The soil sample was from Castel del Monte, near Puglie, and hence the name of the species *S. peucetius*.

The drug is classified as an anthracycline and has similar physicochemical characteristics to rhodomycins, cynerubines, pyrromicins, and rutilantines (DiMarco *et al.*, 1964b; Cassinelli and Orezzi, 1963). Other names for the drug include daunorubicin HCl, rubidomycin, rubomycin C, Cerubidine, and NSC 82151.

Daunomycin consists of a pigmented aglycone (daunomycinone) in glycoside linkage with an amino sugar (daunosamine) (DiMarco *et al.*, 1964b); the structure is depicted in Fig. 1. Total synthesis of daunomycin was reported by Acton *et al.* in 1974.

B. Chemical Properties and Structure-Activity Relationship

Chemical properties necessary for identifying daunomycin are listed in Table I.

The structure–activity relationship of daunomycin has been commented on by Zee-Cheng and Cheng (1970). They found a common structural feature was shared by some nonalkylating antileukemic agents such as aminopterin, anthramycin, 5-azacytidine, camptothecin, cytosine arabinoside, emetine, demecolcine, riboside, methotrexate, streptonigrin, vinblastine, vincristine, and daunomycin. This structural feature is a triangulation between 1 nitrogen and 2 oxygen atoms with rather definite interatomic distances. For daunomycin, the N—O—O triangulation pattern is shown in Fig. 2 with the following interatomic distances:

$$N\text{—}O_1 = 7.05\text{–}10.20\ \text{Å}$$

$$N\text{—}O_2 = 8.36\text{–}11.40\ \text{Å}$$

$$O_1\text{—}O_2 = 2.70\ \text{Å}$$

The relationship of this triangulation pattern and antileukemic activity is substantiated by reports that neither the aglycone of daunomycin alone

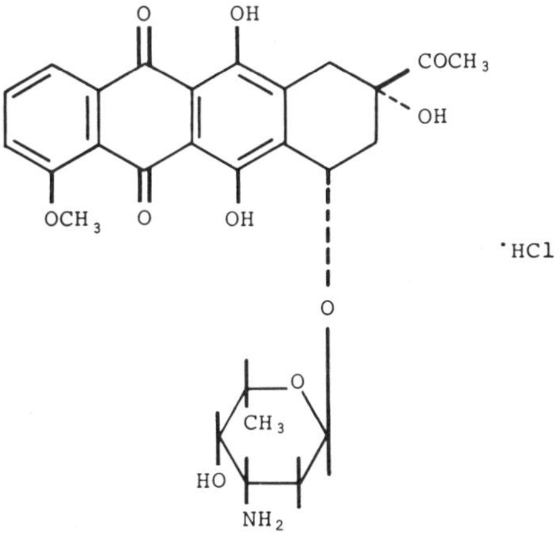

FIG. 1. The structure of daunomycin.

TABLE I

CHEMICAL PROPERTIES OF DAUNOMYCIN

Description
  Red powder or thin red needles
  Melting point, 188°–190°C
  Molecular weight = 563.99 (anhydrous)
The pk_a equals 10.3. The color in aqueous solution varies according to pH of solution: pink at acid pH and blue at alkaline pH.
Elemental composition
  Carbon, 57.5
  Hydrogen, 5.36
  Chlorine, 6.29
  Oxygen, 28.4
Specific rotation
  $[\alpha]_D$ = 253° (reproducibility difficult due to intense color of solution)
Solubility
  In water = 450 mg/ml
  Also soluble in methanol
  Insoluble in chloroform, ether, and benzene
Thin-layer chromatography
  Absorbent—SiO_2
  Solvent system—*sec*-butanol/pyridine/water (1/1/1)
  Detection—visible, UV

(daunomycinone) nor the amino sugar (daunosamine) possesses antileukemic activity.

Other portions of the molecule of daunomycin have been thought to be important for antitumor activity. Daunomycin, adriamycin, rubidazone, and daunomycinone were tested for their ability to inhibit oncornavirus DNA polymerase. All compounds were found to be potent inhibitors of DNA polymerase purified from avian myeloblastosis virus and Rauscher murine leukemia virus. Inhibition was found to be due to the tetracyclic planar ring structure (daunomycine) common to all of these compounds (Schafer and Papas, 1975).

Calendi *et al.* (1965) have found that the amino group of the sugar is necessary for tight binding to the DNA molecule.

C. Other Drugs Equivalent to Daunomycin

Dubost *et al.* (1964) isolated a product having physicochemical and analytical characteristics identical to daunomycin from a culture broth of *Streptomyces coeruleorubidis* and called it rubidomycin. The compounds were determined to be identical by the following studies: elemental analysis; melting point; thin-layer chromatography; ultraviolet spectrum; infrared spectrum; nuclear magnetic resonance; benzoate derivatives of both drugs; and X-ray diffraction patterns.

Rubomycin was produced from *S. coeruleorubidus* and was isolated in the Soviet Union. The drug represents a complex of two chemically related variants, namely, rubomycin B and rubomycin C. Rubomycin C is identical to daunomycin but rubomycin B is different from daunomycin (Gause, 1966).

D. Pharmaceutical Data

Daunomycin is commercially available in Europe but in the United States is available only as an investigational agent through the Investigational Drug Branch of the National Cancer Institute. The product is supplied as a lyophilized cake in vials containing 21.4 mg of daunomycin hydrochloride equivalent to 20 mg of daunomycin base. In addition, the vials also contain 100 mg of mannitol. The intact vials should be stored at room temperature (22°C) protected from light. When reconstituted with 4 ml of sodium chloride for injection, USP, each milliliter of solution contains 5 mg of daunomycin base.

Intact vials are stable for at least 3 years at room temperature (22°C). The reconstituted drug should be used within 8 hours or discarded since the lyophilized cake contains no preservatives.

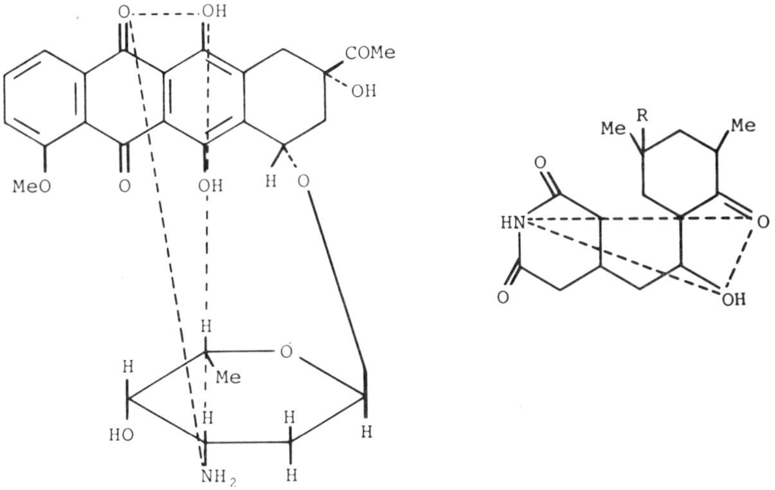

Fig. 2. Triangulation pattern of daunomycin. (From Zee-Cheng and Cheng, 1970, American Pharmaceutical Association. Adapted by permission of the copyright owner.)

III. Biological Properties

Daunomycin possesses an impressive number of biological effects.

A. Antibacterial Activity

Sanfilippo and Mazzoleni (1964) found that *Escherichia coli* Type B was sensitive to daunomycin but *E. coli* K12 was much less sensitive. They ascribed the differences in sensitivities to possible differences in cellular penetration of the daunomycin. Parisi and Soller (1964) found that daunomycin had no effect on growth of *E. coli* B or *E. coli* K12 in concentrations up to 80 μg/ml. When concentrations of up to 300 μg/ml of daunomycin were used, there was a lengthening of the division time to one-half more than normal. The drug has been found to be bacteriostatic against gram-positive organisms especially *Staphylococcus aureus* (Sanfilippo and Mazzoleni, 1964).

Pruzanski and Saito (1974) noted that daunomycin mixed with normal human or leukemic serum did not influence *in vitro* or *in vivo* levels of serum immunoglobulins, lysozyme, or total hemolytic complement. At low doses of daunomycin, there was slight inhibition of bacteriolytic activity of normal sera against *E. coli*. With high doses of daunomycin, there was enhancement of the bacteriolytic activity of normal serum.

B. Antibacteriophage Activity

Daunomycin inhibits the multiplication of bacteriophage (Cassinelli and Orezzi, 1963). It strongly inhibits DNA phages by acting during the replication cycle of the phage and not on absorption, injection, or lysis. The RNA phage growth was unaffected by daunomycin. The antiphage activity was proportional to the concentration of daunomycin. The antiphage activity was partially blocked by DNA but not by nucleotides or nucleosides (Parisi and Soller, 1964; Sanfilippo and Mazzolini, 1964).

C. Antiviral Activity

Daunomycin does not inhibit multiplication of vaccinia, herpes, adenoviruses, or influenza virus (Dubost *et al.*, 1964).

D. Cytotoxic and Antineoplastic Activity

Cytotoxicity and antitumor activity are dealt with in depth in the following sections. Di Marco *et al.* (1964a) reported that daunomycin had marked inhibitory activity on Ehrlich ascites and Sarcoma 180 ascites tumors in mice and also on hepatoma AH130 and Walker carcinoma (see Section V). Rat fibroblast and HeLa and KB cell monolayers in cell cultures treated with daunomycin had marked alterations in the nucleus, nucleoli, and chromosomes with dramatic growth inhibition at 1 μg/ml. The antibiotic also stopped the mitotic activity in cells that have completed the DNA replication cycle and were in G_2 phase (Di Marco *et al.*, 1967).

E. Teratogenic Effect

Daunomycin has been teratogenic in chick embryos treated on the fourth day of incubation but has not been teratogenic in mice or rabbits. The type of malformations in the chick were largely joint deformities, syndactyly, and torsions (Dubost *et al.*, 1964).

F. Immunosuppressive Effect

Gericke and Chandra (1973) found that at low doses, daunomycin stimulates immune responses, with increases in plaque-forming cells in mouse spleen in animals sensitized with sheep red blood cells (SRBC) as well as increases in hemagglutinins to SRBC. At higher doses, there is distinct immunosuppression with the opposite effects in these two systems.

Umezawa *et al.* (1972) noted that timing of SRBC antigen administration was an important factor. If antigen was given 24 hours after daunomycin administration, the number of plaque-forming cells and the hemagglutination titers to SRBC increased, meaning increased immune response. If the antigen was given 24 hours before daunomycin administration, the number of plaque-forming cells decreased, indicating immunosuppression but the hemagglutination titers to SRBC remained the same.

The possibility has been considered that adriamycin is less immunosuppressive than daunomycin and that this difference is in part responsible for the greater therapeutic effects of adriamycin in certain transplantable tumor systems. The immunosuppressive effects of adriamycin and daunomycin were compared using complement-dependent and independent cellular toxicity as an *in vitro* assay of immunity. No significant differences in the effects of adriamycin and daunomycin were seen in that test system (Orsini and Mihich, 1975).

Schwartz (1974) stated that in P388 leukemia in mice, adriamycin has a greater antitumor activity than daunomycin. This therapeutic advantage is lost when the host is pretreated with whole-body radiotherapy. This result suggests that daunomycin is more immunosuppressive than adriamycin.

Daunomycin has been found to have an effect on the hepatitis-associated antigen (HAA). Wands *et al.* (1975) have suggested that antitumor chemotherapeutic agents including daunomycin reduce hepatitis B antibody titers (HBAb). With a decrease in HBAb titers, there is a marked increase in hepatitis B antigen (HBAg) titers, and increase in liver damage is noted. These authors postulated that the appearance of HBAg is related to an inhibition of antibody function, allowing expression of preexisting antigen, or to an inhibition of cellular immunity, allowing viral proliferation.

In summary, depending on dosages used, daunomycin can cause immunosuppression. This may be important in light of tumor antigenicity and increased propensity for infection in patients with cancer.

G. Inhibition of X-Ray Repair

X-Ray repair replication is probably a potential contribution to the repair of cellular sublethal dosages. Drugs that are capable of inhibiting this repair replication may prove useful in combination with X-rays. Both adriamycin and daunomycin block repair replication in L1210 leukemic cells *in vitro*, probably because of their ability to bind to DNA (Lee *et al.*, 1974).

H. Anticoagulant Effect

Komp *et al.* (1974) have postulated that daunomycin might have chemical properties of an anticoagulant nature. They correctly pointed out that interference with fibrin formation by anticoagulation has been associated with decreased implantability of tumor emboli in experimental systems. Daunomycin does not alter the rate of fibrin formation in human plasma, but abnormal fibrin was visible by electron microscopy. Evidence suggested that daunomycin and adriamycin caused loss of fibrin-stabilizing factor activity *in vitro*.

Kubisz and Suranova (1974) found that concentrations of 200 μg/ml of daunomycin are capable of blocking the aggregation of platelets and the availability of platelet Factor 3.

I. Enhancement of Rat Liver Uridine Kinase

Cihak *et al.* (1973) found daunomycin enhanced rat liver uridine kinase activity *in vivo*. This may be of importance since this enzyme catalyzes the phosphorylation of pyrimidine analogs to their corresponding 5′-monophosphates. The absence of uridine kinase in tumor cells is accompanied by resistance to the uridine and cytidine analogs. Perhaps daunomycin, by enhancing uridine kinase activity, may help decrease the emergence of resistant cells.

IV. Modes of Action

A. Mechanisms

1. *Binding to DNA with Complex Formation*

Di Marco *et al.* (1964a) noted that 24 hours after treatment with daunomycin, cultures of rat fibroblasts showed a decrease in growth, in the number of cells in mitosis, and in mitotic index. These decreases were greater at higher doses. A study of the histology of these cells revealed modified nucleic chromatin with a more granular structure and chromosomes that were swollen and fragmented. In cell cultures of HeLa, KB strain, Helius (cancer of larynx), and Walker's carcinosarcoma, daunomycin had a similar action with a decrease in the number of mitoses, change in chromosomes, and a modification of nuclear chromatin and the nucleolus. These investigators concluded that daunomycin had an *in vitro* action on normal and neoplastic cells in both mitosis and mitotic rest.

Ultrastructural studies were done by Dorigotti (1964) who found that, within 2 hours of administration, daunomycin produced specific nucleolar alterations on electron micrographs with fragmentation of the nucleolonema and detachment of nucleolar RNA granules in HeLa cells. In cells followed for 48 hours, there was progressive nucleolar exhaustion with the cytoplasm remaining unchanged.

Simard (1966) noted that daunomycin, proflavin, and ethidium bromide produced identical nuclear and nucleolar lesions in HeLa cells in culture, such as clumping of chromatin with unsticking of nuclear membrane, disappearance of nucleoplasma matrix, and segregation of nucleolar components as treatment progressed. He postulated that the morphological changes might represent the morphological expression for a specific molecular action such as daunomycin intercalation between base pairs of DNA. He also postulated that the secondary inhibition of protein synthesis caused an almost complete loss of nucleoplasmic matrix. He summarized his hypothesis by stating that daunomycin binds to DNA, with a secondary inhibition of DNA-directed RNA synthesis by RNA polymerase.

In the light of the foregoing hypothesis of the binding of daunomycin to DNA, studies were done to prove this reaction. Egorin *et al.* (1974) showed by a fluorescence technique that daunomycin was localized primarily in the nuclei. Daunomycin was present in the deoxynucleoprotein fraction after incubation of hepatic ascites AH 130 cells with a solution of daunomycin. The splitting of deoxynucleoprotein by salt solutions at high ionic strength or treatment with DNAse or trypsin showed the daunomycin was bound to DNA (Di Marco *et al.*, 1964b). Calendi *et al.* (1965) further demonstrated that if daunomycin is added to a solution of DNA, the DNA shows certain physicochemical changes in sedimentation coefficient, in viscosity, in thermal denaturation–renaturation behavior, and in optical rotation. This group of investigators considered different chemical groups as responsible for the linkage between daunomycin and DNA. The rise in viscosity and decrease in sedimentation coefficient suggested changes in the molecular structure of DNA. To produce these changes, a free amino group on the sugar part of the antibiotic was felt to be necessary. Since daunomycin did not produce any changes in viscosity of heat-denatured DNA (single-stranded), daunomycin seems to bind to both strands of the DNA double helix. This binding of daunomycin to DNA with a complex formation is felt to be responsible for the biological activity of daunomycin, including inhibition of RNA and DNA synthesis in animal cells (Rusconi and Calendi, 1964).

Ward *et al.* (1965) noted that daunomycin inhibited RNA synthesis in *E. coli* regardless of the base composition of the DNA template, which firmed up the suggestion that daunomycin intercalates between adjacent base pairs of helical DNA.

Calendi *et al.* (1965) also noted that daunomycin appears to bind with RNA but the physicochemical changes were not the same as those induced in DNA. This complex also requires the presence of the free amino group of the sugar.

2. *Effects of Daunomycin on Nucleic Acid Synthesis*

Rusconi and Calendi (1964) studied the effect of daunomycin on the incorporation of adenine-8-^{14}C by the nucleic acids of hepatoma ascites cells *in vitro* and found inhibition of RNA synthesis. Daunomycin also inhibited the synthesis of RNA and DNA in normally growing *E. coli* cells (Barbieri *et al.* 1964).

Di Marco *et al.* (1965) studied the effect of daunomycin on nucleic acid synthesis *in vitro* in HeLa cell cultures with radioautographic techniques. The mitotic activity and thymidine-^{3}H incorporation into DNA were reduced by daunomycin. They felt this was most likely due to binding of daunomycin to DNA rather than direct effect on the DNA polymerase. In addition, they noted that in cells in interphase the inhibition of incorporation of thymidine-^{3}H into RNA did not exceed 50%. They postulated that the action of daunomycin on DNA and RNA in mitotic cells, and on RNA synthesis in interphase cells, might be two functionally different consequences of the same basic phenomenon, that is, the combination of the antibiotic with the DNA molecule. This combination could prevent the function of DNA as a template for RNA synthesis, and the combination would present a structural change in DNA that makes mitosis difficult.

3. *Effect on DNA and RNA Polymerase*

Zunino *et al.* (1974a,b) studied the effects of daunomycin on *in vitro* activity of *E. coli* DNA-dependent RNA polymerase. They concluded that the inhibition of the RNA polymerase was predominantly due to the interaction of the drug with the template DNA. They also found that the extent of inhibition depended on the base composition and secondary structure of the DNA. In addition, these investigators later showed daunomycin inhibited both DNA and RNA polymerase activity *in vitro*. They found in all cases that adriamycin was more effective than daunomycin in inhibiting DNA synthesis and transcription. In later work, Zunino *et al.* (1975) found that daunomycin and adriamycin possessed some inhibitory activity against bacterial and rat liver DNA polymerase but were greater inhibitors of a viral enzyme (murine sarcoma virus DNA polymerase) than of the bacterial or rat liver polymerase.

In light of recent work showing the resemblance of DNA polymerase in human leukemia cells and the mouse leukemic virus reverse transcriptase, it may be important that the viral DNA polymerase is more sensitive to daunomycin and adriamycin than normal cellular polymerases. This may explain the differential inhibition of tumor cell proliferation (Baxt *et al.*, 1972; Todaro and Gallo, 1973). The greater inhibitory effect of adriamycin against the polymerases tested shows there may be a biochemical basis for the improved therapeutic effectiveness of adriamycin over daunomycin (Zunino *et al.*, 1975).

4. *Effect on Cell Respiration*

Gosalvez *et al.* (1974) studied the effects of daunomycin on respiration of pigeon cardiac mitochondria, rat liver mitochondria, and Ehrlich ascites tumor cells. They found inhibition of reduced nicotinamide adenine dinucleotide (NADH) oxidation at low concentrations and of succinate oxidation at higher concentrations with an accompanying uncoupling of oxidative phosphorylation. The precise importance of these actions in the antitumor activity of daunomycin remain unclear.

In summary, the main mechanism of action of daunomycin appears to be the formation of stable complexes with DNA by intercalation between base pairs. This intercalation produces structural changes that interfere with DNA function in cell mitosis. Daunomycin also causes an inhibition of DNA-dependent RNA synthesis by interfering with the function of DNA as a template for RNA polymerase. The cytotoxic properties of daunomycin also appear to depend on the ability of this drug to interfere with nucleic acid synthesis by inhibiting both DNA and RNA polymerase. This inhibition also appears related to the formation of a complex between daunomycin and DNA.

B. Phase Specificity

With synchronized mouse fibroblast cells in tissue culture (L929), daunomycin was found to have the greatest inhibitory effect on cell growth when the drug was administered during the later stages of cell division, S, G_2, and M_1. These findings were consistent with those of other investigators who observed the maximum effect of the drug in late S phase, the least during G_1 (Kim *et al.*, 1968; Silvestrini *et al.*, 1970).

In contrast to the preceding findings, Linden *et al.* (1974) showed that when daunomycin was applied in the S phase, the cells were not influenced by the daunomycin, probably indicating that DNA synthesis of cells, having already started, is not disturbed by daunomycin. Daunomycin given in the late S or in the G_2 phase caused an accumulation of L929 mouse fibroblast cells in the G_2 phase (G_2 block). Daunomycin treatment in the G_1 phase also produced an arrest in the G_1 phase.

Di Marco *et al.* (1965) noted that daunomycin inhibited mitotic activity in cells but felt the drug inhibited not only cells in S phase but cells in G_2 or M phases also.

Very recently, Arlin *et al.* (1975) found that, in patients with acute leukemia who were given a single injection of daunomycin, there were variable effects on bone marrow blasts. In 3 of 7 patients the blasts were blocked in G_2, in 1 they accumulated in S and G_2, and in 3 there was very little change in the frequency of distribution of blasts in the various cell cycles. Despite the variability of accumulation of blasts in specific phases, all patients had a marked reduction in marrow blasts.

In summary, the bulk of data suggests daunomycin is not a cell-cycle phase-specific agent since it may inhibit cell progress in many of the phases.

C. Resistance to Daunomycin

Riehm and Biedler (1971) studied *in vitro* Chinese hamster cells that were resistant to daunomycin after exposure to that antibiotic. They felt that reduced permeability of the cell membrane to the drug was predominantly responsible for resistance. In later work, they showed that Tween 80, a surface-active, nonionic detergent, caused a marked potentiation of the daunomycin effect on cells resistant to daunomycin. Increased uptake of radioactively labeled daunomycin was documented and was directly related to the concentration of the detergent (Riehm and Biedler, 1972).

Dano *et al.* (1972) found cellular uptake of daunomycin was less in resistant lines of Ehrlich ascites tumor cells *in vitro,* but the difference was too small to account for the differences of daunomycin inhibition of nucleic acid synthesis in sensitive and resistant cells. Synthesis of DNA and RNA was inhibited in both sensitive and resistant cells. The preferential inhibition of transfer RNA was less pronounced in the resistant cells than in the sensitive cells, thus indicating the lack of sensitivity of transfer RNA may be an important reason for development of resistance.

V. Experimental Antitumor Activity

Daunomycin has exhibited antitumor effects in a wide variety of experimental tumors.

Di Marco *et al.* (1964c) found that daunomycin had an inhibitory effect in 10 out of the 12 animal tumor systems tested. With a daily dose of 1 to 2 mg/kg intraperitoneally, it had marked inhibitory effect on ascites tumors (Yoshida AH130 hepatoma, Walker 256 carcinoma, Ehrlich carcinoma, Sarcoma 180, and Oberling-Guérin-Guérin (OGG) myeloma) and remarkably increased the average survival time of tumor-bearing mice and rats. It also inhibited the growth of solid tumors (Ehrlich carcinoma, 41.1% inhibition; Sarcoma 180, 42.2%; Walker carcinoma, 66.1%; OGG myeloma, 70.8–85.2%; and methylcholanthrene-induced sarcoma, 67%).

Venditti *et al.* (1966) reported the activity of daunomycin against L1210 mouse leukemia. In mice with L1210, increases in life-span of 50–56% were obtained with daily doses of 0.7–2.0 mg/kg. They determined that the optimal dose of daunomycin was 3.0 mg/kg/day. Later data on the L1210 system are summarized in Table II. No schedule dependency is apparent from these data. In advanced L1210 leukemia, daunomycin was less but still effective. Daunomycin was also active in a subline L1210/C95 which was resistant to 6-mercaptopurine, methotrexate and cyclophosphamide.

TABLE II

DAUNOMYCIN VERSUS MOUSE LEUKEMIA L1210[a]

i.p., once; day 1	i.p., q.d.; day–death	i.p., q.d.; days 1–3, 8–10, 15–17
50 (5.0)	34 (1.0)	45 (2.0)
31 (8.0)	56 (0.7)	
43 (13)	27 (0.5)	i.p., q.d.; days 1–5, 11–15, etc.
50 (2.5)	59 (2.0)	56 (1.0)
50 (5.0)	61 (2.0)	31 (1.0)
47 (4.0)	68 (2.0)	
45 (4.0)	30 (0.5)	s.c., q.d.; days 1–5, 11–15, etc.
22 (4.0)	54 (2.0)	62 (4.0)
39 (8.0)		36 (4.0)
55 (8.0)		
54 (5.0)		
i.p., q.d.; day 1–3	i.p., q.2d.; day 1–death	i.p., once; day 2
36 (4.0)	25 (4.0)	47 (8.6)
i.p., q.d.; days 1–5	i.p., q.4d.; days 1–9	i.p., q.d.; days 2–16
47 (2.0)	56 (5.0)	43 (2.3)
i.p., q.d.; days 1–7	i.p., q.3h.; day 1 only	i.p., q.4d.; days 2–16
50 (1.0)	45 (8.0/8)	41 (5.7)
48 (2.0)	62 (8.0/8)	
i.p., q.d.; days 1–9	i.p., q.3h.; days 1, 5, 9	i.p., q.2d.; days 2–16
39 (1.7)	27 (4.0/8)	42 (3.7)
45 (1.5)	62 (4.0/8)	
28 (0.6)		
27 (2.0)		
50 (1.0)		
i.p., q.d.; days 1–10	i.p., q.3h.; days 1, 9	i.p., q.3h.; q.4d.; days 2–16
55 (2.0)	40 (8.0/8)	36 (7.4/8)

[a] Each set of figures under each schedule shows the maximum increase in lifetime over controls from a wide range of doses. The dose at which the maximum increase was observed (optimal dose) in milligrams per kilogram per day is shown in parentheses. When the mice received more than one injection per day the dosage is shown as the total dose per day/the number of injections per day. Limited oral testing continued to produce erratic and non-reproducible results that are not shown.

Daunomycin is effective against intraperitoneally implanted B16 melanoma with some schedules capable of curing some mice. However, the drug is not active against subcutaneously implanted B16 melanoma.

When two-drug combinations were tested in the early or advanced L1210 system, enhanced effectiveness was observed with 1,2 bis(3,5-dioxopiperazin-1-yl)propane (ICRF-159) plus daunomycin. Daunomycin or adriamycin given in combination with ICRF produced increases in life-spans of 170 and 172%, respectively (Kline, 1974).

Woodman (1974) did point out that the maximum dose of daunomycin tolerated by nonleukemic mice could be greatly increased if they were treated simultaneously with ICRF-159. Of special note was that leukemic mice could receive a dose of daunomycin higher than the optimal therapeutic dose for treatment with daunomycin alone and, as a result, exhibit a higher response rate.

Further study of the reversal of daunomycin toxicity by ICRF-159 indicated that the reversal occurred whether ICRF-159 is given several hours before or after the daunomycin. The reversal of toxicity was not influenced by incubating ICRF-159 with daunomycin prior to injection, but the activity in L1210 was less with this incubated mixture. The maximally tolerated dose of intraperitoneal adriamycin could not be increased by therapy with ICRF-159.

The following are other combinations of note that include daunomycin:

A. Cytosine Arabinoside (Ara-C) + Daunomycin

Edelstein *et al.* (1974) found that when these two agents are given together, the degree of cell kill, using a leukemic spleen colony assay system, was less than additive. When daunomycin was given before Ara-C the resulting cell kill was additive. If daunomycin was given 2–40 hours after Ara-C a marked increase in cell kill occurs reaching a maximum when the two agents are given 15 hours apart. Ara-C did potentiate the lethality of daunomycin. The mechanism for this is unknown, but it may be that Ara-C partially synchronizes the leukemic cells in the cell cycle, killing those in S phase and blocking others in the G_1-S where lethality of daunomycin is appreciable.

B. VP16-213 (NSC 141540) + Daunomycin

The combination of 4′-demethyl-1-*O*-[4,6-*O*-(ethylidene)-β-D-glucopyranosyl] epipodophyllotoxin (VP16-213) with daunomycin was less than additive, so far as antineoplastic activity in the L1210 system is concerned (Dombernowsky and Nissen, 1975).

C. L-Asparaginase + Daunomycin

With 500 units per kilogram of L-asparaginase and 0.5 mg/kg of daunomycin administered 6 hours apart on days 1, 2, and 3, with daunomycin given first and asparaginase given last, there was a 100% survival of mice with L5178Y leukemia at 50 days and a greater than 400% increase in mean survival time (Nahas, 1974).

D. Daunomycin + Ara-C + 6-Mercaptopurine

This three-drug combination was used in L1210 system by Hoshino *et al.* (1972). The combination was active and the investigators point out that this combination is also active in the treatment of human leukemia in Japan.

VI. Animal Toxicity

A. Quantitative Toxicity

Five animal species (mouse, rat, hamster, monkey, and dog) have been studied for single- and repeated-dose toxicity.

In the mouse, the LD_{50} has been 3.08–5.00 mg/kg via i.p. dosage, and 17.3–20 mg/kg via the i.v. route (Di Marco *et al.*, 1964b,c; Dubost *et al.*, 1964; Morrison, 1967). Delayed deaths were noted with the i.p. dosage with diarrhea and distention suggesting peritonitis. This heightened toxicity by the intraperitoneal versus the intravenous route may arise from the strong local inflammatory effects of the drug. Rat data show a similar trend with LD_{50} of 8 mg/kg i.p. and 13–15 mg/kg with i.v. injections. Early studies in 1967 had defined the LD_{50} in dogs for a single i.v. dose at 5 mg/kg with death on days 4 and 6. If doses were given every day for 9–12 days, the LD_{50} was between 0.5 and 1.0 mg/kg. Studies done with weekly dosing showed an LD_{50} of 2–3 mg/kg/week. Deaths were secondary to thrombocytopenia with multiple hemorrhages (Morrison, 1967).

All of the foregoing studies lead to the determination of the highest nontoxic dose or maximally tolerated dose in the beagle dog which was less than 0.5 mg/kg, or less than 10 mg/m^2, i.v. daily for 12 days (see Table III).

Monkey toxicology data are shown in Table III. With 3-day courses repeated every 6 days for 5 courses, the highest nontoxic dose (HNTD) was 0.5 mg/kg (6 mg/m^2). In green monkeys, the total dose, regardless of priming or maintenance dose, was the limiting factor as 12 of 15 monkeys died after a total dose of 14–19 mg/kg. In addition, delayed

TABLE III

IMPORTANT DOSAGE LEVELS OF DAUNOMYCIN IN DOGS AND MONKEYS

Dose schedule	Dogs		Monkeys		
	LD_{50}[a]	HNTD[b]	LD[a]	TDH[c]	HNTD[b]
Single i.v.	5 mg/kg	—	—	—	—
i.v., q.d., × 9–12	0.5–1.0 mg/kg	0.5 mg/kg/day (10 mg/m²/day)			
i.v., q. week	2–3 mg/kg	—	—	—	—
i.v. × 3 days, rest 3 days, repeat × 5	—	—	2.0 mg/kg (24 mg/m²)	1.0 mg/kg (12 mg/m²)	0.5 mg/kg (6 mg/m²)

[a] Lethal dose (LD): the lowest dose to produce drug-induced death in any animals during the treatment or observation period.

[b] Highest nontoxic dose (HNTD): the highest dose at which no hematological, chemical, clinical, or pathological drug-induced alterations occurred; doubling this dose produces the aforementioned alterations.

[c] Toxic dose high (TDH): the lowest dose to produce drug-induced pathological alterations in hematological, chemical, clinical, or morphological parameters; doubling this dose produces lethality.

deaths were a consistent finding, with 14 of 15 animals dying 20 or more days after the last injection of drug. The monkey was considered the most sensitive species (Morrison, 1967).

B. Qualitative Toxicity

In both the dog and the monkey the qualitative toxicities included the following:

1. *Bone Marrow*

At all levels of drug dosage there were degrees of leukopenia and anemia. Reversibility of these parameters was demonstrable at the 0.5-mg/kg/day dose in the dog, whereas at a dose of 1.0 mg/kg/day, granulocytopenia and thrombocytopenia developed with resultant pyrexia.

2. *Gastrointestinal*

At 2 mg/kg/day of drug there were hemorrhagic lesions in the intestinal tracts of all the monkeys. Emesis was often seen.

3. *Hepatic*

Elevations of SGOT, SGPT, and alkaline phosphatase were seen in both dogs and monkeys receiving toxic doses. In the dog, the primary histological finding was a fine vacuolization of hepatocytes and sinusoidal dilatation. The livers of the monkeys demonstrated fat accumulation.

4. *Kidney*

Both species showed abnormalities in renal function tests with elevated blood urea nitrogen (BUN) and creatinine. The histopathological changes in the dog were an accumulation of periglomerular debris and cloudy swelling of tubular epithelium.

Of interest, in light of these findings in the higher animals, were the findings of Sternberg and Phillips (1967) and Walski (1974) who reported on the development of a biphasic intoxication and nephrotic syndrome in rats. With a single i.v. dose of 20 mg/kg of daunomycin, the first toxicity phase appeared in the first week with cell renewal system damage (i.e., lymphoid, GI, and bone marrow damage). A second toxic phase began in the second week with rats showing proteinuria, hyperlipemia, tissue edema, and glomerular damage. A nephrotic syndrome with progressive renal damage was noted. Fluorescent microscopy revealed selective localization of daunomycin in glomerular nuclei (Sternberg, 1970). On electron microscopy studies, there was fusion of foot processes, and the basement membrane structure was completely obliterated. These changes have been named *daunomycin nephrosis*.

Lamberts *et al.* (1973) studied the oxygen uptake and carbohydrate metabolism of isolated glomeruli of rats with daunomycin-induced nephrotic syndrome. The results indicated an inhibition in the production of acetyl–coenzyme A from pyruvate and of succinyl–coenzyme A from α-ketoglutarate.

5. *Cardiopulmonary*

Pulmonary edema was seen in either the gross pathology and/or histopathology of all monkeys, and in the dogs receiving 3 mg/kg/week. There were no apparent signs of dyspnea, tachycardia, or edema in these animals. The pathology of the hearts showed cardiac enlargement, and histopathological examination revealed myofibrolysis of the heart and pulmonary edema. The monkey was, therefore, considered a good model for cardiac toxicity prediction (toxicology data on file, Investigational Drug Branch, NCI).

Studies were undertaken to look directly at the cardiac toxicity. A single dose of 50 mg/kg was required to produce atrioventricular dissociation in anesthetized dogs. To effect EKG changes in cats, 40–50 mg/kg daunomycin was required, and single intraperitoneal doses of 50 mg/kg resulted in hamster EKG changes. The EKG changes were characterized by atrioventricular dissociation, with slower atrial than ventricular rates. Necropsy findings were unremarkable, and no evidence of microscopic damages was observed in animals showing EKG changes (toxicology data on file, Investigational Drug Branch, NCI).

6. *Other*

Transient decreases in magnesium, calcium, and blood sugar were noted at all dosage levels, but these effects spontaneously reverted to normal in each instance. Alopecia was noted in areas of injection in the dog along with local sloughing of the skin.

C. Toxic Effects in the Rabbit

Maral *et al.* (1967) reported that daunomycin given chronically to rabbits for 3 months caused myocardial degeneration and fibrosis. Jaenke (1974) followed this with more extensive studies. He gave New

Zealand rabbits 2.43–3.0 mg/kg/week of daunomycin. Doses greater than 3.0 mg/kg/week (33 mg/m^2) resulted in uniformly high death losses within 10–16 days from thrombocytopenia.

Myocardial lesions consisting of focal myofiber degeneration were present and progressed to severe myofiber degeneration and necrosis when total doses greater than 350 mg/m^2 of daunomycin were administered. Adriamycin could be given to 250–340 mg/m^2 before this necrosis appeared. Jaenke concluded that the specific myocardial toxicity of adriamycin in the rabbit was greater than that of daunomycin. Some animals developed congestive heart failure on the daunomycin.

The earliest myofiber alterations appeared to be extensive vacuolization within the myocardial cells, especially of the elements of the transverse tubular systems and sarcoplasmic reticulum. There were also focal dilatations in the outer mitochondrial envelope.

Jaenke (1974) postulated that perhaps the daunomycin also interferes with normal renewal processes of the myocardial cell because of interference with protein synthesis leading to gradual atrophy of the cell.

D. Perfusion Studies

Fischerman and Olsen (1974) performed extracorporeal gastric perfusion in 8 pigs with 2 mg/kg daunomycin for 30 minutes. They found that daunomycin caused minor and major ulcerations of the mucosa and submucosa but not sufficient to cause perforation with peritonitis. All 8 pigs healed a surgical anastomosis. They saw no systemic toxicity with the perfusion.

VII. Metabolism and Disposition

A. *In Vitro* Studies

The products of mild acid hydrolysis (0.2*N* HCl for 1 hour at 90°C) of daunomycin HCl are a red aglycone, daunomycinone, and an amino sugar daunosamine, as seen in Fig. 3 (Arcamone *et al.*, 1964a,b).

Daunomycin (D_1) is converted to daunorubicinol (D_2) by a cytoplasmic enzyme, daunorubicin reductase, in rat tissue homogenates with reduced nicotinamide adenine dinucleotide phosphate (NADPH) as a cofactor (Fig. 4). The daunorubicinol is then converted to its aglycone (D_3) by the rat tissue homogenates (Bachur, 1971; Bachur and Cradock, 1970; Bachur and Gee, 1971; Huffman and Bachur, 1972). Daunorubicin reductase isolated from rat liver by Feldsted *et al.* (1974) has a molecular weight of 39,591 with an isoelectric point of 6.3 and strictly requires NADPH for a cofactor.

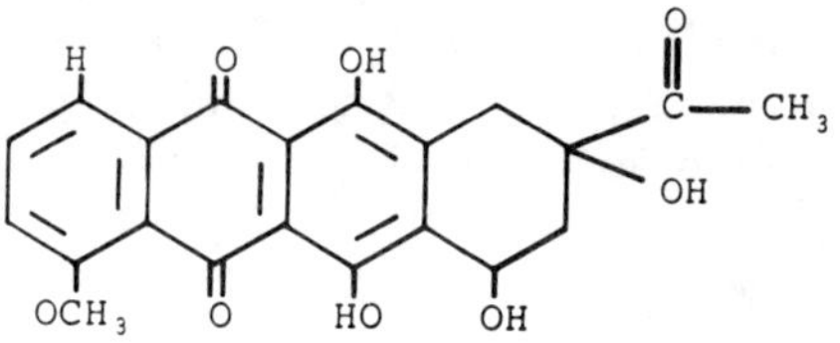

Daunomycinone

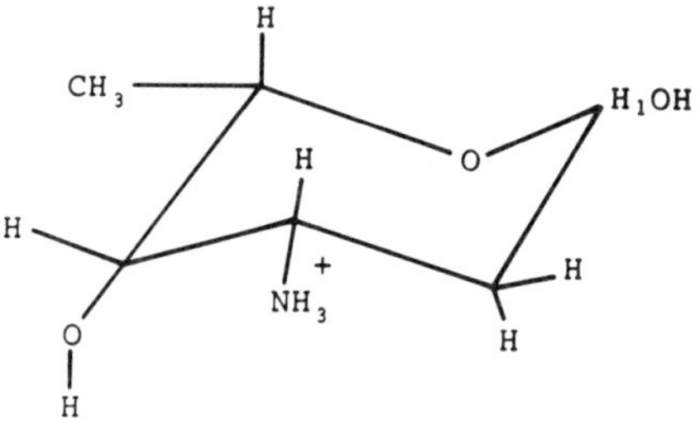

Daunosamine

FIG. 3. The products of mild acid hydrolysis of daunomycin, namely, daunomycinone and daunosamine.

Hematological Daunorubicin Metabolism

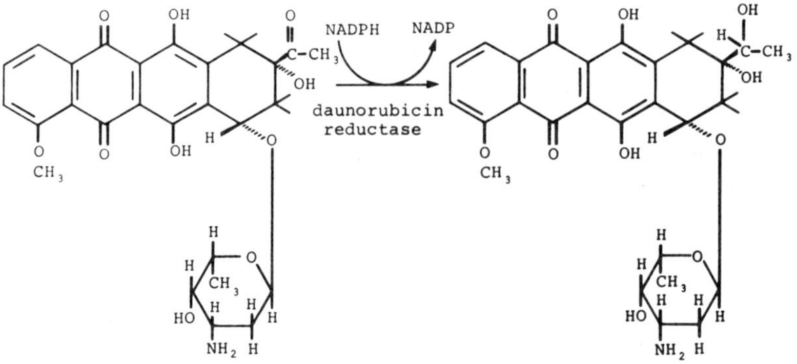

NADPH NADP

daunorubicin reductase

Daunomycin (Daunorubicin) (D_1)

Daunorubicinol (D_2)

FIG. 4. Daunorubicin reductase reaction. (From Huffman and Bachur, 1972. Adapted by permission of the copyright owner.)

Asbell *et al.* (1972) studied the metabolism of daunomycin in the rat liver and found it metabolized to deoxydaunorubicin aglycone which was converted to deoxydaunorubicinol aglycone, but in the rat kidney daunomycin was converted from $D_1 \rightarrow D_2 \rightarrow D_x$. Structures of these compounds are detailed elsewhere (Bullock *et al.*, 1972; Takanashi and Bachur, 1975).

Huffman and Bachur (1972) found that intact human blood elements, as well as their homogenates, could convert daunomycin to daunorubicinol (see Fig. 4). The activity of the elements in their ability to do this can be ranked as: lymphocyte > whole white blood cell (WBC) > bone marrow cells > red blood cells (RBC) > platelets. The active enzyme was daunorubicin reductase. In both leukocytes and erythrocytes, the activity is cytoplasmic, heat-labile, and requires NADPH but not molecular oxygen.

The only metabolite observed from the action of the blood elements on daunomycin is D_2. Of considerable interest is the metabolism by the platelet. The demonstration of metabolism of a foreign molecule, daunomycin, by platelets is unique.

Huffman *et al.* (1971) have shown that daunomycin is capable of being metabolized by human leukemic myeloblasts *in vitro* into D_2. Once formed, the D_2 shows a longer plasma and urinary $t_{1/2}$ than the parent compound daunomycin (see in following).

B. Metabolism in Rodents

Studies have been performed in mice and rats using both a fluorescent and an isotopic method for daunomycin levels.

The plasma concentration of daunomycin, as measured by fluorometric and isotopic methods, decreased rapidly and remained nearly constant at low levels 20 minutes after intravenous administration in the mouse and the rat. This rapid disappearance suggested a localization of drug in tissues and/or rapid excretion (Rusconi *et al.*, 1968; Finkel *et al.*, 1964; Yesair *et al.*, 1972). Ten percent of the radioactivity of the administered radioactively labeled daunomycin was excreted in the urine, and 30–40% in the feces of rats within 4 days (Rusconi *et al.*, 1968).

Yesair *et al.* (1972) studied the feces of rats by a fluorescent method and found the feces contained little (less than 5%) of the fluorescence of the administered dose of daunomycin. This difference between the isotope method and the fluorescent method suggested that the intestinal flora metabolized daunomycin to nonfluorescent products.

Yesair *et al.* (1972) took the experiment one step further and cannulated the bile ducts of rats and mice and found that biliary excretion of daunomycin (as measured by fluorescent methods) in rats and mice was extensive and equivalent to urinary excretion.

Attempts have been made to differentiate the drug and metabolites appearing in the rodent urine and bile by using thin-layer chromatography. In normal rats given daunomycin, thin-layer chromatography on the urine and bile has shown two fluorescent species (Yesair *et al.*, 1972): one species was daunomycin and the other was named D_2 and corresponded to daunorubicinol (D_2) as described by Bachur and Gee (1971). Similar patterns were noted in both urine and bile.

Daunomycin was excreted into the bile and urine, initially to a greater degree than the metabolite, but at 2 hours the D_2 represented greater than 50% of the daunomycin equivalent and by 24 hours the metabolite was 2 times the concentration of the daunomycin (Yesair *et al.*, 1972). Of note is that the D_2 was equivalent in antileukemic activity to daunomycin in the P388 leukemic system.

The distribution of daunomycin and its metabolite, D_2, was also studied by Yesair *et al.* (1972) in tissues of rats. High tissue levels were seen in the rat kidney, liver, heart, and small intestine. Tissue distribution was similar in the mouse except for the rapid decrease in daunomycin equivalents in mouse liver at the end of 24 hours. The major drug species in the tissues of the mouse after i.v. daunomycin were daunomycin and D_2 with the percent of daunomycin greater at earlier times, and D_2 greater than daunomycin 6 hours after administration.

As already stated, Bachur and Gee (1971) reported that homogenates of rat liver converted daunomycin to aglycones of daunomycin and its metabolite, D_2. Yesair *et al.* (1972) noted that rat tissues allowed to stand at room temperature converted D_1 and D_2 to the aglycone which they labeled D_x. This aglycone, D_x, also appeared in rat and mouse tissues exposed to hypobaric stress.

Herman *et al.* (1969) have noted that hamsters, in contrast to rats, are very susceptible to daunomycin-induced cardiotoxicity, and Yesair *et al.* (1972) noted that hamsters produced D_x in small amounts under normal conditions. They postulated along with Mhatre *et al.* (1972) that this new aglycone (D_x), not the aglycone of D_1 or D_2, was the cardiotoxic metabolite of daunomycin. This metabolite, D_x, was increased in amount under anaerobic conditions and, hence, perhaps could be higher in the critically ill, acidotic, and hypoxic patients (Yesair *et al.*, 1972).

C. Metabolism in the Rabbit

The rabbit has been an important test animal because only the rabbit has been shown to develop a cardiomyopathy associated with chronic administration of the anthracyclines (Jaenke, 1974). As a result, the pharmacokinetics of daunomycin have been studied extensively in the rabbit. Rabbits with cannulated bile ducts were given 5 mg/kg of daunomycin i.v. and monitored. Bile flow or urine output was not affected by the drug, but respiration and heart rate were transiently increased after administering the drug, with return to normal within 2 hours. The 30-minute samples of plasma contained significant amounts of daunorubicinol with a peak at 30 minutes and values exceeding daunomycin after that period for the rest of the determinations (Bachur *et al.*, 1974).

With falling plasma levels, the drug and its metabolites appeared in the bile and urine. Seventeen percent of the administered daunomycin appeared in the bile primarily as daunorubicinol (84%). Unchanged daunomycin and aglycone metabolites were 1.3 and 0.2% of the drug fluorescence in the bile. In an 8-hour urine collection, the rabbits excreted 2% of the daunomycin administered. The fluorescence in the urine was accounted for by 90% daunorubicinol, 6.2% polar metabolites, and 2% aglycones (Bachur *et al.*, 1974).

When the tissues of rabbits given daunomycin were examined, most of the tissues contained daunorubicinol as the major fluorescent species. Aglycone levels were minimal except in the kidney, liver, small intestine, and a small amount in the heart.

Bachur *et al.* (1974) pointed out that the tissues with active anthracycline metabolism, as well as excretory function, contained a significant aglycone concentration. They postulated that the daunomycin may be metabolized intracellularly to daunorubicinol, which is more polar and remains intracellularly longer. They did not feel the aglycone concentrations measured in the heart were the main cause of cardiotoxicity in the rabbits.

D. Metabolism in the Dog

In the dog, the plasma level of daunomycin equivalent, as measured by fluorescence, decreased rapidly and was similar to the rat and mouse. Excretion of daunomycin and its fluorescent metabolites in the urine and bile showed 8% of the intravenous dose was present in a 4-hour urine collection, whereas less than 1% was present in a 4-hour bile collection. Therefore, daunomycin biliary excretion was much less than urinary excretion in the dog (Yesair *et al.*, 1972).

The drug species in the urine were differentiated into daunomycin and its metabolite, D_2. Initially, daunomycin represented a large percentage of the urinary species, but with progression of time the proportion of the metabolite D_2 increased (Yesair *et al.*, 1972).

Table IV shows tissue concentration of daunomycin obtained from dog tissues assayed after i.v. daunomycin injection. In measurements of kidney, heart, and liver tissues for daunomycin and daunomycin metabolites, there was only a small percentage (less than 20%) of daunomycin with the remainder being metabolite.

Conclusions obtained from animal pharmacology include the following:

1. In the mouse, rat, and dog, daunomycin is cleared rapidly from the plasma, deposited in tissue, extensively metabolized, and slowly excreted with biliary excretion being equivalent to urinary excretion in rats, but less than urinary excretion in the dog.
2. In normal rats, dogs, and mice the distribution of daunomycin in tissues was similar.
3. Daunomycin was metabolized only to D_2 in normal tissue of rats, mice, and dogs. The D_2 has antitumor activity in the P388 system equivalent to daunomycin.
4. Under anaerobic conditions, a second metabolite, an aglycone D_x, was noted which causes cardiotoxicity in a sensitive species, the hamster, and may be of importance in the acidotic and hypoxic patient.

E. Metabolism and Pharmacokinetics in Man

Through the use of the fluorescent assay technique and the isotopic method with tritiated daunomycin, Alberts *et al.* (1971) did an elegant study on the pharmacokinetics of daunomycin in man. Patients with various solid tumors were given 80 or 120 mg/m^2 of daunomycin as a single injection.

TABLE IV

Concentration of Daunomycin and Metabolites in Dog Tissue

Tissue	Concentration (μg/gm tissue)
Kidney	39
Liver	37
Heart	18
Gastrointestinal	22
Lung	37
Spleen	22
Muscle	6
Adipose	5
Brain	1

By fluorescence studies the disappearance of the drug from plasma is slow. This curve was biphasic with an initial short plasma $t_{1/2}$ of 45 minutes and with a second long plasma $t_{1/2}$ of 55 hours.

The excretion in the urine for the 80-mg/m^2 dose was 7.5% in the first 24 hours and 2.3% during the second 24 hours. Most of the fluorescence in the urine was not extractable by toluene, indicating that most of the excreted drug was not aglycone. Except for the day of administration the daily fractional excretion was nearly constant (Alberts *et al.*, 1971).

Fecal fluorescence could not be measured because of interfering materials. The tissues of 2 patients who had received daunomycin 16 and 19 hours before death were examined post-mortem for daunomycin fluorescence. The concentrations were highest in the kidney, spleen, liver, and lung. Daunomycin was still present in tissue extracts of 2 other patients who died 11 and 12 days after drug administration.

Alberts *et al.* (1971) also used radioisotope techniques to study 3 patients and showed that the short plasma $t_{1/2}$ was the same as that determined by the fluorescence method, but the isotope technique gave a mean long plasma $t_{1/2}$ of 104 hours which was twice that determined by the fluorescence method. The difference was thought to be due in part to a nonfluorescent metabolite of the drug as red cells and white cells can metabolize daunomycin rapidly.

Fecal collections on 1 patient showed 20% of the initial radioactivity in the 7-day stool collection.

Analysis of plasma samples by thin-layer chromatography after daunomycin administration revealed four metabolites that coincided with daunomycin (D_1), daunomycinone (D_4), and two other metabolites, D_2 and D_3. Thin-layer chromatography of urine, bile, and tissue samples showed similar metabolites with D_1 and D_2 the predominant materials present.

Di Fronzo and Bonadonna (1970) gave daunomycin-^{3}H to 6 patients at doses of 1 mg/kg. In all 6 cases the whole blood levels of radioactivity were higher than plasma levels during the first 6–8 hours after administration. Radioactivity in all white blood cells was very low and undetectable after that time. The $t_{1/2}$ of the drug in the body (as calculated from radioactivity in stools and urine) was 171–226 hours. After intraperitoneal injection, there was a rapid fall in ascitic radioactivity with plasma levels of radioactivity that rose after 2 hours and remained stable for 4 days. Concentrations of radioactivity were also measured in cerebrospinal fluid. After i.v. administration in 1 patient, cerebrospinal fluid was obtained at 15 and 90 minutes. No radioactivity was noted, indicating daunomycin does not appear to cross the blood–brain barrier.

Urinary excretion was noted to be 16–40% of the injected radioactivity. Fecal excretion was measured in 4 patients. Three patients excreted

20–30% of administered radioactivity in the first day, and 1 patient excreted only 6% of the injected dose.

Takanashi and Bachur (1974, 1975) studied the urinary metabolites of adriamycin and daunomycin. The most prominent adriamycin metabolite in human urine is adriamycinol (A_2) after adriamycin administration, and daunorubicinol (D_2) is obtained after daunomycin administration. Other metabolites present in the urine after daunomycin administration include daunorubicinol aglycone, deoxydaunorubicinol aglycone, deoxydaunorubicin aglycone, demethyldeoxydaunorubicinol aglycone, demethyldeoxydaunorubicinol aglycone 4-*O*-sulfate, demethyldeoxydaunorubicinol aglycone 4-*O*-glucuronide, and deoxydaunorubicinol aglycone glucuronide. Other metabolites have been purified but not identified. The metabolites indicate the importance of carbonyl reduction, reductive glycosidic cleavage, *O*-demethylation, *O*-sulfation, and *O*-glucuronidation in anthracycline metabolism. Since D_2 has biological activity in the P388 system, it will be of importance to determine the biological and toxicologic activities of the metabolites of daunomycin.

Of additional note is that, recently, a radioimmunoassay technique has been developed to measure 2 pmoles of daunomycin equivalent per milliliter of plasma or urine (Van Vunakis *et al.*, 1974; Bachur *et al.*, 1977). This should help refine drug assay techniques.

The conclusions drawn from the human studies are as follows:

1. Daunomycin is very likely fixed by body tissues within a short period of time after administration, but daunomycin has a second plasma $t_{1/2}$.
2. Because of the secondary plasma $t_{1/2}$ with sustained blood levels of drug after a single dose, it would make more sense pharmacologically to administer the drug in a single large dose rather than in 3–5 doses on successive days.
3. The total output of daunomycin and its metabolites in the urine is low; therefore, there is probably significant biliary excretion of the drug (feces indicate this as well as measurements on human bile).
4. The major metabolites in the human, daunomycin and daunorubicinol are both cytotoxic in the P388 and L1210 systems, whereas the other metabolites, D_3 and D_4, are inactive in the animal tumor systems (Alberts *et al.*, 1971; Di Marco, 1967; Huffman and Bachur, 1972).

VIII. Clinical Studies

The initial studies with daunomycin began in 1965. Since that time information in clinical trials involving 5613 patients studied by cooperative oncology groups and independent investigators has been accumulated by the Investigational Drug Branch of the NCI.

In this section when discussing response rates certain terminology will apply. Partial remission (PR) denotes a greater than 50% measurable decrease in tumor areas, lasting a minimum of 1 month or the occurrence of an M_2 marrow (5–25% blasts) in the case of leukemias. Complete remission (CR) denotes complete disappearance of measurable disease or an M_1 marrow (less than 5% blasts) lasting a minimum of 1 month.

A. Phase I Studies

A Phase I study is a toxicology study designed to determine the maximum dose of drug tolerated by man. The Phase I studies of daunomycin did not proceed in the usual manner. Highest escalated doses and maximally tolerated doses were not consistently obtained, and most studies proceeded immediately to Phase II trials.

In 1965, Bertazzoli began using a daily schedule of daunomycin. The patients were treated until leukopenia intervened. Total doses per course of drug ranged from 25–400 mg with daily doses ranging from 5–40 mg. (information on file at the Investigational Drug Branch of the NCI).

Bernard *et al.* (1967) reported using daunomycin in a daily regimen of 1–2 mg/kg for 3–8 days. That regimen was successful in treating acute leukemia and generated a great deal of enthusiasm. Bone marrow aplasia was seen in all patients who responded to the drug with incipience of aplasia between the tenth and twentieth days of treatment and lasting a mean of 10 days. In addition Bernard *et al.* (1967) noted cardiac toxicity occurring in 2 patients who received more than 40 mg/kg total dose. Transient alopecia was reported with oral ulceration and stomatitis. The recommended dose for acute lymphocytic leukemia (ALL) was 1–2 mg/kg/day for 2–8 days with discontinuation when the WBC count was less than 1500, and 2 mg/kg/day for 5–8 days for acute myelogenous leukemia (AML) patients.

Tan *et al.* (1967) reported the early Phase I and II studies in the United States. They studied 25 evaluable patients with acute leukemia. They found the following regimen as the maximally tolerated dose for children with leukemia: 1 mg/kg/day for 4–5 days with a 3-day rest, then 1–1.5 mg/kg for 1 day, followed by 3 days' rest, and then by 2 mg/kg once to twice a week. In 34 children with solid tumors treated by Tan *et al.* (1967), the recommended dose was 1 mg/kg/day for 6–8 days with a decrease in dose if they had previously received chemotherapy or radiotherapy. The following dosage regimen was recommended for adults: 0.8 mg/kg/day for 4 days, rest for 5–10 days, then resume at 0.5–0.8 mg/kg every 1–2 days, after which increase to 0.8–1 mg/kg every 2–3 days until evidence of toxicity.

Tan *et al.* (1967) did note that in childhood leukemia the daunomycin produced high percentages of complete remissions plus partial remissions in 10 of 12 previously untreated patients (83%) and in 5 of 13 patients (38%), refractory to other forms of therapy. The remissions were of brief duration, but were maintained in some patients by a weekly or twice weekly maintenance regimen.

It is of interest that bona fide Phase I trials using weekly, monthly, and continuous infusion methods of administration have not been attempted.

B. Phase II and III Studies

1. *Acute Leukemias*

Daunomycin has been most extensively tested and has shown its greatest activity in the treatment of acute leukemias. Because of the importance of age and cell type in the prognosis of the leukemias, distinctions for these important prognostic variables will be made.

a. Daunomycin Alone for ALL in Children. To date in cooperative or large group studies there have been 180 children with ALL treated with daunomycin alone. (Many studies do not specify if children patients have ALL or AML and assessments of those studies cannot be performed.) There have been 68 CR (36%) and 20 PR (11%) for an overall response rate of 47% (Table V). Most of these patients have been previously treated.

TABLE V

Daunomycin as Single-Agent Therapy for Children with Acute Lymphocytic Leukemia

Dose		No. of evaluable	Complete response		Partial response		
(mg/m²)	Schedule[a]	patients	No.	(%)	No.	(%)	Reference[b]
30	Daily × 5	29	5	17	2	7	(1)
37[c]	Daily × 5	21	7	29	11	43	(2)
37[c]	Daily × 5	6	4	66	1	17	(3)
37–74[c]	Daily × 5	36	21	58	4	11	(4)
45	Daily × 5	21	7	33	1	3	(5)
45	Daily × 5	28	9	32	0	0	(1)
60	Daily × 5	39	15	38	1	3	(1)
Total		180	68	38	20	11	

[a] All drug was given intravenously.

[b] Key to references: (1) Jones *et al.* (1971); (2) Massimo *et al.* (1968); (3) Jacquillat *et al.* (1966); (4) Bernard *et al.* (1967); (5) Jones *et al.* (1972).

[c] Calculated by conversion factor of 37 from milligrams per kilogram to milligrams per square meter.

In analyzing these collected studies one can see that daunomycin has been used over a relatively narrow dose range with complete remissions induced in 17–66% of patients. The duration of remission was 19 days to 1 year with occasional remissions lasting longer.

It is difficult to determine the most effective dosage regimen for treatment of ALL in children. The Acute Leukemic Group B (ALGB) study 6611 did show the 60 mg/m^2 daily for 5 days had better remission induction rates than the 30 mg/m^2 daily for 5 days (41 versus 24%) but the difference was not statistically significant or impressive between the 60 mg/m^2 daily for 5 days and the 45 mg/m^2 daily for 5 days regimens. This study (Jones *et al.*, 1971) did conclude, however, that generally there were higher response rates with higher dosages of daunomycin.

Jones *et al.* (1971) also noted that there was a relationship between response and total dose of the drug (Table VI). The range of 60–140 mg/m^2 showed particular sensitivity to the drug, but the 220–240 and 300 mg/m^2 group was therapeutically superior to the lower dosages. However, they found remission duration was independent of the dosage. The severity and duration of peripheral pancytopenia were about the same at all three dosage levels. Of note was that 12 of the patients responding to daunomycin had CNS leukemia during the course of their therapy, indicating that daunomycin did not cross the blood–brain barrier.

One can conclude that daunomycin is an effective agent in inducing remissions in childhood ALL even in patients previously treated with vincristine and prednisone. Clearly, combination chemotherapy was indicated to attempt even greater success.

b. Daunomycin plus Other Drugs for Childhood ALL. Table VII represents a summary of the various combinations of daunomycin with other drugs in the treatment of ALL in children. It is not within the

TABLE VI

EFFECT OF INCREASING TOTAL DAUNOMYCIN DOSE ON RESPONSE[a]

Total dose (mg/m^2)	% CR + PR[b]
60–140	36.4
150–200	18.2
225–250	45.0
300	42.0

[a] Data from Jones *et al.* (1971).

[b] CR, complete remission; PR, partial remission.

TABLE VII

INVESTIGATIONS OF DAUNOMYCIN COMBINED WITH OTHER CHEMOTHERAPEUTIC AGENTS FOR TREATMENT OF CHILDHOOD ACUTE LYMPHOCYTIC LEUKEMIA

Drug(s) (plus daunomycin)	References[a]
Prednisone	(1) (2) (3) (4)
Prednisone, vincristine	(2) (5) (6) (7) (8) (9) (10)
Prednisone, vincristine, L-asparaginase	(11)
Prednisone, vincristine, methotrexate	(12)

[a] Key to references: (1) Jaffe *et al.* (1974); (2) Jones *et al.* (1972); (3) Holton *et al.* (1968); (4) Holton *et al.* (1969); (5) Haghbin *et al.* (1974); (6) Verzosa and Fite (1971); (7) Vietti *et al.* (1971); (8) Jacquillat *et al.* (1973); (9) Mathé *et al.* (1967); (10) Pavlovsky *et al.* (1973); (11) Acute Leukemia Group B study; (12) Acute Leukemia Group B study in progress.

scope of this review to determine which regimen is best, but the combinations have been summarized to show what has been used.

The contribution of prednisone to the response rates in patients receiving prednisone plus daunomycin is difficult to assess. Howard and Tan (1967) noted an M_1 marrow in 5 of 7 patients resistant to conventional therapy who were treated with both drugs. Holton *et al.* (1969) noted 39 CR and 10 PR in 60 children with advanced leukemia (82%). When patients who had one previous course of prednisone were eliminated, a 57% response rate was computed (17 out of 30).

Using daunomycin + prednisone + vincristine, Mathé *et al.* (1967) reported 11 CR in 11 patients with previously untreated ALL. These findings were confirmed by Bernard *et al.* (1968), whereas Vietti *et al.* (1971) and Holton (1969) noted somewhat lower response rates.

The best-controlled study comparing daunomycin to daunomycin + prednisone to daunomycin + prednisone + vincristine was conducted by the ALGB in their 6801 study. All patients had been previously treated with vincristine and prednisone and had relapsed on those drugs. Their total remissions (CR + PR) for the various treatment regimens were daunomycin alone, 38%; daunomycin + prednisone, 45%, and daunomycin + prednisone + vincristine, 44%. In that study the addition of prednisone or vincristine and prednisone to daunomycin did not improve the frequency of remission induction. Furthermore, the severe hematologic toxicity reactions induced by the daunomycin alone were not significantly altered by the addition of prednisone (Jones *et al.*, 1972).

c. Daunomycin Alone for ALL in Adults. In 1972, Bloomfield *et al.* noted that up to then there had been only nine papers that included reports of adults with ALL treated with daunomycin and other drugs, and there were no reports on using daunomycin alone for treating adult ALL. This is surprising in light of the extensive use of daunomycin in childhood ALL.

In the very few adult patients with ALL who were treated with daunomycin alone, response rates have varied from 0–66% (Tan *et al.*, 1967; Malpas and Scott, 1968; Baudo *et al.*, 1968).

d. Daunomycin plus Other Drugs for Adult ALL. In contrast to the small number of adult ALL patients treated with daunomycin alone, there have been many combination regimens with daunomycin used to treat that disease. The combinations employed have included daunomycin plus prednisone (Bloomfield *et al.*, 1972); daunomycin plus L-asparaginase (Bodey *et al.*, 1974); and daunomycin plus vincristine plus prednisone (Mathé *et al.*, 1973; Pavlovsky *et al.*, 1973).

The number of patients in each of the studies is very small and the only conclusions that can be drawn is that the combination regimens are active in adult ALL, even in patients resistant to other treatment. However, the optimal regimen has not yet been determined.

e. Daunomycin Alone for AML in Children. Table VIII details the response to daunomycin of a total of 83 children with AML. Some of the patients had been previously treated. Daunomycin produced an overall response rate of 58%.

The ALGB protocol 6706A compared the 60 mg/m^2 daily for 5 days administration versus the twice weekly schedule versus the weekly schedule. There was a greater percent of remissions induced by the repeated daily and twice weekly courses (66% and 60%, respectively) than by the weekly dosage (35% remissions). The 5-day regimen was declared the most active; however, there was a longer duration of survival in the twice weekly and weekly dosage regimens than in the daily administration for 3, 5, or 7 days. There was some question whether this increase in survival might have been secondary to a decrease in drug-related deaths because the intermittent dose was less toxic (Weil *et al.*, 1973).

The ALGB 6706 study had originally determined that, in childhood AML, the daily treatment for 3 or 5 days was better than that repeated for 7 days. The latter regimen was declared too toxic by that study group. They also noted that good results were exceptional in adults and were more frequent in children. Results were also better in the previously untreated patient. The gratifying activity of daunomycin in childhood AML also led to combination work.

f. Daunomycin plus Other Drugs for Childhood AML. Combination regimens used in childhood AML include daunomycin plus prednisone

TABLE VIII

DAUNOMYCIN AS SINGLE-AGENT THERAPY FOR CHILDREN WITH ACUTE MYELOCYTIC LEUKEMIA

Dose		No. of evaluable	Complete response		Partial response		
(mg/m²)	Schedule[a]	patients	No.	(%)	No.	(%)	Reference[b]
37[c]	Daily × 5	6	2	33	2	33	(1)
60	Weekly	14	3	21	2	14	(2)
60	Twice weekly	10	5	50	1	10	(2)
60	Daily × 3	7	4	57	1	14	(2)
60	Daily × 5	6	4	66	0	0	(2)
60	Daily × 5	3	0	0	1	33	(2)
60	Daily × 7	3	1	33	0	0	(2)
74[c]	Daily × 3–5	16	11	69	2	13	(3)
74[c]	Daily × 3–10	18	8	44	2	11	(4)
Total		83	38	45	11	13	

[a] All drug was given intravenously.

[b] Key to references: (1) Massimo *et al.* (1968); (2) Weil *et al.* (1973); (3) Boiron *et al.* (1969); (4) Bernard *et al.* (1967).

[c] Calculated by conversion factor of 37 from milligrams per kilogram to milligrams per square meter.

(Jaffe *et al.*, 1974; Holton *et al.*, 1969), daunomycin plus cytosine arabinoside (Rai *et al.*, 1975), daunomycin plus 5-azacytidine (children's cancer group study CCG 242), daunomycin plus vincristine plus prednisone (Pavlovsky *et al.*, 1973), and daunomycin plus prednisone plus vincristine plus cytosine arabinoside (Ara-C) plus 6-mercaptopurine (Eppinger-Helft *et al.*, 1975). At this point in time the only two regimens that appear superior to daunomycin alone are the daunomycin plus Ara-C combination and the daunomycin plus 5-azacytidine combination. However, no direct comparative trials between these combinations and daunomycin alone have been carried out.

g. Daunomycin Alone for AML in Adults. In this review a total of 609 adult patients with AML have been treated with daunomycin alone (Table IX). There has been an overall response rate of 38% (29% CR and 9% PR). The patients have been both previously treated and untreated.

There are many schedules for treating adult AML. The ALGB did a study of 60 mg/m² of daunomycin given daily for 3, 5, and 7 days. They found that the total remission rates in adults were approximately equal, but that the 7-day injection could seldom be tolerated secondary to severe marrow aplasia. They also noted good results were exceptional in patients over 60 years of age, and results were better in the previously untreated patients (Weil *et al.*, 1973).

TABLE IX

DAUNOMYCIN AS SINGLE-AGENT THERAPY FOR ADULT ACUTE MYELOCYTIC LEUKEMIA

Dose (mg/m^2)	Schedule[a]	No. of evaluable patients	Complete response No.	Complete response (%)	Partial response No.	Partial response (%)	Reference[b]
37[c]	Daily × 5	7	1	14	1	14	(1)
60	Weekly	55	8	15	5	9	(2)
60	Twice weekly	52	8	15	6	12	(2)
60	Daily × 3	144[d]	61	42	19	7	(3)
60	Daily × 3	37	9	24	1	3	(2)
60	Daily × 3	22	11	50	0	0	(4)
60	Daily × 5	46	8	17	6	13	(2)
60	Daily × 5	56	17	30	6	11	(2)
74[c]	Daily × 3–5	48	24	50	6	13	(5)
74[c]	Daily × 5	19	3	16	1	5	(6)
60	Daily × 7	28	21	21	3	11	(2)
60 *or* 180	Daily × 5 Daily × 1	14[e]	2	14	2	14	(7)
180	Daily × 1	16[d]	4	25	1	6	(8)
180	Daily × 1	16[e]	2	33	1	17	(8)
Total		609	177	29	55	9	

[a] All drug was given intravenously.

[b] Key to references: (1) Bezwoda *et al.* (1974); (2) Weil *et al.* (1973); (3) Wiernik *et al.* (1975); (4) Wiernik and Serpick (1972); (5) Boiron *et al.* (1969); (6) Malpas and Scott (1968); (7) Lippman *et al.* (1972); (8) Green *et al.* (1972).

[c] Calculated by conversion factor of 37 from milligrams per kilogram to milligram per square meter.

[d] Previously untreated.

[e] Previously treated with daunomycin and other agents.

Lippman *et al.* (1972) tried large intermittent doses of 180 mg/m^2/day in patients who had and had not already received daunomycin. Responses in 4 of 14 patients were restricted to those patients who received greater than 300 mg/m^2 of the drug and who had not been previously exposed to lower-dose levels of the drug. None of the 8 patients who had received daunomycin before responded to the higher dose of daunomycin. They concluded that previous exposure to daunomycin at lower-dose levels substantially reduced the chance of subsequent response with high-dose level therapy. They also noted that dose levels greater than 600 mg/m^2 were fraught with irreversible cardiac failure (2 patients died of intractible congestive heart failure) and the high dose gave severe leukopenia and chemical phlebitis. The dermal phlebitis was a major cause of death in their series.

Greene *et al.* (1972) also used a single large dose of daunomycin on the suggestion in pharmacokinetic studies that persistent serum levels seen after one large dose might be equivalent to the usual schedule of daily smaller doses. As an added facet to their study they measured the levels of daunomycin reductase which is the enzyme that mediates the conversion of daunomycin to daunorubicinol. This metabolic conversion is common to all tissues.

The complete remission rate in the high-dose treated patients was 40% overall with 5 of 16 (31%) of previously untreated and 3 of 6 (50%) previously treated patients responding. Of note was that the clinical response correlated closely with *in vitro* determination of peripheral leukemic myeloblast daunorubicin reductase activity. Thirteen patients had enzyme analysis, and those patients responding to daunomycin in the high-dose schedule had the highest myeloblast to erythrocyte daunorubicin reductase ratios. The serum ratio for 4 patients who achieved complete remission was 44.5 ± 3.0 which was greater than the level (20.9 ± 9.9) for patients that failed to respond. The ratio apparently had no relationship to sex or previous therapy.

These investigators also noted that in patients over 60 years of age there was an inverse relationship between age and daunorubicin reductase levels. There was no such correlation among normal controls, however, so no statements could be made to point to a possible reason for the poor response to daunomycin therapy in patients older than 60 years of age. They noted that daunorubicinol penetrates the cells less readily than daunorubicin and that the daily dose may allow a higher concentration of daunorubicinol in leukemic cells by providing higher plasma levels of daunomycin to serve as a substrate for intracellular daunorubicin reductase. They also observed that previously treated patients had a prolonged bone marrow depression well beyond that seen in previously untreated patients.

A number of studies have compared daunomycin alone to other drug combinations used for treating AML. Wiernik and Serpick (1972) compared daunomycin given for 3 consecutive days with a 6-mercaptopurine + vincristine + methotrexate + prednisone (POMP) regimen and obtained a 50% CR rate with the single agent and a 28% CR rate with the multiple-agent regimen.

Wiernik and Schimpff (1975) later compared daunomycin alone versus daunomycin + pyrimethamine + Ara-C, and thioguanine (DDTA) for the treatment of acute nonlymphocytic leukemia. Forty-nine percent of patients treated with daunomycin alone and 46% of patients treated with DDTA had a complete remission. Median survival was superior for daunomycin compared to DDTA. The DDTA-treated patients did have a longer diagnosis to CNS leukemia interval than did the daunomycin patients, but the pyrimethamine did not reduce the incidence of CNS leukemia.

h. Daunomycin plus Other Drugs for Adult AML. Because of the activity of daunomycin alone in AML, it was placed in combination with other agents active in the disease. The most frequently used combinations are listed in Table X.

Daunomycin + Ara-C has been a popular combination with overall response rates of 25–79% in various series (Table X). Glucksman *et al.* (1973) noted that the 2-day course of daunomycin (45 mg/m²/day) and a 5-day infusion of Ara-C (100 mg/m²/day) produced subtotal bone marrow response. Yates *et al.* (1973) proposed an extension of drug administration of daunomycin for 3 days and Ara-C for 7 days to produce adequate marrow suppression after a single course to get earlier remissions. Response rates with the extended administration have been as high as 62–77% (Yates *et al.*, 1973; Rai *et al.*, 1975).

A number of investigators feel that the daunomycin + Ara-C program is the combination of choice for induction of remission in adults with

TABLE X

DAUNOMYCIN COMBINED WITH OTHER CHEMOTHERAPEUTIC AGENTS FOR TREATMENT OF ADULT ACUTE MYELOCYTIC LEUKEMIA

Drug(s)[a] (plus daunomycin)	Reference[b]
Ara-C	(1) (2) (3) (4) (5) (6) (7)
L-Asp	(8)
Ara-C + 6TG	(9)
VCR + Pred	(10) (11)
VCR + Ara-C	(12)
Ara-C + L-Asp	(3)
VCR + Pred + L-Asp	(10)
VCR + Pred + Ara-C + 6MP	(13)
Pred + Ara-C + 6MP + 6TG	(14)
VCR + Ara-C + 6TG + MTX + CTX + Pred	(15)
VCR + Ara-C + 6TG + MTX + CTX + Pred + hydroxyurea	(15)

[a] Ara-C, cytosine arabinoside; L-Asp, L-asparaginase; 6TG, 6-thioguanine; VCR, vincristine; Pred, prednisone; 6MP, 6-mercaptopurine; CTX, cyclophosphamide; MTX, methotrexate.

[b] Key to references: (1) Friend *et al.* (1974); (2) Yates *et al.* (1973); (3) Crowther *et al.* (1970); (4) Bernard *et al.* (1974); (5) Freeman *et al.* (1973); (6) Crowther *et al.* (1973); (7) Brincker (1972); (8) Bodey *et al.* (1974); (9) Wiernik *et al.* (1975); (10) Gerhartz *et al.* (1973); (11) Pavlovsky *et al.* (1973); (12) Rosenthal and Maloney (1972); (13) Eppinger-Helft *et al.* (1975); (14) Stavem and Gjemdal (1974); (15) Brincker (1975).

AML. However, the European Organization for Research and Treatment of Cancer (EORTC) did a controlled study of Ara-C versus Ara-C + 6-thioguanine (6-TG) versus Ara-C + daunomycin and found no statistically significant difference in induction of complete remission (25, 30, and 31%, respectively). There were also no statistical differences in survival, and the Ara-C + daunomycin regimen was probably the most toxic (Malpas *et al.,* 1974). Even with that piece of evidence, the daunomycin + Ara-C combination is still popular and used for remission induction.

Cytosine arabinoside + 6-TG has been a common regimen for remission induction in AML. As noted in Table X some studies have added daunomycin to these two drugs. The ALGB study 7221 was a randomized controlled study of daunomycin versus Ara-C + 6-TG versus Ara-C + 6-TG + daunomycin (D+A+T). The CR rates were 42, 44, and 59%, respectively. An additional 7, 7, and 6% of patients achieved partial remissions. No important differences in toxicity were noted among the daunomycin, Ara-C + 6-TG and daunomycin + Ara-C + 6-TG regimens and they concluded that D+A+T *may* be superior to daunomycin or Ara-C + 6-TG for remission induction. They did not mention if this difference in response was significant (Wiernik *et al.*, 1975).

Crowther *et al.* (1970) compared Ara-C + daunomycin versus Ara-C + daunomycin + L-asparaginase and noted that the L-asparaginase did not add to the remission rates obtained by daunomycin + Ara-C alone. The toxicities were considerably greater in the group treated with L-asparaginase.

The Southwestern Chemotherapy Group study 560/561 compared Cytoxan + vincristine + Ara-C + prednisone (COAP) versus daunomycin + vincristine + Ara-C + prednisone (DOAP) versus vincristine + Ara-C + prednisone (OAP). They noted that CR for AML patients on an OAP regimen was 41%, and 53% for COAP and DOAP (no significant difference in response). Median remission durations were as follows: DOAP, 47 weeks; COAP, 40 weeks; OAP, 35 weeks. The DOAP regimen median survival was slightly longer, but not significantly different from the COAP or OAP regimens (Southwestern Oncology Group data).

In conclusion, daunomycin is an effective agent for the treatment of AML in adults. Combination chemotherapy with Ara-C gives significantly greater remission rates than daunomycin used alone. At the present time this combination is probably the program of choice for the induction of remission in AML.

i. Daunomycin for Treatment of Rare Leukemias of Children and

Adults. Daunomycin has been used alone and in combination for treating the less common leukemias. Remissions have been attained in chronic myelogenous leukemia in blast crisis (Bernard *et al.*, 1967; Fennelly *et al.*, 1974), in acute plasma cell leukemia (Yates *et al.*, 1973), in erythroleukemia (Bloomfield *et al.*, 1974), in eosinophilic leukemia (Marcovitch *et al.*, 1973), in acute monocytic leukemia of children (Komiyama *et al.*, 1973), and in acute promyelocytic leukemia, alone (Bernard *et al.*, 1967, 1973) and in combination with heparin (Nomura *et al.*, 1974).

j. Daunomycin for Maintenance Therapy in Leukemia. Daunomycin has been used for maintenance therapy of leukemia in remission. Humphrey *et al.* (1975) reported on 70 patients with ALL maintained after remission induction on either methotrexate biweekly alone or methotrexate biweekly plus daunomycin monthly. There was not significant difference between the distribution of remission times for the two maintenance arms (median 147 and 162 days, respectively).

Several investigators have warned that daunomycin should not be used in maintenance regimens because it can cause cardiotoxicity at large cumulative doses (Jones *et al.*, 1971).

2. *Solid Tumors*

Although daunomycin has received extensive testing for the treatment of leukemias, it has not been adequately studied in most of the solid tumors of children and adults.

a. Adult Solid Tumors. There is a paucity of information regarding the activity of daunomycin in the solid tumors of adults (see Table XI).

TABLE XI

ACTIVITY OF DAUNOMYCIN IN SOLID TUMORS[a]

Tumor	No. of studies	Evaluable patients	No. of responses
Breast	1	2	0
Lung	4	19	2
Gastrointestinal	5	54	6
Melanoma	6	10	2
Sarcoma	5	59	8
Hodgkin's lymphoma	3	20	3
Non-Hodgkin's lymphoma	5	25	3
Ovary	4	5	0
Renal	8	8	1
Testicular	8	8	0

[a] Data from Von Hoff *et al.* (1976*b*). Adapted by permission of the copyright owner.

Adult solid tumors have been treated with the drug (Tan *et al.*, 1967; Kenis and Brule, 1970), but only a few studies have enough data to call this drug active or inactive in the adult solid tumors (Von Hoff *et al.*, 1976b; Weiss and Cantor, 1976). It would be of interest to have further trials of daunomycin in the adult solid tumors, so that the activity of daunomycin could be compared to its analog, adriamycin, which has a broad antitumor spectrum.

b. Pediatric Solid Tumors. Daunomycin has been used to treat neuroblastoma in a number of trials using daily for 3 days and weekly schedules (Samuels *et al.*, 1971; Evans *et al.*, 1974; Sutow *et al.*, 1970; Tan *et al.*, 1967). Response rates in this tumor have ranged from 0 to 100% with a cumulative response rate of 16% in 119 patients (all partial remissions). Daunomycin might have a place in the treatment of patients with advanced neuroblastoma who are no longer responsive to more effective agents (Samuels *et al.*, 1971).

A variety of other pediatric solid tumors have had trials using daunomycin therapy. These include rhabdomyosarcoma (Tan *et al.*, 1967; Evans *et al.*, 1974), osteogenic sarcoma (Evans *et al.*, 1974), Ewings sarcoma (Tan *et al.*, 1967), and other miscellaneous tumors (Tan *et al.*, 1967; Evans *et al.*, 1974; Massimo *et al.*, 1968). However, an insufficient number of patients have been evaluated to draw any conclusions about the activity of the drug in those tumors.

C. Toxicity in Man

The Investigational Drug Branch has received toxicity reports on 1156 patients receiving daunomycin. These patients were treated with five different dosage schedules: single, weekly, every 4 days, and daily. The overall percent of each of the toxicities noted in the 1156 patients is summarized in Table XII. Each major toxicity will be discussed in detail.

1. *Hematologic Side Effects*

Leukopenia has consistently been the immediate dose-limiting toxicity of daunomycin. The leukopenia is dose-related with the usual day of nadir on days 8–10 on a daily for 3 days administration (Jaffe *et al.*, 1974; Burns, 1975). Recovery takes place on an average of 2–3 weeks, but leukopenia has lasted longer in patients who have had previous daunomycin therapy.

Thrombocytopenia ($<50{,}000/mm^3$) has been noted in 54% of patients. The nadir of thrombocytopenia has been 4–15 days after starting therapy with recovery in 2–3 weeks.

TABLE XII

TOXICITIES SECONDARY TO DAUNOMYCIN IN 1156 PATIENTS[a]

Toxicity	% Incidence
Leukopenia (< 1500/mm^3)	65
Thrombocytopenia (< 50,000/mm^3)	54
Anemia	4.6
Cardiotoxicity	1.96
EKG changes	0.80
Congestive heart failure	1.16
Nausea	27
Vomiting	37
Diarrhea	25
Mucositis	15
Fever	33
Phlebitis	30
Skin rash	6
Alopecia	35

[a] Data from Von Hoff *et al.* (1976a). Adapted by permission of the copyright owner.

Anemia has not been a particular problem with daunomycin administration except in one study where daunomycin was administered to patients with neuroblastoma (Sutow *et al.*, 1970).

2. *Cardiotoxicity*

The first report of congestive heart failure in patients receiving daunomycin was made by Karnofsky in 1966 (Livingston and Carter, 1970). Since that time there have been several reports of its occurrence (Halazun *et al.*, 1974; Holton *et al.*, 1968, 1969; Tan *et al.*, 1965, 1967; Holland and Glidewell, 1972; Bernard *et al.* , 1967; Jones *et al.* , 1971; Bernard, 1967; Weil *et al.*, 1973; Mathé *et al.*, 1967; Massimo *et al.*, 1968; Jacquillat *et al.*, 1973; Gilladoga *et al.*, 1976). Although the drug-induced cardiotoxicity is a well-known phenomenon, there has been a paucity of details regarding its relation to total dose, its time of onset, and its impact on administration of the drug.

A recent analysis by the Investigational Drug Branch carefully analyzed the 110 cases of daunomycin-induced cardiotoxicity reported since 1966 (Von Hoff *et al.*, 1977). That analysis indicated there were two distinct types of cardiotoxicity: drug-induced EKG changes and congestive heart failure or cardiomyopathy.

The EKG changes seen with daunomycin do not appear to be related to the total dose of drug administered and do not seem to presage the development of congestive heart failure. The EKG abnormalities consisted of nonspecific ST-T wave changes, low voltage of the QRS complex, and a myriad of other less common abnormalities (Halazun *et al.*, 1974; Von Hoff *et al.*, 1977). The EKG changes were less common in children than in the adult population receiving daunomycin.

The congestive heart failure secondary to daunomycin usually presents with a sudden onset of tachycardia, dyspnea, hepatomegaly ventricular gallop, cyanosis, and finally full blown congestive heart failure. Chest X-rays will frequently show increased cardiothoracic ratios (Raskin *et al.*, 1973).

The incidence of congestive heart failure is definitely related to the total dose of daunomycin administered, with a higher risk of cardiomyopathy as the total dose of daunomycin is increased. Figure 5 demonstrates the dose–response curve for incidence of heart failure secondary to daunomycin. There is a 1.5% incidence of development of congestive heart failure at a total dose of 600 mg/m^2 and a 12% incidence at 1000 mg/m^2. Von Hoff *et al.* (1977) have shown that children might be more susceptible to the development of drug-induced congestive heart failure than adults. Other observers have concluded the opposite (Bonadonna *et al.*, 1969; Malpas and Scott, 1969).

Drug-induced cardiomyopathy is a devastating complication. Eighty-four percent of patients were in complete remission from their leukemia or tumor at the time of onset of congestive heart failure and 74% of the patients with the cardiomyopathy died as a result of that complication (Von Hoff *et al.*, 1977).

At the present time the only sure way to avoid the cardiomyopathy is to limit the total dose of drug administered. As can be seen in Fig. 5 the risk of cardiomyopathy increases as the total dose of daunomycin increases. There does not seem to be a precise cutoff point of a total dose of daunomycin that should never be exceeded under any circumstances, but rather there is a continuum of increasing risk with a rather abrupt increase in risk beginning at 1100 mg/m^2 total dose.

Careful cardiac monitoring is essential for the patient receiving daunomycin.

3. *Gastrointestinal*

Nausea and vomiting are seen with administration of daunomycin and seem to be dose related. At doses of 180 mg/m^2/day of daunomycin, there is nearly a 100% incidence of nausea and vomiting which persists for 3–7 days suggesting an accumulation of the drug (Greene *et al.*, 1972).

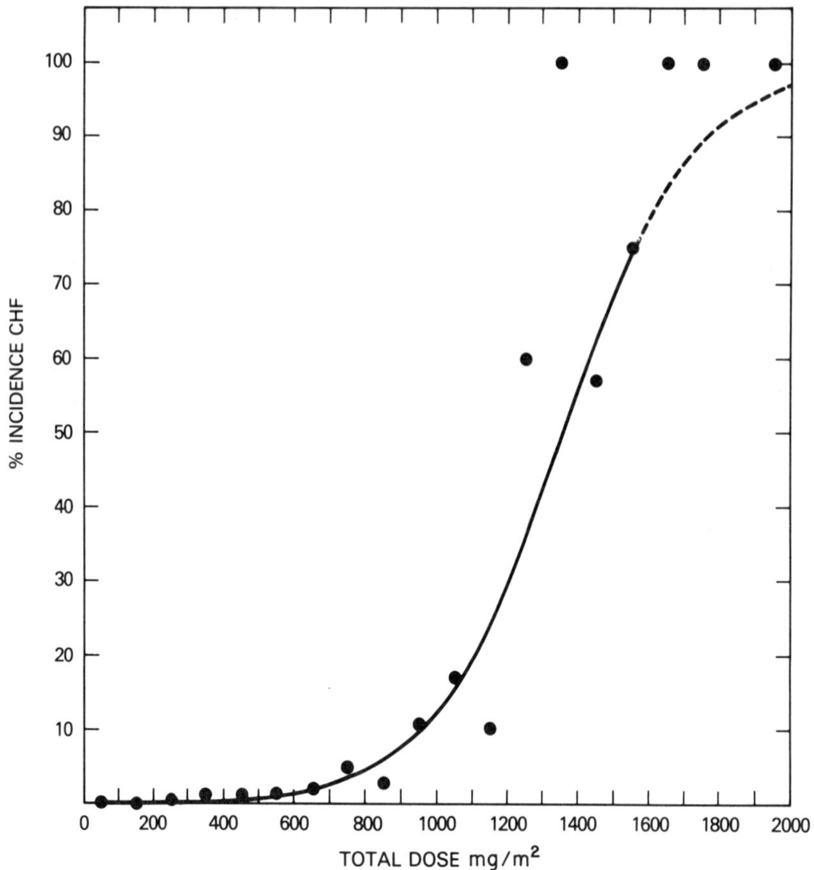

FIG. 5. Congestive heart failure (CHF) in patients receiving daunomycin (5613 patients; 65 cases of CHF). (From Von Hoff *et al.*, 1977. Adapted by permission of the copyright owner.)

Anorexia and diarrhea are noted occasionally. Bloody diarrhea with a cleavage of the mucosa from the underlying muscular layer of the intestine has been noted in a child and ascribed to daunomycin (Massimo *et al.*, 1968).

Oral mucosal lesions have been noted in some patients and usually disappear when the drug is stopped (Green *et al.*, 1972).

4. *Fever*

Fever thought secondary to daunomycin has been reported by several investigators (Tan *et al.*, 1967; Green *et al.*, 1972; Wiernik and Serpick,

1972). It usually returns to base-line within 24 hours after discontinuation of drug.

5. *Phlebitis*

Tan *et al.* (1967) noted pain, necrosis, and fibrosis at extravasation sites of daunomycin. Chemical phlebitis with high-dose daunomycin was a major cause of death in 8 of 14 patients given the drug because of secondary infection at the necrotic injection site (Lippman *et al.*, 1972). Vietti *et al.* (1971) reported 1 case of brawny edema of an entire arm and lateral chest wall after an infusion of daunomycin.

6. *Skin and Allergic Reactions*

A generalized rash has been seen in 6% of patients receiving daunomycin. There have been a number of reports of urticarial reactions with daunomycin administration (Crowther *et al.*, 1973; Vietti *et al.*, 1971).

Freeman (1970) reported angioneurotic edema of the lips and eyes and urticaria on the trunk and extremities in a patient who received 60 mg/m^2 of daunomycin after he had had prior monthly daunomycin and prednisone for reinduction. This patient recovered in 2 hours.

7. *Alopecia*

This side-effect has been noted in both children and adults. The alopecia has ranged from a thinning to alopecia totalis. Regrowth of scalp hair usually occurs within 2 months (Tan *et al.*, 1967).

8. *Other*

Less common toxicities reported to the Investigational Drug Branch were headache, red urine (1 report), seizures (2 reported cases related to primary disease, sepsis or the drug), abnormal liver function tests (6 cases), and elevations in BUN (2 cases).

One case of hepatomegaly ascribed to daunomycin occurred in a patient with AML and was reported to the Investigational Drug Branch. The postmortem examination showed fatty metamorphosis, severe bile stasis, multifocal necrosis, and hepatocellular degeneration consistent with drug toxicity. No other drugs could be implicated at that time.

One case of renal tubular dysfunction with hypocalcemia and hypercalciuria allegedly secondary to daunomycin has been reported.

IX. Summary and Conclusions

Daunomycin is an antitumor antibiotic of the anthracycline family which was introduced into clinical trials in 1965. The drug possesses antibacterial, immunosuppressive, cytotoxic, and antineoplastic effects. It also inhibits X-ray repair and perhaps coagulation systems.

The mechanism of action of daunomycin appears to be the formation of stable complexes with DNA by intercalation between base pairs producing structural changes that interfere with DNA function in cell mitosis. It also inhibits DNA-dependent RNA synthesis by interfering with the formation of DNA as a template for RNA polymerase. The drug is not a cell-cycle phase-specific agent since it may inhibit cell progress in many of the phases of the cell cycle.

Daunomycin exhibits antitumor effects in the L1210, C1498, Sarcoma 180, P388, and B16 melanoma systems. Combinations with ICRF-159 seem to increase the antitumor effect of daunomycin substantially in these systems. Many other promising combinations have been noted in animal tumor systems.

Animal toxicology studies have shown the monkey to be the most sensitive species. Toxic effects of the drug were noted on the bone marrow, gastrointestinal system, liver, and kidneys. Cardiac toxicity was noted in the monkey, but the hamster and rabbit seem to be the best experimental models for this toxicity.

After injection into the mouse, rat, or dog, daunomycin is cleared rapidly from the plasma, deposited in tissue, extensively metabolized, and slowly excreted with biliary excretion being equivalent to urinary excretion in rats but less than urinary excretion in the dog.

In the human, daunomycin is fixed by the body tissues within a short period of time after administration of the drug, but a second plasma half-life is present with more sustained blood levels of the drug. The total output of daunomycin and its metabolites in the urine is low. Therefore, there is probably significant biliary excretion of the drug. The major urinary metabolites in the human are daunomycin and daunorubicinol which are both cytotoxic in the P388 and L1210 mouse leukemia systems.

Clinical trials with daunomycin have been ongoing since 1965 using a variety of dosages and schedules. The present review involves information accumulated on 5613 patients studied by clinical cooperative groups and independent investigators.

The responses of the various human tumor types have been analyzed. Daunomycin alone has been active in acute lymphocytic leukemia of adults and children and acute myelogenous leukemia of adults and children. When used in certain combinations in these diseases, it has equal or greater activity depending on the disease treated. Daunomycin also seems to possess activity in monocytic, promyelocytic, and chronic myelogenous leukemia in blast crisis. The drug does not, however, appear to have a place in maintenance therapy of any disease.

Daunomycin has not had promising activity in adult solid tumors, although trials have not been extensive enough to make this conclusion in most of the signal solid tumors. It does appear to have documented activity in neuroblastoma of children.

Toxicities seen with daunomycin include leukopenia and thrombocytopenia which can be severe. Nausea, vomiting, anorexia, diarrhea, mucositis, fever, phlebitis, rash, alopecia, and other less frequent toxicities have been noted.

Of major importance is the cardiotoxicity associated with daunomycin. The EKG changes that are seen with daunomycin administration appear to be unrelated to the total dose of drug administered and do not presage the development of congestive heart failure. The drug-induced cardiomyopathy is definitely total dose-related and is often a fatal complication.

In conclusion, daunomycin is a compound with definite clinical activity in human acute leukemia. The major obstacle to its chronic use in patients is the drug-induced cardiomyopathy. Future work with the drug should include exploration of its activity in adult solid tumors and a search for methods of making the drug less cardiotoxic.

References

Acton, E. M., Fujiwara, A. N., and Henry, D. W. (1974). *J. Med. Chem.* **17,** 659–660.

Alberts, D. S., Bachur, N. R. , and Holtzman, J. L. (1971). *Clin. Pharmacol. Ther.* **12,** 96–104.

Arcamone, F., Di Marco, A., Gaetani, M., and Scotti, T. (1961). *G. Microbiol.* **9,** 83–90.

Arcamone, F., Franceschi, G., Orezzi, P., Cassinelli, G., Barbieri, W., and Mondelli, R. (1964a). *J. Am. Chem. Soc.* **86,** 5334–5335.

Arcamone, F., Cassinelli, G., Orezzi, P., Franceschi, G., and Mondelli. R. (1964b). *J. Am. Chem. Soc.* **86,** 5335–5336.

Arlin, Z., Fried, J., and Clarkson, B. (1975). *Proc. Am. Assoc. Cancer Res.* **16,** 180.

Asbell, M. A., Schwartzbach, E., Bullock, F. J., and Yesair, D. W. (1972). *J. Pharmacol. Exp. Ther.* **182,** 63–69.

Bachur, N. R. (1971). *J. Pharmacol. Exp. Ther.* **177,** 573–578.

Bachur, N. R. and Cradock, J. C. (1970). *J. Pharmacol. Exp. Ther.* **175,** 331–337.

Bachur, N. R. and Gee, M. (1971). *J. Pharmacol. Exp. Ther.* **177,** 567–572.

Bachur, N. R. Hildebrand, R. C., and Jaenke, R. S. (1974). *J. Pharmacol. Exp. Ther.* **191,** 331–340.

Bachur, N. R., Riggs, C. E., Jr., Green, M. R., Langone, J. J., Van Vunakis, H., Levine, L. (1977). *Clin. Pharmacol. Ther.* **21,** 70–77.

Barbieri, P., Di Marco, A., Mazzoleni, R., Menozzi, M., and Sanfilippo. A. (1964). *G. Microbiol.* **12,** 71–82.

Baudo, F., Camera, G., Cipriani, D., de Cataldo, F., Pensabene, A., Tiso, R., and Bussi, L. (1968). *Oncology* **22,** 67–73.

Baxt, W., Hehlman, R., and Spiegelman, S. (1972). *Nature (London), New Biol.* **240,** 72–76.

Bernard, J. (1967). *Cancer Res.* **27,** 2565–2569.

Bernard, J., Jacquillat, C., Boiron, M., Najean, Y., Seligmann, M., Tanzer, J., Weil, M., and Lortholary, P. (1967). *Presse Med.* **75,** 951–955.

Bernard, J., Boiron, M., and Jacquillat, C. (1968). *Proc. Congr. Int. Soc. Hematol., 12th, 1967,* p. 5.

Bernard, J., Weil, M., Boiron, M., Jacquillat, C. M., Flandrin, G., and Gemon, M. F. (1973). *Blood* **41,** 489–496.

Bezwoda, W. R., Lynch, S. R., Sacks, P., Gale, D., Bothwell, T. H., and Stevens, K. (1974). *S. Afr. Med. J.* **48,** 963–967.

Bloomfield, C. D., Brunning, R. D., and Kennedy, B. J. (1972). *Cancer* **30,** 47–55.

Bloomfield, C. D., Brunning, R. D., and Kennedy, B. J. (1974). *Ann. Intern. Med.* **81,** 746–750.

Bodey, G. P., Hewlett, J. S., Coltman, C. A., Jr., Rodriguez, V., and Freireich, E. J. (1974). *Cancer* **33,** 626–630.

Boiron, M., Jacquillat, C., Weil, M., Tanzer, J., Levy, D., Sultan, C., and Bernard, J. (1969). *Lancet* **1,** 330–333.

Bonadonna, G., Monfardini, S., Marmont, A. M., Damasio, E., and Rossi, F. (1969). *Lancet* **1,** 837–838.

Brincker, H. (1972). *Scand. J. Haematol.* **9,** 657–664.

Brincker, H. (1975). *Scand. J. Haematol.* **14,** 35–41.

Bullock, F. J., Bruni, R, J., and Asbell, M. A. (1972). *J. Pharmacol. Exp. Ther.* **182,** 70–76.

Burns, C. P. (1975). *Cancer Chemother. Rep.* **59,** 757–760.

Calendi, E., Di Marco, A., Reggiani, M., Scarpinato, B., and Valentini, L. (1965). *Biochim. Biophys. Acta* **103,** 25–49.

Cassinelli, G., and Orezzi, P. (1963). *G. Microbiol.* **11,** 167–174.

Cihak, A., Vesely, J., and Harrap, K. R. (1974). *Biochem. Pharmacol.* **23,** 1087–1094.

Crowther, D., Bateman, C. J. T., Vartan, C. P., Whitehouse, J. M. A., Malpas, J. S., Hamilton Fairley, G., and Scott, R. B. (1970). *Br. Med. J.* **4,** 513–517.

Crowther, D., Powles, R. L., Bateman, C. J., T., Beard, M. E. J., Gauci, C. L., Wrigley, P. F. M., Malpas, J. S., Hamilton Fairley, G., and Scott, R. B. (1973). *Br. Med. J.* **1,** 131–137.

Dano, K., Frederiksen, S., and Hellung-Larsen, P. (1972). *Cancer Res.* **32,** 1307–1314.

Di Fronzo, G., and Bonadonna, G. (1970). *Rev. Eur. Etud. Clin. Biol.* **15,** 314–320.

Di Marco, A. (1967). *Pathol. Biol.* **15,** 897–902.

Di Marco, A., Gaetani, M., Dorigotti, L., Soldati, M., and Bellini, O. (1964a). *Cancer Chemother. Rep.* **38,** 31–38.

Di Marco, A., Gaetani, M., Orezzi, P., Scarpinato, B. M., Silvestrini, R., Soldati, M., Dasdia, T., and Valentini, L. (1964b). *Nature (London)* **201,** 706–707.

Di Marco, A., Soldati, M., Fioretti, A., and Dasdia, T. (1964c). *Cancer Chemother. Rep.* **38,** 39–47.

Di Marco, A., Silvestrini, R., Di Marco, S., and Dasdia, T. (1965). *J. Cell Biol.* **27,** 545–550.

Di Marco, A., Boretti, C., Rusconi, A., and Silvestrini, R. (1967). *Proc. Int. Cancer Congr., 9th, 1966* p. 376.

Dombernowsky, P., and Nissen, N. I. (1975). *Proc. Am. Assoc. Cancer Res.* **16,** 167.

Dorigotti, L. (1964). *Tumori* **50,** 117–135.

Dubost, M., Ganter, P., Maral, R., Ninet, L., Pinnert, S., Preud'homme, J., and Werner, G. H. (1964). *Cancer Chemother. Rep.* **41,** 35–36.

Edelstein, M., Vietti, T., and Valeriote, F. (1974). *Cancer Res.* **34,** 293–297.

Egorin, M. J., Hildebrand, R. C., Cimino, E. F., and Bachur, N. R. (1974). *Cancer Res.* **34,** 2243–2245.

Eppinger-Helft, M., Pavlovsky, S., Suarez, A., Sackmann Muriel, F., Hidalgo, G., Pavlovsky, A., and Vilaseca, G. (1975). *Cancer* **35,** 347–353.

Evans, A. E., Baehner, R. L., Chard, R. L., Jr., Leikin, S. L., Pang, E. M., and Pierce, M. (1974). *Cancer Chemother. Rep.* **58,** 671–676.

Feldsted, R. L., Gee, M., and Bachur, N. R. (1974). *J. Biol. Chem.* **249,** 3672–3679.

Fennelly, J. J., O'Connell, L. G., Cahalane, S. F., Keane, T., Gorman, A., and McBride, A. (1974). *Ir. J. Med Sci.* **143,** 129–136.

Finkel, J. M., Knapp, K. T., and Mulligan, L. T. (1969). *Cancer Chemother. Rep.* **53,** 159–164.

Fischerman, K., and Olsen, J. (1974). *Acta Chir. Scand.* **140,** 143–146.

Freeman, A. I. (1970). *Cancer Chemother. Rep., Part 1* **54,** 475–476.

Freeman, C. B., Harris, R., Geary, C. G., Leyland, M. J., MacIver, J. E., and Delamore, I. W. (1973). *Br. Med. J.* **4,** 571–573.

Friend, J. H., Giles, C., and Richardson, S. G. N. (1974). *J. Clin. Pathol.* **27,** 53–54.

Gause, G. F. (1966). *Chem. Ind. (London)* pp. 1506–1513.

Gerhartz, H., Bleihofer, B., Engelbert, B., Paulisch, R., and Schneider, J. (1973). *Proc. Int. Symp. Comp. Leuk. Res. 5th, 1972* Vol. 5 (30) pp. 1142–1146.

Gericke, D., and Chandra, P. (1973). *Z. Krebsforsch.* **79,** 277–281.

Gilladoga, A. C., Manuel, C., Tan, C. T. C., Wollner, N., Sternberg, S. S., and Murphy, M. L. (1976). *Cancer* **37,** 1070–1078.

Gluckman, E., Basch, A., Varet, B., and Dreyfus, B. (1973). *Cancer* **31,** 487–491.

Gosalvez, M., Blanco, M., Hunter, J., Miko, M., and Chance, B. (1974). *Eur. J. Cancer* **10,** 567–574.

Greene, W., Huffman, D., Wiernik, P. H., Schimpff, S., Benjamin, R., and Bachur, N. (1972). *Cancer* **30,** 1419–1427.

Grein, A., Spalla, C., Di Marco, A., and Canevazzi, G. (1963). *G. Microbiol.* **11,** 109–118.

Haghbin, M., Tan, C. C., Clarkson, B. D., Mike, V., Burchenal, J. H., and Murphy, M. L. (1974). *Cancer* **33,** 1491–1498.

Halazun, J. F., Wagner, H. R., Gaeta, J. F., and Sinks, L. F. (1974). *Cancer* **33,** 545–554.

Herman, E. H., Schein, P., and Farmar, R. M. (1969). *Proc. Soc. Exp. Biol. Med.* **130,** 1098–1102.

Holland, J. F., and Glidewell, O. (1972). *Cancer* **30,** 1480–1487.

Holton, C. P. (1969). *Proc. Am. Assoc. Cancer Res.* **10,** 40.

Holton, C. P., Lonsdale, D., Nora, A. H., Thurman, W. G., and Vietti, T. J. (1968). *Cancer* **22,** 1014–1017.

Holton, C. P., Vietti, T. J., Nora, A. H., Donaldson, M. H., Stuckey, W. J., Jr., Watkins, W. L., and Lane, D. M. (1969). *N. Engl. J. Med.* **280,** 171–174.

Hoshino, A., Kato, T., Amo, H., and Ota, K. (1972). *Adv. Antimicrob. Antineoplast. Chemother., Proc. Int. Congr. Chemother., 7th, 1971* Vol. 2, pp. 777–779.

Howard, J. P., and Tan, C. (1967). *Proc. Am. Assoc. Cancer Res.* **8,** 32.

Huffman, D. H., and Bachur, N. R. (1972). *Cancer Res.* **32,** 600–605.

Huffman, D. H., Benjamin, R. S., and Bachur, N. R. (1971). *Clin. Res.* **19,** 493.

Humphrey, G. B., Fernbach, D. J., Razek, A. A., Stuckey, W. J., Komp, D., and George, S. (1975). *Cancer Chemother. Rep.* **59,** 395–399.

Jacquillat, C. , Boiron, M., Weil, M., Tanzer, J., Najean, Y., and Bernard, J. (1966). *Lancet* **2,** 27–28.

Jacquillat, C., Weil, M., Gemon, M. F., Auclerc, G., Loisel, J. P., Delobel, J., Flandrin, G., Schaison, G., Izrael, V., Bussell, A., Dresch, C., Weisgerber, C., Rain, D., Tanzer, J., Najean, Y., Seligmann, M., Boiron, M., and Bernard, J. (1973). *Cancer Res.* **33,** 3278–3284.

Jaenke, R. S. (1974). *Lab. Invest.* **30,** 292–304.

Jaffe, N., Traggis, D. G., and Das, L. (1974). *Cancer Chemother. Rep.* **58,** 661–665.

Jones, B., Holland, J. F., Morrison, A. R., Lee, S. L., Sinks, L. F., Cuttner, J., Rausen, A., Kung, F., Pluss, H. J., Haurani, F. I., Patterson, R. B., Blom, J., Burgert, O. E., Jr., Moon, J. H., Chevalier, L., Sawitsky, A., Albala, M. M., Forcier, R. J., Falkson, G., and Glidewell, O. (1971). *Cancer Res.* **31,** 84–90.

Jones, B., Cuttner, J., Levy, R. N., Patterson, R. B., Kung, F., Pleuss, H. J., Falkson, G., Treat, C. L., Haurani, F., Burgert, E. O., Jr., Rosner, F., Carey, R. W., Lukens, J., Blom, J., Degnan, T. J., Wohl, H., Glidewell, O., and Holland, J. F. (1972). *Cancer Chemother. Rep.* **56,** 729–737.

Kenis, Y., and Brule, G. (1970). *Eur. J. Cancer* **6,** 155–156.

Kim, J. H., Gelbard, A. S., Djordjevič, B., Kim, S. H., and Perez, A. G. (1968). *Cancer Res.* **28,** 2437–2442.

Kline, I. (1974). *Cancer Chemother. Rep. , Part 2* **4,** 33–43.

Komiyama, A., Eguchi, M., Tsukada, M., Hanamura, K., and Akabane, T. (1973). *Med. J. Shinshu Univ.* **17,** 115–125.

Komp, D. M., Lyles, R. L., Jr., Boyd, T. H., III, Stoner, G. E., and Cox, B. J. (1974). *Pediatr. Res.* **8,** 75–81.

Kubisz, P., and Suranova, J. (1974). *Vnitr. Lek.* **20,** 573–578.

Lamberts, B., Buss, H., and Heintz, R. (1973). *Clin. Nephrol.* **1,** 81–85.

Lee, Y. C., Byfield, J. E., Bennet, L. R., and Chan, P. Y. M. (1974). *Cancer Res.* **34,** 2624–2633.

Linden, W. A., Baisch, H., Canstein, L. V., Konig, K., and Canstein, M. V. (1974). *Eur. J. Cancer* **10,** 647–651.

Lippman, M., Zager, R., and Henderson, E. S. (1972). *Cancer Chemother. Rep.* **56,** 755–760.

Livingston, R. B., and Carter, S. K. (1970). *Chemother. Fact Sheet* March, pp. 1–20.

Malpas, J. S., and Scott, R. B. (1968). *Br. Med. J.* **3,** 227–229.

Malpas, J. S., and Scott, R. B. (1969). *Lancet* **1,** 469–470.

Malpas, J., Mathé, G., and Hayat, M. (1974). *Eur. J. Cancer* **10,** 413–418.

Maral, R., Bourat, G., Ducrot, R., Fournel, J., Ganter, P., Julou, L., Koenig, F., Myon, J., Pascal, S., Pasquet, J., Populaire, P., de Ratuld, Y., and Werner, G. H. (1967). *Pathol. Biol.* **15,** 903–908.

Marcovitch, H., Cain, F., and Havard, C. W. H. (1973). *Br. J. Clin. Pract.* **27,** 185–188.

Massimo, L., Fossati-Guglielmoni, A., Monig, A., and Fortuna, E. (1968). *Helv. Paediatr. Acta* **23,** 315–333.

Mathé, G., Schwarzenberg, L., Schneider, M., Schlumberger, J. R., Hayat, M., Amiel, J. L., Cattan, A., and Jasmin, C. (1967). *Lancet* **2,** 380–382.

Mhatre, R. M., Herman, E. H., Huidobro, A., and Waravedekar, V. S. (1970). *Pharmacologist* **12,** 243.

Morrison, R. K. (1967). Toxicology Report to NCI, Jan. 1967.

Nahas, A. (1974). *Proc. Am. Assoc. Cancer Res.* **15,** 49.
Nomura, T., Komiya, M., Kashiwagi, H., Onozawa, Y., and Tahoue, K. (1974). *Thromb. Diath. Heamorrh., Suppl.* **60,** 271–279.
Orsini, F. R., and Mihich, E. (1975). *Proc. Am. Assoc. Cancer, Res.* **16,** 130.
Parisi, B., and Soller, A. (1964). *G. Microbiol.* **12,** 183–194.
Pavlovsky, S., Penalver, J., Eppinger-Helft, M., Sackmann-Muriel, F., Bergna, L., Suarez, A., Vilaseca, G., Pavlovsky, A. A., and Pavlovsky, A. (1973). *Cancer* **31,** 273–279.
Pruzanski, W., and Saito, S. (1974). *J. Natl. Cancer Inst.* **52,** 643–647.
Rai, K. R., Holland, J. F., and Glidewell, O. (1975). *Proc. Am. Assoc. Cancer Res.* **16,** 265.
Raskin, M. M., Rajurkar, M. G., and Altman, D. H. (1973). *Am. J. Roentgenol., Radium Ther. Nucl. Med.* [N.S.] **118,** 68–71.
Riehm, H., and Biedler, J. L. (1971). *Cancer Res.* **31,** 409–412.
Riehm, H., and Biedler, J. L. (1972). *Cancer Res.* **32,** 1195–1200.
Rosenthal, D. S., and Maloney, W. C. (1970). *N. Engl. J. Med.* **286,** 1176–1178.
Rusconi, A., and Calendi, E. (1964). *Tumori* **50,** 261–266.
Rusconi, A., Di Fronzo, G., and Di Marco, A. (1968). *Cancer Chemother. Rep.* **52,** 331–335.
Samuels, L. D., Newton, W. A., Jr., and Heyn, R. (1971). *Cancer* **27,** 831–834.
Sanfilippo, A., and Mazzoleni, R. (1964). *G. Microbiol.* **12,** 83–92.
Schafer, M. P., and Papas, T. S. (1975). *Proc. Am. Assoc. Cancer. Res.* **16,** 11.
Schwartz, H. S. (1974). *Cancer Chemother. Rep.* **58,** 55–62.
Silvestrini, R., Di Marco, A., and Dasdia, T. (1970). *Cancer Res.* **30,** 966–973.
Simard, R. (1966). *Cancer Res.* **26,** 2316–2328.
Stavem, P., and Gjemdal, T. (1974). *Acta Med. Scand.* **196,** 121–125.
Sternberg, S. S., (1970). *Lab. Invest.* **23,** 39–51.
Sternberg, S. S., and Philips, F. S. (1967). *Proc. Am. Assoc. Cancer Res.* **8,** 64.
Sutow, W. W., Fernbach, D. J., Thurman, W. G., Holton, C. P., and Watkins, W. L. (1970). *Cancer Chemother. Rep., Part 1* **54,** 283–289.
Takanashi, S., and Bachur, N. R. (1974). *Proc. Am. Assoc. Cancer Res.* **15,** 76.
Takanashi, S., and Bachur, N. R. (1975). *J. Pharmacol. Exp. Ther.* **195,** 41–49.
Tan, C., Taska, H., and DiMarco, A. (1965). *Proc. Am. Assoc. Cancer Res.* **6,** 64.
Tan, C., Tasaka, H., Yu, K. P., Murphy, M. L., and Karnofsky, D. A. (1967). *Cancer* **20,** 333–353.
Todaro, G. J., and Gallo, R. C. (1973). *Nature (London)* **244,** 206–209.
Umezawa, I., Komiyama, K., and Kasamatsu, M. (1972). *Kitasato Arch. Exp. Med.* **45,** 181–191.
Van Vunakis, H., Langone, J. J., Riceberg, L. J., and Levine, L. (1974). *Cancer Res.* **34,** 2546–2552.
Venditti, J. M., Abbott, B. J., Di Marco, A., and Goldin, A. (1966). *Cancer Chemother. Rep.* **50,** 659–665.
Verzosa, M., and Fite, A. (1971). *Cancer Chemother. Rep., Part 1* **55,** 79–82.
Vietti, T. J., Starling, K., Wilbur, J. R., Lonsdale, D., and Lane, D. M. (1971). *Cancer* **27,** 602–607.
Von Hoff, D. D., Rozencweig, M., and Slavik, M. (1976a). *Kanser* **6,** 1–16.
Von Hoff, D. D., Rozencweig, M., Slavik, M., and Muggia, F. M. (1976b). *J. Am. Med. Assoc.* **236,** 1693.
Von Hoff, D. D., Layard, M., Slavik, M., and Muggia, F. M. (1977). *Am. J. Med.* **62,** 200–208.
Walski, M. (1974). *Ann. Med. Sect. Pol. Acad. Sci.* **19,** 155–156.

Wands, J. R., Chura, C. M., Roll, F. J., and Maddrey, W. C. (1975). *Gastroenterology* **68,** 105–112.

Ward, D. C., Reich, E., and Goldberg, I. H. (1965). *Science* **149,** 1259–1263.

Weil, M., Glidewell, O. J., Jacquillat, C., Levy, R., Serpick, A. A., Wiernik, P. H., Cuttner, J., Hoogstraten, B., Wasserman, L., Ellison, R. R., Gailani, S., Brunner, K., Silver, R. T., Rege, V. B., Cooper, M. R., Lowenstein, L., Nissen, N. I., Haurani, F., Blom, J., Boiron, M., Bernard, J., and Holland, J. F. (1973). *Cancer Res.* **33,** 921–928.

Weiss, A. J., and Cantor, R. I. (1976). *Cancer Treat. Rep.* **60,** 1667–1670.

Wiernik, P. H., and Schimpff, S. C. (1975). *Proc. Am. Assoc. Cancer Res.* **16,** 236.

Wiernik, P. H., and Serpick, A. A. (1972). *Cancer Res.* **32,** 2023–2026.

Wiernik, P. H., Glidewell, O., and Holland, J. F. (1975). *Proc. Am. Assoc. Cancer Res.* **16,** 82.

Woodman, R. J. (1974). *Cancer Chemother. Rep., Part 2* **4,** 45–52.

Yates, J. W., Wallace, H. J., Jr., Ellison, R. R., and Holland, J. F. (1973). *Cancer Chemother. Rep.* **57,** 485–488.

Yesair, D. W., Schwartzbach, F., Shuck, D., Denine, E. P., and Asbell, M. A. (1972). *Cancer Res.* **32,** 1177–1183.

Zee-Cheng, K. Y., and Cheng, C. C. (1970). *J. Pharm. Sci.* **59,** 1630–1634.

Zunino, F., Di Marco, A., Zaccara, A., and Luoni, G. (1974a). *Chem.-Biol. Interact.* **9,** 25–36.

Zunino, F., Gambetta, R., and Di Marco, A. (1974b). *Biochem. Pharmacol.* **24,** 309–311.

Zunino, F., Gambetta, R., Di Marco, A., Zaccara, A., and Luoni, G. (1975). *Cancer Res.* **35,** 754–760.

Drug Information Services

CONSTANTINE J. GILLESPIE

Library
National Institutes of Health
Bethesda, Maryland

I. Introduction

The essential aim of drug information is to encourage the appropriate use and to discourage the inappropriate use of drugs (Herxheimer, 1974). To this end many information sources and services have been applied. There is great variation in the kind of information offered by these services: some provide only references to journal articles or books that contain varying degrees of mention of the drug in question; others give factual information about the drug, i.e., names for the drug, dosages, indications, unwanted effects, precautions, and often also give bibliographic references that substantiate this information; still others provide factual abstracts along with the bibliographic reference.

The means of presentation of the drug information also assume many forms. Conventional book publications serve some, card files serve others, and computerized data banks serve still others. Each medium has its own advantages and disadvantages and it is not possible to say that one form is always better than another. Each must be looked at separately, keeping in mind the purpose that it is intended to serve and the audience for whom it is intended.

Computer technology has resulted in the creation of many services that could not have even been attempted a few years ago. Credit must be given to workers in the computer field who have made such great contributions to information science and who have been responsible for most of the services to be reported in this chapter.

We present in the following a description of some of the major information sources that are available to scientists in the drug field.

II. Drug Information Retrieval Systems

There are currently available many computerized information retrieval systems that can provide valuable service to scientists in the areas of pharmacology, chemotherapy, toxicology, and oncology. Most of these systems are outgrowths of published abstracting and indexing services that have a long history of dedicated and comprehensive application to the literature of their scientific disciplines. Although these major systems are geared to the literature of medicine, chemistry, or biology, they also contain much information that relates to drugs and their use. Access to these on-line systems is through typewriter-like data communications terminals that connect directly to computers using ordinary telephone lines.

The following are some of the advantages of on-line retrieval systems: rapid retrieval of information or bibliographic citations; the ability to modify searching strategy in response to the retrieval results in order to get greater or lesser specificity, as desired; and, the ability for a user to browse through segments of the data base when he cannot clearly define his needs. The disadvantages of on-line retrieval systems include the need for well-trained search analysts in order to get the best results, although persons with a minimal amount of training and experience can often get adequate results with simple questions; high costs for computer connect charges, telephone communication charges, and equipment purchase or rental; and, difficulties with the search vocabulary, whether the system uses a controlled vocabulary or a free-text-searching vocabulary.

Descriptions follow for some specific on-line retrieval systems that have great value for gathering drug information.

A. MEDLINE

In operation since 1971, MEDLINE (*MED*LARS on-*Line*) is the sophisticated outgrowth of the MEDLARS (*Med*ical *L*iterature *A*nalysis and *R*etrieval *S*ystem) searching system that operated in a batch mode so effectively from 1966 to 1971. MEDLINE, a data base that was built and is maintained by the National Library of Medicine, contains references to more than 2.6 million citations from approximately 3000 worldwide biomedical journals. The data base begins in 1966 and is made up of a series of 3-year segments, each separately searchable.

The MEDLINE segment contains citations only for the years 1975, 1976, and 1977, and, as of August 15, 1977, contained 751,013 citations. Earlier coverage is provided by back-file segments for 1966–1968 with 545,463 citations, for 1969–1971 with 649,346 citations, and for 1972–1974 with 671,116 citations. In addition, a data base containing only the current month's citations, called SDILINE (*S*elective *D*issemination of *I*nformation on-*Line*), is used to provide current awareness service for interested requesters. The MEDLINE file is updated with approximately 20,000 new citations each month and the SDILINE file is replaced each month.

Access to MEDLINE is afforded by a variety of typewriter-like terminals connected to computers either in Bethesda, Maryland, or in Albany, New York, using ordinary telephone lines and the nationwide TYMNET or TeleNet communications networks.

Requesters may retrieve citations from the MEDLINE files on their subjects of interest by entering terms from article titles and/or abstracts or by entering any of 14,000 medical subject headings listed in the National Library of Medicine's controlled vocabulary, *Medical Subject Headings* (MeSH), either singly or in combination using the Boolean operators, AND, OR, and AND NOT. Subject headings may be further refined by the use of some 68 qualifiers designed to pinpoint specific aspects of a subject. For example, if only the untoward or harmful effects of a drug are desired, then any or all of the qualifiers "adverse effects," "poisoning," and "toxicity" may be used in conjunction with the drug name to get only these aspects. Searches may be limited to certain age groups, experimental animals (including very specific animals such as nude mice or inbred WF rats), languages, years of publication, journals or specific authors, since these are all searchable elements. Citations may be printed on-line right at the user's terminal while he waits, or off-line and mailed to the user from the computer center the following day. This latter procedure is more economical when more than just a few dozen citations have been retrieved. Users may select a print format varying from a complete record of the citation, including subject headings and abstract (if present), to a brief identification of the author(s), title, and source journal, sufficient to enable the user or his librarian to find the original article.

The MEDLINE service is available at more than 500 medical libraries, medical schools, government agencies, and companies in the United States, as well as at locations in Canada, the United Kingdom, France, Mexico, Iran, the World Health Organization in Geneva, South Africa, and Sweden.

Subscribers to the MEDLINE service pay the National Library of Medicine $15 for each hour of computer connect time between 10:00 A.M. and 5:00 P.M. (Eastern Time) and $8 for each hour of connect time at all other times. A fee of 10¢ is also charged for each page of off-line printout that is requested. The subscribing institutions may recover these costs as well as the cost of their search analyst's time from their customers.

1. Advantages

The value and advantages of the MEDLINE system go far beyond the very reasonable price that the National Library of Medicine charges for the use of its system. First, with respect to the searching vocabulary, MEDLINE is the only major information retrieval service that uses a controlled vocabulary in its search strategy. This vocabulary (MeSH) has the decided advantage of eliminating the synonym problem for the user by indexing the particular concept under a designated term even though the author might have used a synonym for that concept in his article. For example, articles on the tranquilizer Equanil are indexed under the generic term "meprobamate," and the user of MEDLINE does not need to be concerned with the dozens of other brand names for meprobamate (e.g., Arcoban, Bamate, Meprospan, Meprotabs, Miltown, Tranmep) that an author might have used. The problems of synonyms, whether they be drug names, disease names, or anatomical sites, are avoided because they have all been brought together by MeSH under the one synonym deemed to be the most widely used.

Nevertheless, problems do exist with controlled vocabularies, namely the problem of the new concept that is appearing in the literature for the first time for which the controlled vocabulary has no heading. This is especially true of drugs and the MEDLINE indexers are forced to index such new drugs under broad group terms such as "antibiotics" or "analgesics & antipyretics" or "tranquilizing agents." This makes retrieval of specific drugs difficult, if not impossible, because the specific drug desired is grouped with many other specific drugs that are not wanted.

However, several years ago the National Library of Medicine took steps to diminish this problem. They created indexes to all the significant words in the titles and abstracts of articles, thus making all of these words directly searchable. Now if you wish to retrieve citations on Meprospan, for example, you merely add the qualifier TW (for Text Word) after the word you want, i.e., MEPROSPAN (TW), and the system will retrieve any citation in which the word Meprospan was used in the title or abstract. This feature gives users of the MEDLINE system the best of both worlds: a controlled vocabulary for easy dependable searching of well-known existing concepts, and natural language, text word searching for very specific concepts not yet recognized by the controlled vocabulary. These are powerful capabilities that contribute to more exact searching and greater relevance in retrieval.

As stated earlier, most other searching systems rely on natural language, text word searching almost exclusively for their retrieval, making it mandatory for their users to think of many synonyms and alternate forms of expression to maximize their retrieval and minimize the missing of relevant citations.

Another very valuable feature of the MEDLINE searching system is the hierarchical coding scheme that has been provided for all MeSH terms. Each MeSH term has been placed into one or more categories that bring together all similar kinds of terms, i.e., anatomical terms (Category A), organism terms (Category B), disease terms (Category C), chemical and drug terms (Category D), etc. Within each category there are subcategories that give more specific hierarchical arrangements. For example, Category A, Anatomical Terms, has as one of its subcategories, A7, Anatomy—Cardiovascular System. A segment of this subcategory appears in Table I.

A MEDLINE search calling for heart valves as one of its parameters is easily satisfied by the expression: EXPLODE A7.541.510 or just EXPLODE HEART VALVES. This statement will retrieve any citations that have been indexed with any of the seven heart valve terms that begin with this alphanumeric character string in their hierarchical "tree" number. It avoids the necessity for inputting each of the seven terms separately in English.

This "explosion" capability is even more dramatic and beneficial in other instances where the hierarchical tree structure contains dozens of subject heading terms indented under a broad grouping. Take, for example, the term POISONS (D5.569.612) with 40 specific headings

TABLE I

SEGMENT OF *Medical Subject Headings*—TREE STRUCTURES

(A7) Anatomy—Cardiovascular System	
HEART	A7.541
ENDOCARDIUM	A7.541.207
FETAL HEART	A7.541.278
DUCTUS ARTERIOSUS	A7.541.278.395
TRUNCUS ARTERIOSUS	A7.541.278.930
HEART ATRIUM	A7.541.358
HEART CONDUCTION SYSTEM	A7.541.409
ATRIOVENTRICULAR NODE	A7.541.409.147
BUNDLE OF HIS	A7.541.409.273
PURKINJE FIBERS	A7.541.409.683
SINO-ATRIAL NODE	A7.541.409.819
HEART SEPTUM	A7.541.459
HEART VALVES	A7.541.510
AORTIC VALVE	A7.541.510.110
CHORDAE TENDINEAE	A7.541.510.240
MITRAL VALVE	A7.541.510.507
PAPILLARY MUSCLES	A7.541.510.619
PULMONARY VALVE	A7.541.510.738
TRICUSPID VALVE	A7.541.510.893
HEART VENTRICLE	A7.541.560
MYOCARDIUM	A7.541.704
PERICARDIUM	A7.541.795

indented under it; ANTIBIOTICS (D20.85) with more than 200 more specific headings indented under it; and, NEOPLASMS, EMBRYONAL AND MIXED (C4.557.537) with 35 specific neoplasms indented under it. The one tree number in each of these cases allows all of the indented terms to be searched quickly, efficiently, and economically.

2. *Disadvantages*

Disadvantages and shortcomings also exist in the MEDLINE system. One of these relates to the tree structures and explosion capability that I have just outlined above as such a worthwhile feature. Subcategory C4, Diseases—Neoplasms presents a problem because so often requesters want information on a particular facet of cancer, pertaining to any kind of cancer. They cannot limit their search request to just leukemias or just sarcomas or just adenomas; they want any and all kinds of neoplasms. Subcategory C4 contains some 387 distinct cancer terms, and to satisfy a requester who wants all cancers would require use of the statement: EXPLODE C4. But the MEDLINE programs cannot accommodate such an explosion because there are too many terms in the explosion and there would be more citations retrieved than the system could handle.

One solution has been to break the explosion into a series of smaller explosions: EXPLODE C4.182, EXPLODE C4.557, etc. But this is tedious and expensive because it is time-consuming, and it does not really work completely satisfactorily. The final solution that I have adopted (but which creates some other problems of its own) for searches that require the inclusion of all cancer terms is to run them in the OFFSEARCH mode. With the MEDLINE file (covering the years 1975–1977) OFFSEARCH allows the user to input his search formulation at the data communications terminal in an on-line mode but to have the search itself actually run in a batch mode at a later time that evening after the system has completed its normal operating hours. In this OFFSEARCH mode, most very large-scale explosions that are not possible in the on-line mode can be accomplished. The danger with most offsearches, especially one involving all of the cancer terms, is that you do not know how big your retrieval will be and you have no opportunity at running time to modify your strategy to improve the results of the search. This requires very careful search formulation by the search analyst and preliminary examination of the printed *Index Medicus* and *Cumulated Index Medicus* (the published equivalents of the MEDLINE files) to estimate expected retrieval and to adjust accordingly. A useful safeguard with offsearches is to formulate very tightly for maximum relevance on the initial search and then to repeat the search with a broader formulation if the results of the first search are too narrow. The MEDLINE system has a built-in default condition that limits the printout from any offsearch to a maximum of 500 citations; thus, if the search retrieved more than this, only the first 500 would be printed.

It is important to mention at this point that the OFFSEARCH mode is the *only* way in which the MEDLINE back files for the years 1966 through 1974 can be searched. These precautions of careful formulation and of advance research to get accurate estimates of expected retrievals are important for efficient economic searching.

A further disadvantege of MEDLINE is the inability to specify the sequence of the output received. The results of a search are printed out on the basis of the last citations entered into the data base being the first citations printed out. This is true when the printout is either on-line or off-line. (Keep in mind, however, that input of indexed citations is not strictly chronological because of variations in receipt dates for journals and delays and gaps often experienced with foreign journals.) In some instances, it would be desirable to have the citations arranged in alphabetical order by the senior author's last name or in alphabetical order by the title of the journal in which the article was published. No print options for output sequencing are available nor are any anticipated. There are useful options, of course, as to how much or how little of each record is to be printed. During on-line searching it is often advantageous, even necessary, to just look at the titles of articles and nothing else to see if you are retrieving the right kind of material. Adjustment can then be made in the search strategy.

When all is said and done, however, MEDLINE is an information retrieval system with tremendous value, ease of searching, rapid interaction, economy of use, and great potential for very sophisticated searching in the hands of a well-trained information specialist.

B. TOXLINE

The TOXLINE (*Tox*icology on-*Line*) system is another of the National Library of Medicine's computerized data bases. This one, developed by the Toxicology Information Program, contains more than 645,000 references to published human and animal toxicity studies, effects of environmental chemicals and pollutants, adverse drug reactions, and analytical methodology. The data bases contain full bibliographic citations, almost all with abstracts, from 10 component files. Five of these files are from major secondary indexing and abstracting services and five are specialized small collections of material. There are two TOXLINE data bases, the first covering literature from 1971 to 1977, and the second (called TOXBACK) covering literature prior to 1971. As with the MEDLINE data bases for literature prior to 1975, the TOXBACK file also can only be searched in the OFFSEARCH mode explained earlier.

A description of each of the TOXLINE component files follows.

1. *Chemical-Biological Activities (CBAC)*

This biweekly computer-readable file covering over 13,000 primary journals is compiled and published by the Chemical Abstracts Service (CAS). It contains citations and abstracts covering the scientific literature on the interactions of chemical substances with biological systems *in vivo* and *in vitro*. For the years 1965 through 1974, CBAC contained abstracts only from Sections 1–5 of *Chemical Abstracts*. These five sections of the total of twenty sections of biochemistry appearing in *Chemical Abstracts* cover the topics: pharmacodynamics, hormone pharmacology, biochemical interactions, toxicology, and agrochemicals. In 1975, CBAC coverage was expanded to include Sections 62, 63, and

64 of *Chemical Abstracts* on the topics: essential oils and cosmetics, pharmaceuticals, and pharmaceutical analysis, respectively. CBAC was published as a separate journal from 1965 to 1971 but thereafter was only included within the regular issues of *Chemical Abstracts* and also was issued as a magnetic-tape file to interested users with their own computer facilities. All CBAC records contain *Chemical Abstracts* Registry Numbers.

2. *Toxicity Bibliography (TOXBIB)*

The TOXBIB file is a subset of *Index Medicus* and also, therefore, a subset of the MEDLINE files. It contains citations dealing with the adverse effects, toxicity or poisoning caused by drugs and chemicals, as well as disease conditions induced by many chemical substances. The bibliographic citations in TOXBIB are indexed with terms taken from *Medical Subject Headings*, but they are searched as single terms since TOXLINE is a free-text-searching system. There are no *Chemical Abstracts* Registry Numbers for the citations in TOXBIB.

3. *International Pharmaceutical Abstracts (IPA)*

The IPA file is a product of the American Society of Hospital Pharmacists and has been published since 1964 as an international periodical devoted to all phases in the development and use of drugs. As a monthly publication it covers more than 1000 primary journals providing citations and abstracts that reflect new trends and developments in pharmacy. The IPA also cover the following categories: pharmaceutical technology; institutional pharmacy practice; adverse drug reactions; toxicity; investigational drugs; drug evaluations; drug interactions; biopharmaceutics; pharmaceutics; drug stability; pharmacology; preliminary drug listing; pharmaceutical chemistry; drug analysis; drug metabolism and body distribution; and pharmacognosy.

The IPA records in TOXLINE begin with 1970 material, the year that the American Society of Hospital Pharmacists established its computerized abstracting and indexing system for IPA. These records are also enriched with searchable subject index terms as APPENDED terms in the abstract field. The IPA records do not contain *Chemical Abstracts* Registry Numbers.

4. *Abstracts on Health Effects of Environmental Pollutants (HEEP)*

The HEEP file is a compilation of abstracts and reference citations to published papers emphasizing the effects on human health of environmental chemicals or substances, other than medicinals. The data are derived from *Biological Abstracts* and from *BioResearch Index*. The HEEP records in TOXLINE contain abstracts, bibliographic citations, and *Chemical Abstracts* Registry Numbers .

5. *Pesticides Abstracts (PESTAB)*

This monthly publication of the Environmental Protection Agency began in January 1974 but was formerly known as *Health Aspects of Pesticides Abstracts Bulletin* (HAPAB) for the years 1967–1973. Both PESTAB and its predecessor, HAPAB, contain citations and abstracts covering published reports on the epidemiological effects of pesticides on humans. The publication represents a monthly review and indexing of more than 500 domestic and foreign primary journals. This file in TOXLINE has had *Chemical Abstracts* Registry Numbers added to it.

6. *Environmental Mutagen Information Center (EMIC) File*

The Environmental Mutagen Information Center was established at the Oak Ridge National Laboratory for the purpose of collecting, organizing, and disseminating published information on chemical mutagenesis. Information in the EMIC file is either pertinent to the testing of chemicals in one of the many available mutagenic assay systems or contains data useful for understanding the known or suspected mutagenic activity of environmental chemical agents. The file currently contains more than 17,000 citations for articles published primarily since 1968 in about 1600 publication sources. Entries in the EMIC file contain bibliographic details as well as key words relating to chemicals, organisms, and systems studied. The file has also been enriched with *Chemical Abstracts* Registry Numbers.

7. *Hayes File on Pesticides*

This file is a collection of 10,043 citations to published articles on the health aspects of pesticides compiled by Dr. W. J. Hayes, Jr. It essentially constitutes the earlier years (1940–1966) of HAPAB. The original cards of this file are maintained by the Environmental Protection Agency in its Atlanta, Georgia, offices. The Hayes file contains no abstracts or *Chemical Abstracts* Registry Numbers.

8. *Toxic Materials Information Center (TMIC) File*

The TMIC file contains 4553 records on various toxic substances that have been compiled by the Toxic Materials Information Center at the Oak Ridge National Laboratory.

9. *Environmental Teratology Information Center (ETIC) File*

This file contains 8803 records on various environmental teratogenic substances that have been compiled by the Environmental Teratology Information Center at the Oak Ridge National Laboratory.

10. *Teratology (TERA)*

This is a closed file of 5984 records for the years 1971–1974 which was purchased from IFI/Plenum Data Corporation and represents a portion of the references compiled since 1963 by Weinstein (1976). The references deal with congenital malformations caused by a variety of agents, especially those induced by chemicals, drugs, pesticides, diseases, stress, and environment. Methods and techniques for studying teratogenesis are also included as are those aspects of embryology, reproduction, and genetics that lead to a better understanding of the development of the malformations. Recent references to mutagenicity and screening tests for carcinogenicity have been added, too.

11. *File Size*

Tables II and III give the components, sizes, and years of coverage for the TOXLINE and TOXBACK data bases, respectively.

12. *Searching the Data Bases*

Searching the TOXLINE data bases presents some of the same difficulties that are encountered in any free-text-searching system, namely synonyms and the need to express the concepts you are trying to retrieve in different ways in order to avoid missing desired information. Naturally, the TOXLINE data bases are full of drug and chemical names with all of their attendant multiple names. To diminish this problem, the National Library of Medicine's Specialized Information Services, in collaboration with the Chemical Abstracts Service, created the CHEMLINE (*Chem*ical Dictionary on-*Line*) file. An interactive chemical dictionary file, CHEMLINE provides a mechanism whereby some 550,000 chemical substance names representing more than 243,373 unique chemicals can be searched and retrieved on-line. This file contains *Chemical Abstracts* Registry Numbers, molecular formulas, preferred chemical nomenclature, generic and trivial names derived from the *Chemical Abstracts* Registry Nomenclature File, and a limited number of Wiswesser line notations. In addition, each Registry Number record in CHEMLINE contains, where applicable, ring information including number of rings, ring sizes, ring elemental analysis, and component line formulas.

TABLE II

TOXLINE FILE COMPONENTS[a]

File components[b]	No. of records	Years of coverage
CBAC	217,468	1971–July 1977
TOXBIB	92,057	1971–Aug. 1977
IPA	32,221	1971–July 1977
HEEP	68,765	1971–July 1977
HAPAB/PESTAB	15,831	1971–April 1977
EMIC	11,302	1971–1976
ETIC	8,803	1950 to present
TERA	5,984	1971–1974
TMIC	2,013	1971–1974
Total	456,134	

[a] As of August 15, 1977.

[b] CBAC, *Chemical-Biological Activities*; TOXBIB, *Toxicity Bibliography*; IPA, *International Pharmaceutical Abstracts;* HEEP, *Abstracts on Health Effects of Environmental Pollutants;* HAPAB, *Health Aspects of Pesticides Abstracts Bulletin;* PESTAB, *Pesticides Abstracts;* EMIC, Environmental Mutagen Information Center; ETIC, Environmental Teratology Information Center; TERA, Teratology; TMIC, Toxic Materials Information Center.

The user searches CHEMLINE, employing the same terminal that is available for TOXLINE or MEDLINE searching, by entering a chemical name, generic name, trivial name, company identification name, or its equivalent molecular formula. If any of these names is found in CHEMLINE, then a record can be printed out giving the *Chemical Abstracts* Registry Number and synonyms that are then used as search terms when entering the TOXLINE files. Users of TOXLINE should always search CHEMLINE first when a chemical is part of the search strategy. If the exact name of a chemical substance is not known, a search may be conducted using the Boolean operator AND to connect those fragments of the name, ring analysis terms, and/or molecular formula that are known. As before, these retrieved records serve to provide chemical names that can then be used in the search of the TOXLINE data bases.

Although the TOXLINE data bases are described as toxicology data bases, all of the records in these data bases do not address toxicologic aspects. It is necessary for the user to enter search terms for "poisoning," "toxicity," "untoward effects," or "unwanted effects," etc., to coordinate with the desired chemical names in order to get at the needed kind of information. Just to enter the chemical names alone will be futile because, in many instances, there will be far more records in the system than a user could afford to print out or be able to wade through if he did print them all out. Obviously, if a search on a chemical substance name by itself retrieves a small number of references, then it is unnecessary to go through additional complicated searching when a scanning of the retrieval by eye will be sufficient to select the useful references.

A minor irritant with TOXLINE retrievals is the presence of duplicate citations. Since different services have contributed to the component files, it is not uncommon for two or three of them to have indexed the same article. No attempt is made by the National Library of Medicine to eliminate such duplicate entries.

TABLE III

TOXBACK FILE COMPONENTS[a]

File component[b]	No. of records	Years of coverage
CBAC	91,223	1965–1970
TOXBIB	60,229	1966–1970
IPA	8,611	1970
HEEP	3,500	pre-1971
HAPAB	7.275	1966–1970
EMIC	5,765	1968–1970
HAYES	10,043	1930–1970
TMIC	2,540	pre-1971
Total	189,186	

[a] As of August 15, 1977.

[b] CBAC, *Chemical-Biological Activities*; TOXBIB, *Toxicity Bibliography*; IPA, *International Pharmaceutical Abstracts*; HEEP, *Abstracts on Health Effects of Environmental Pollutants;* HAPAB, *Health Aspects of Pesticides Abstracts Bulletin;* EMIC, Environmental Mutagen Information Center; HAYES, Hayes File on Pesticides; TMIC, Toxic Materials Information Center.

C. CANCERLINE

The National Cancer Institute, through its International Cancer Research Data Bank Program, and in cooperation with the National Library of Medicine, has created the CANCERLINE (*Cancer* on-*Line*) file of more than 90,000 citations dealing with all aspects of cancer. The sources of these citations are articles from scientific and biomedical journals that have been abstracted for *Carcinogenesis Abstracts* for

1963–1976, and for *Cancer Therapy Abstracts* for 1974–1976 (as well as its predecessor, *Cancer Chemotherapy Abstracts*, for 1967–1973). Since 1975, other articles related to cancer that are not included in these two abstracting journals have also been processed for addition to the data base. In all, more than 2000 worldwide journals are now being screened for additional cancer articles to be included in CANCERLINE. All citations in CANCERLINE have abstracts with them.

Since CANCERLINE is one of the National Library of Medicine's (NLM) family of computerized data bases, it is accessed by the same communications terminals used for MEDLINE and is available at all the world-wide locations where MEDLINE is available.

In contrast to MEDLINE, CANCERLINE does not use a controlled vocabulary for retrieving citations (although a hierarchical classification of approximately 1000 categories is now being developed). One may retrieve citations on a given subject by entering the desired terms as they are likely to appear in the titles or abstracts of articles in the data base or by searching on any assigned index terms. Terms may be entered singly or in combination by means of the Boolean operators AND, OR, and AND NOT. In addition to words in titles and abstracts, other parameters, such as author names, year of publication, secondary sources (i.e., *Carcinogenesis Abstracts* or *Cancer Therapy Abstracts*), languages, or primary journal titles, may be used to modify the retrieval. As with all the MEDLINE files, the printouts from the file may be tailored by the requester to give a complete record with the abstract or just brief identification of the authors, title, and source journal.

An associated file of the International Cancer Research Data Bank Program is the CANCERPROJ file. It is an on-line data base containing more than 15,000 summaries of ongoing cancer research projects for the years 1976–1977. These summaries have been provided by cancer researchers in many countries. CANCERPROJ is available as one of the additional data bases on the NLM computer and is searched in a free-text mode as is CANCERLINE. However, CANCERPROJ may also be searched using index terms assigned by the Smithsonian Science Information Exchange (SSIE), the contractor who developed the CANCERPROJ file. The CANCERPROJ file will cover cancer research in progress for the most recent 2 years and will always contain between 12,000 and 16,000 summaries.

Another new data base in the International Cancer Research Data Bank is CLINPROT (*Clin*ical Cancer *Prot*ocols). It contains 834 summaries of clinical investigations of new therapeutic agents and procedures. Most of the protocols are those supported by the Division of Cancer Treatment of the National Cancer Institute; others, however, have been supplied by major United States cancer centers and by sources outside the United States. CLINPROT is updated every 3 months but will remain a very small, highly specialized data base.

1. *Advantages*

One of the major advantages of the CANCERLINE file is that it contains abstracts for all of its 90,464 citations. This allows abstracts to be printed out easily so that a researcher can decide quickly if a retrieved article is potentially useful to him. However, it is uneconomical to print out abstracts at the terminal in an on-line mode; it is much better to have them included with the off-line printouts.

The abstracts also provide an advantage in searching because all of the significant words in the abstract are directly searchable. This improves the possibility of retrieving desired concepts since there is much more detail on the content of the article available in the abstract than there is in just the title of the article or in assigned index terms.

2. *Disadvantages*

In the past a serious disadvantage of CANCERLINE has been the lack of very recent citations in the file. However, the National Cancer Institute is now requiring its contractors to make substantial improvements in this area. The extent of this improvement can be shown by an actual request for information on "estrogen or progesterone receptors in human breast cancer." The CANCERLINE search was formulated as follows:

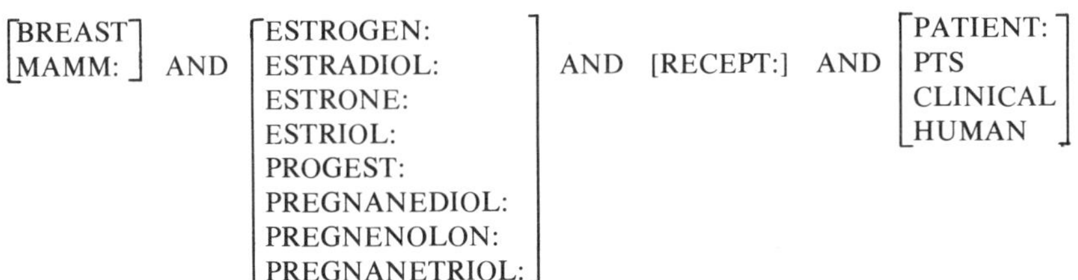

The colon was used as a truncation symbol to retrieve additional terms with variant endings: ESTROGENS, ESTROGENIC, PROGESTERONE, PROGESTATIONAL, PROGESTOGENS, etc. For a citation to be retrieved it must have included at least one term from each of the four groups above. Since all of CANCERLINE is devoted to cancer articles, it was not necessary to include cancer terms (CANCER, NEOPLASMS, TUMORS, etc.) in the search strategy. This search was run in November 1976 and was repeated in August 1977. When the search was first run it retrieved 65 citations, all of them relevant. Forty of these citations (61.5%) were dated 1974 or later, while 27 citations (41.5%) were dated 1975 or 1976. The same search in August 1977 retrieved 205 citations, a 215% increase over the earlier retrieval. More important, however, this later search contained 181 citations (88.3%) which were dated 1974 or later, and 106 citations (51.7%) which were dated 1976 or 1977. These figures all represent substantial improvements both in the total number of citations retrieved and in their recency of publication.

As a further comparison this same search was run against the MEDLINE file for 1975–1977. The search strategy in MEDLINE required that at least one term from each of the following four groups of terms be present for a citation to be retrieved:

[BREAST NEOPLASMS] AND [EXPLODE D6.472.265
EXPLODE D6.472.798]

AND [RECEPTORS, DRUG
RECEPTORS, ESTROGEN
RECEPTORS, HORMONE
RECEPTORS, PROGESTERONE] AND [HUMAN]

The hierarchical tree numbers represent, respectively, all the estrogen terms (11 different terms) and all the progestational hormone terms (seven terms) that exist in *Medical Subject Headings*. One hundred and ninety citations were retrieved by this MEDLINE strategy.

Comparison of this MEDLINE retrieval with the latest CANCERLINE retrieval shows the MEDLINE search retrieving 182 citations (95.8%) with publication dates of 1974 or later, and 97 citations (51.1%) with publication dates of 1976 or 1977. The latest CANCERLINE search with its figures of 88.3% and 51.7%, respectively, compares very favorably with this MEDLINE search.

The problem of recency of citation is an important one, and it is being vigorously attacked by the developers of the CANCERLINE file as one that is of vital concern to researchers. Statistics on updates to the CANCERLINE file indicate an improvement in this area. From August to November 1976, three updates to the CANCERLINE file added 7662 citations, of which 3844 citations (50.2%) had a 1976 publication date. The results of the recent CANCERLINE search on "estrogen or progesterone receptors in human breast cancer," mentioned above, show an even more dramatic improvement in currency.

Another serious disadvantage of CANCERLINE is its size, i.e., the number of citations that it contains. As of August 15, 1977, CANCERLINE contained 90,464 citations with abstracts. For a 15-year file that

TABLE IV

CANCER CITATIONS IN MEDLINE FILES[a]

File segment	Total citations	Cancer citations	Percentage
1966–1968	545,463	48,629	8.92
1969–1971	649,346	65,614	10.10
1972–1974	671,116	69,588	10.37
1975–1977	751,013	80,518	10.72
Total	2,616,938	264,349	10.10

[a] As of August 15, 1977.

deals with a subject as important as cancer, on which so much research is being conducted, and which generates so much literature, this is completely inadequate. By contrast, the MEDLINE files from January 1966 through September 1977 contain a total of 2,616,938 citations, of which 264,349 citations, or 10.1%, relate to some aspect of cancer (Table IV). The MEDLINE files contain 2.9 times more cancer citations than the entire CANCERLINE file. Furthermore, when you consider that MEDLINE covers a 12-year period in contrast to the 15-year period covered by CANCERLINE, the file size differences are even more pronounced, with MEDLINE averaging 22,029 cancer citations added per year whereas CANCERLINE averages only 6030 records added per year. On this basis there are 3.6 times more cancer citations in MEDLINE than in CANCERLINE. However, because of the recent improvements made in updating CANCERLINE, additions to the file have been scheduled at an average rate of more than 20,000 abstracts per year. In actual fact, almost 33,000 new records have been added since November 1976.

When the topic that is being searched is one on which very little literature exists, then the file size is even more critical. Whereas CANCERLINE may not contain anything on the topic, a larger file may contain at least a few relevant citations.

File size is important too, if a comprehensive search on a topic is needed. Another actual request was for citations on "BCG immunization and melanoma." This is a straightforward request that can be searched easily in CANCERLINE. It requires only the coordination of BCG AND MELANOMA: (again, the colon is a truncation symbol allowing any character string beginning with the letters MELANOMA to be retrieved, namely melanoma, melanomas, melanomatous). This strategy retrieved 282 relevant records. The same search run in MEDLINE called for either BCG VACCINE or BCG VACCINATION to be

"ANDed" with MELANOMA. One hundred and thirty-six citations were retrieved, and these, too, were all relevant. However, these 136 citations were retrieved from a 33-month file, whereas the 282 CANCERLINE records were retrieved from a 15-year file. Thus, the size of the file searched is important if the user needs a complete search and the most recent articles that have been published.

For the years 1963 to 1975 the sources of citations in CANCERLINE were only the abstracting publications that dealt with carcinogenesis and cancer therapy. Consequently, CANCERLINE is mostly slanted toward these two areas of the cancer literature, although admittedly they are extremely important areas. This points up another disadvantage of CANCERLINE: there are other important areas of cancer that are being studied and are of interest to scientists that were not included in CANCERLINE prior to 1975. An information retrieval system dealing with cancer should cover all areas of cancer, but CANCERLINE did not begin this full coverage until 1975 when additional sources of cancer-related articles were sought out. This is an important and useful step that the CANCERLINE developers have taken, and over the next few years, as more of the full cancer literature gets into the CANCERLINE data base, CANCERLINE should become an extremely valuable file.

Expansion of the CANCERLINE file many times over is the key to its becoming an information retrieval service that is truly worthy of its name. It must include as much of the cancer literature as possible. It must be broadened to cover all of the cancer literature for the years prior to 1975 just as it is now beginning to do for the recent literature. Granted, it would not be cost-effective to have a contractor go back and abstract all of the missed cancer literature for the past 10 or 12 years, but it would be effective and economical to take the 264,349 cancer citations that already exist in the MEDLINE data bases back to 1966 and add them to the CANCERLINE file (just as 152,286 toxicology citations were taken out of the MEDLINE files and added to the TOXLINE files; Section II,B,2). Even though abstracts are included with only a few thousand of these 264,349 cancer citations, they would still be of great value to researchers by giving them a cancer file that was fully comprehensive.

Moreover, CANCERLINE's currency must be improved dramatically. The major reason behind a computerized information retrieval system is speed: fast retrieval of the most recent literature. It is hardly of great value to get rapid retrieval of old references.

These improvements must be made to justify the creation and maintenance of the CANCERLINE file. If these improvements cannot be made then the cancer researcher must go to other sources for his cancer literature needs.

D. Lockheed DIALOG

Lockheed Information Systems has been operating its very successful DIALOG information retrieval service for many years now. Lockheed has a large number of data bases available for on-line searching; however, only a few of these data bases are of value to users of drug information. The thirty-five DIALOG data bases cover a wide range of subject areas in science, technology/engineering, social sciences, and business/economics. No other on-line information retrieval service offers as many data bases, and for many of these data bases DIALOG is the only service offering on-line access to them.

A surprising feature is that the approximately 12 million total citations in these data bases are all continuously and simultaneously available for on-line searching. The data bases in the subject areas of science are the ones most likely to be of value to researchers in drug fields, and these are described in the following.

1. *BIOSIS Previews*

The BIOSIS Previews offers worldwide coverage of the life sciences as presented in *Biological Abstracts* and *BioResearch Index*, publications of the BioSciences Information Service. Coverage of BIOSIS Previews is from January 1972 to date with approximately 1,150,000 citations available and an additional 20,000 citations added each month.

2. *Chemical Abstracts Condensates (CHEMCON)*

CHEMCON contains bibliographic data and key-word phrases from the literature of chemistry and chemical engineering. This is supplied by the Chemical Abstracts Service, and, for coverage from January 1972 to date, it contains approximately 1,556,000 citations with an additional 26,000 citations added each month.

3. *Chemical Abstracts Subject Index Alert (CASIA)*

CASIA contains general subject index headings and *Chemical Abstracts* Registry Numbers for the documents covered by CHEMCON. Provided by the Chemical Abstracts Service, CASIA coverage began in January 1973 and contains 1,156,000 citations with an additional 26,000 citations added each month.

4. *Chemical Abstracts Chemical Name Dictionary (CHEMNAME)*

This dictionary contains *Chemical Abstracts* Registry Numbers, *Chemical Abstracts* index names, molecular formulas, and synonyms for chemical substances that are covered in CASIA. CHEMNAME contains 1,150,000 entries and is augmented by 25,000 new entries each month.

5. *SCISEARCH*

SCISEARCH is the on-line equivalent of the *Science Citation Index* that is published by the Institute for Scientific Information of Philadelphia. It is a multidisciplinary index to the literature of all areas of science and technology containing more than 1,200,000 citations from January 1974 to date. It is updated monthly with 42,000 additional citations. The unique feature of this data base is that it allows searching on the relationship between published articles and other articles that have cited those published articles in their lists of references. Citation indexing is based on the simple concept that an author's references to previously recorded information identify much of the earlier work that is pertinent to the subject of his present document (Weinstock, 1971). Just as *Science Citation Index* is the only major index based on the principle of citation indexing, SCISEARCH is the only data base that can be searched using the same principle.

6. *Advantages and Disadvantages*

Lockheed DIALOG has the advantage of offering many data bases to users via quick on-line access. However, to use these data bases efficiently and economically requires a thorough understanding of the published equivalents of the on-line files. This means that to make effective use of BIOSIS Previews, for example, a searcher must know a great deal about *Biological Abstracts*, what it contains, how it is indexed, how the indexes are constructed, how titles are augmented, how taxonomic names are handled, what the CROSS and Biosystematic codes mean, etc. In other words, thorough knowledge of the published product means that the user can conduct a search of the on-line data base with a minimum of guesswork.

The reason that this thorough knowledge is so essential is because on-line searching of DIALOG data bases is so expensive. Costs are based on the time that the user is connected to the DIALOG computer while conducting his search. For BIOSIS Previews this charge is $65 per hour of computer connect time; for CHEMCON, $45 per hour; for SCISEARCH, $70 per hour. In addition to these connect time charges, there is an $8 per hour or $10 per hour charge for usage of one of two nationwide communications networks that link the user's telephone to the DIALOG computer in Palo Alto, California. A simple, fairly straightforward search can be expected to take about 15 minutes, on the average. In the BIOSIS Previews file, a 15 minute search would cost about $1.25 per minute, or $18.75; a 15 minute search of SCISEARCH would cost $1.33 per minute or about $19.95. The cost of any citations or records printed off-line (at 10¢ each) would be in addition to these connect charges.

Obviously, with charges such as these a user would have to be very cautious in his searching and do a lot of preliminary scanning of printed indexes before sitting at the terminal. He would also need to have his search strategy planned out in advance in substantial detail. Such steps are essential to minimize costs and maximize results.

However, even with these precautions, searchers using DIALOG are often surprised with the results. Surprised because the strategy they have worked out and entered into the computer yields zero results. They must then try alternative approaches to get at the citations they want, but have to do so in an inefficient and expensive manner. They enter different synonyms for the concepts they wish to retrieve in the hope that the data base contains some posting on that concept. In addition, they must browse through segments of the file looking for clues to the concepts they want. They must also try different coordinations of terms than those they tried originally. The end result is a search that was expected to take 10 or 15 minutes being dragged out to an hour or more, and possibly still yielding little or no results. At the high rates charged by DIALOG, such a search can easily run to more than $100.

The two factors of high cost and the difficulty of searching some Lockheed data bases are the two greatest disadvantages of this searching system.

E. SDC Search Service

The System Development Corporation (SDC) of Santa Monica, California, offers on-line computer access to almost thirty different bibliographic data bases in many different subject fields. Most of these data bases, in areas such as education, physics, and petroleum, are not of interest to those engaged in drug research. The data bases that are of value to drug researchers are essentially the same ones that are offered by Lockheed Information Systems, i.e., BIOSIS Previews and CHEMCON. However, SDC does provide coverage of several other data bases that should be considered in seeking drug information.

1. *Pharmaceutical News Index (PNI)*

This data base is an index to items in four weekly publications: *Drug Research Reports* (The Blue Sheet); *FDC Reports* (The Pink Sheet); the

Pharmaceutical Manufacturers Association Newsletter; and the *Washington Drug and Device Letter.* This data base differs from others that have been described above in that it is not a bibliographic data base of authored scientific articles. It is a data base to published items, but these four newsletters contain hundreds of short reports that deal with major health bills; individual drug company's sales and earnings analyses; Food and Drug Administration recalls and court actions; convention coverage; legislative actions; *Federal Register* notices and hearings; and recent requests for proposals. Coverage began in January 1974 for *FDC Reports,* and in December 1975 for the other publications. There are approximately 13,700 items in the data base with 600 new items added monthly.

2. *Smithsonian Science Information Exchange (SSIE)*

The SSIE data base covers on-going and recently completed research projects in the life, physical, and social sciences. Some drug research projects are included in the data base. Reports on research in progress are included from over 1300 funding organizations, including government organizations at all levels, nonprofit associations, academic institutions, some foreign organizations, and, private industry. The data base, beginning with fiscal year 1974, contains 262,400 reports and is updated with an additional 9000 reports each month.

Other services from SSIE are offered by other organizations and are mentioned elsewhere in this chapter, i.e., CANCERPROJ (Section II,C), and *TOX-TIPS* and *Toxicology Research Projects Directory* (Section III,A,3 and 4).

3. *Ringdoc*

The Ringdoc data base covers over 400 of the world's scientific journals, providing extensive coverage of the pharmaceutical literature. Access to the citations is possible by means of key-words as well as by coded data that represent various chemical fragments. The file contains 466,600 citations dating from July 1964 and has 10,000 added each month. Rates for use of this file must be obtained from the owner of the file, Derwent Publications, Ltd., London, England, and usage is available only to those organizations that subscribe to the published Ringdoc service.

4. *Advantages and Disadvantages*

The searching system used by the SDC Search Service is the Orbit III retrieval system. Present users of MEDLINE will find this a great advantage since the National Library of Medicine uses the same retrieval system for their data bases. A user need not learn a new searching language to use the SDC data bases.

Again, the disadvantages are the same as those already mentioned: high charges for access to the data bases and difficulties in the use of free-text-searching systems.

F. Bibliographic Retrieval Services, Inc.

In May of 1976, a new company was organized to provide on-line access to some of the same bibliographic data bases provided by organizations listed in the foregoing. Mention is made here of Bibliographic Retrieval Services, Inc. (BRS) of Schenectady, New York, because they charge substantially less for access to the same data bases that are offered by other organizations at a higher charge. The BRS offers access to the following data bases that have been described already: MEDLINE (Section II,A); BIOSIS Previews (Section II,D,1); and CHEMCON (Section II,D,2). In addition, BRS offers access to some other scientific data bases which are not of direct interest to researchers in the drug field.

The BRS pricing schedule is based on the number of connect-time hours contracted for in a month. For example, not-for-profit educational institutions and governmental agencies would pay $13 per hour of connect time for access to any of the data bases if they contracted for a minimum of 40 hours of usage per month. If they contracted for only 20 hours of usage per month, their rate would be $16 per hour. However, added to these connect-hour charges is an hourly fee for use of the TeleNet Communications Network and a royalty fee paid to the data base supplier. Thus, a user of the BIOSIS Previews file would pay a maximum of $34.40 per hour if he contracted for a minimum of 40 hours per month or he would pay a maximum of $37.40 per hour for a minimum of 20 hours per month.

The BRS searching system uses a modification of IBM's on-line retrieval program called STAIRS (*St*orage *a*nd *I*nformation *R*etrieval *S*ystem). It has many useful features and is an effective searching program. No superiority in searching through BRS is claimed over searching through the National Library of Medicine, Lockheed DIALOG, or other systems. It can be confusing to a user, however, if he subscribes to several different systems, because he has to learn the searching systems of each and keep them clear and separate in his mind. The same advantages and disadvantages exist in searching through BRS that exist in the searching of any natural language data base.

The prices charged by BRS represent a substantial advantage to users and have stimulated price competition resulting in some reductions for the users of other data bases. Both Lockheed DIALOG and System Development Corporation announced new rate structures effective January 1, 1977, that provided reduced usage rates. However, the new rate schedules are complex, and it is not possible to compare prices among the three companies without going into very detailed explanations. Competition has largely been lacking heretofore, and a user who wanted access to particular data bases had no alternative but to pay the price. Now, the thousands of organizations making use of on-line data bases will be able to shop for the data base supplier who provides them with the greatest benefits at the most reasonable rates. Furthermore, the small organizations that could not afford access to any on-line systems may well be able to do so now.

III. Toxicology Information Services

For years now, there has been a growing interest in toxicity data on substances to which humans, animals, and plants are exposed. Governmental, industrial, and academic organizations have shown increasing interest and need for these data. A report by a panel of the President's Science Advisory Committee (1966) stressed the ever-increasing problems of harmful chemicals and made recommendations regarding toxicological information.

A. Toxicology Information Program

One of the recommendations of the President's panel was for the establishment of a computer-based system for handling toxicologic information. It was this report which led, in 1967, to the creation of the Toxicology Information Program at the Department of Health, Education and Welfare's (DHEW) National Library of Medicine (Cosmides, 1976).

Program Objectives

General objectives of the program are (1) to create computer-based toxicology data banks from the scientific literature and from the files of collaborating industrial, academic, and governmental agencies; and (2) to establish toxicology information services for the scientific community.

The first objective is being reached by the building of a number of computerized toxicology data bases, either independently or in collaboration with other organizations. One of these is the Toxicology Data Bank, an on-line interactive data retrieval system that will contain evaluated data on selected chemicals to which humans are exposed and which present actual or potential health hazards (Oxman *et al.*, 1976). Collected data will include chemical and physical properties and analytical methods; animal and human toxicology (e.g., overdose treatment, drug interactions, carcinogenesis information); production, uses, and shipment methods; environmental hazards; and explosive and fire potential. Another example is the Product Composition File, a planned on-line system that will contain use, composition, and toxicity data for some 19,000 commercial products listed in the handbook, *Clinical Toxicology of Commercial Products* (National Library of Medicine, 1975).

Under the sponsorship of the Toxicology Information Subcommittee of the DHEW Committee to Coordinate Toxicology and Related Programs, the Toxicology Information Program is charged with coordinating toxicology information activities throughout DHEW and among other federal agencies (Kissman, 1976). To this end, the following projects have been initiated.

1. Establishment of a Laboratory Animal Data Bank that collects and disseminates in an on-line file, base-line values for selected strains of unmanipulated control animals.
2. Organization of a Toxicology Document and Data Depository that will publish, mostly via microform, documents and data files that, because of size, complexity, or format, are not now published in journals.
3. Publication of *TOX-TIPS*, a monthly current awareness bulletin for the exchange of information on projected long-term toxicology testing of compounds by industry and government agencies (Laney, 1976). The intent is to allow toxicological investigators to help one another avoid costly duplication of long-term safety testing of chemicals and other substances by filling in a simple form describing their research project and sending it to the *TOX-TIPS* editor. The notice is also forwarded to the Smithsonian Science Information Exchange for inclusion in their data base as well. In addition to a summary of their project, toxicological investigators must include the name of the test compound, the species and strain of the test animal, the route of administration, and the planned duration of the test.
4. Publication of a quarterly *Toxicology Research Projects Directory* to disseminate descriptions, taken from the files of the Smithsonian Science Information Exchange, of ongoing research projects in toxicology. Each quarterly issue contains approximately 2500 project descrip-

tions classified into chapters and subchapters. An extensive subject index is included as well as indexes to investigators, performing organizations, supporting organizations, and master grant numbers. Its indexes are useful in surveying the research on a topic being conducted by different organizations for an overview of ongoing research in the broad field of toxicology.

5. Establishment of a Chemical Monograph Referral Center, operated by the Consumer Product Safety Commission, to collect and distribute information about plans for the preparation of monographs on chemical compounds.

The computerized information systems called for by the panel report of the President's Science Advisory Committee (1966) exist already or are being built, but the information and data in these systems come almost entirely from the published scientific literature. Few inroads have been made in funneling the toxicologic information in the files of government agencies or industrial companies into publicly accessible retrieval systems (Cosmides, 1976).

The second objective of the Toxicology Information Program, to provide toxicology information service to the scientific community, is presently being implemented in three ways.

a. Query Response through the Toxicology Information Response Center (TIRC). The TIRC was founded in 1971 at the Oak Ridge National Laboratory to establish a national and international source of toxicology information (Huff *et al.,* 1976). It provides information to all individuals on a variety of chemical classes: food additives, environmental pollutants, pharmaceuticals, industrial chemicals, and other substances of toxicologic concern. As an information analysis center, TIRC acquires, selects, stores, retrieves, evaluates, analyzes, and synthesizes comprehensive literature packages according to a user's specific request or a current need. Moreover, it provides extensive toxicology information assistance and services to the scientific, administrative, and public communities. Requesters may ask for specific published toxicology data; individualized literature searches; topical bibliographies; annotated and/or key-worded bibliographies; state-of-the art reviews; custom searches of computerized data bases; access to over 650 bibliographic collections generated annually; use of the toxicology reference library in the center; or selected reports available from the National Technical Information Service (Miller *et al.,* 1974).

The center utilizes various information sources such as on-line access to MEDLINE, TOXLINE, CHEMLINE, CANCERLINE (all described in the foregoing), and computerized data bases of the Oak Ridge National Laboratory itself. Center personnel also consult published secondary sources such as *Biological Abstracts, Chemical Abstracts, Excerpta Medica, Index Medicus,* and *ERDA Research Abstracts,* in fulfilling requests for toxicology information.

Searches are accomplished for requesters under a direct cost recovery system. The rate for domestic search requests is $20 per hour with a $25 minimum charge; foreign search requests are charged $25 per hour with a $30 minimum charge. Computer-associated charges, reproduction costs, as well as use fees for copyrighted materials are in addition to the hourly rates.

b. Publications. In this area the Toxicology Information Program has sponsored or created a number of journals and monographs. Among these are *Toxicity Bibliography*, a quarterly publication containing bibliographic references with MeSH terms derived from the MEDLARS data base; *Abstracts on Health Effects of Environmental Pollutants,* a monthly abstract journal and magnetic-tape service prepared jointly with the BioSciences Information Service; *A Directory of Information Resources in the United States: General Toxicology* prepared in cooperation with the National Referral Center of the Library of Congress; and *Drug Interactions—An Annotated Bibliography with Selected Excerpts.* In addition, state-of-the-art reviews written by experts on topics of current interest are sponsored by the Toxicology Information Program and published in various scientific journals.

c. On-Line Interactive Retrieval Services. The Toxicology Information Program provides on-line retrieval service through its TOXLINE, TOXBACK, and CHEMLINE files, which were described in detail in previous sections.

B. National Institute for Occupational Safety and Health

The National Institute for Occupational Safety and Health (NIOSH) has the responsibility for assuring safe and healthful working conditions for every working man and woman in the United States (Christensen, 1976a). Toxic responses of workers to substances in their work environment are of special concern to NIOSH, and it must make a concerted effort to identify these substances and to recommend corrective actions.

The NIOSH prepares criteria documents on hazardous chemical and physical agents to which workers may be exposed. Recommendations are made to the Department of Labor for standards to protect workers against these hazards. Each criteria document provides, when appropriate, an environmental workplace limit; recommendations for medical examinations and clinical tests, recordkeeping, engineering, and control procedures; personal protective clothing and devices; and methods for informing the employee of the workplace hazard. Many criteria documents have been prepared on substances ranging from ammonia to zinc oxide; many others are being prepared or are planned for future years.

A section of the Occupational Safety and Health Act requires that NIOSH provide "at least annually a list of all known toxic substances by generic, family or other useful grouping and the concentrations at which such toxicity is known to occur." To fulfill this mandate NIOSH is producing the Registry of Toxic Effects of Chemical Substances. The scope of the registry includes all chemicals as well as data selected according to specific criteria; unevaluated toxicity data; and standards and reviews for toxic substances. The total data base is designed for on-line computer capability and is updated monthly. It is also updated annually and published in book form (Christensen, 1976b). Each entry contains: (1) chemical substance prime name; (2) *Chemical Abstracts* Registry Number; (3) molecular weight; (4) molecular formula; (5) Wiswesser line notations; (6) synonyms (including other chemical names, trade names, common or generic names, or codes); (7) toxic dose data (including qualifying toxic dose; route of exposure or administration; species exposed; description of exposure; units of dose measurement; and, notations descriptive of the toxicology); (8) cited reference; (9) aquatic toxicity (relative toxicity to aquatic life); (10) reviews (either threshold limit values or cancer reviews); (11) standards and regulations (as promulgated in United States laws or by agencies); and (12) NIOSH criteria documents.

The registry has many potential uses. As a reference tool it allows users to locate toxicity data, chemical prime name, and synonyms for compounds when only a trade name or common name is used. Users may also obtain information about relative toxicity, toxicology from reviews, and aquatic toxicity, as well as to determine quickly if there are relevant U.S. standards for a particular compound. Compounds may be delineated by the physical descriptors and definitions for each compound, and relative acute toxicity can be determined quickly in cases of accidental exposure.

The registry also helps in starting a bibliography for toxicology studies and as a current awareness tool to avoid duplication of effort. Toxicologic data can be gathered from the registry and research gaps can be identified. In addition, occupational health requirements can be anticipated from data in the registry.

Occupational health professions can use the registry as a guide for establishing safer workplace standards, for evaluating workplace hazards, and for preparing material safety data sheets.

The NIOSH itself uses the registry for identifying potential hazards in the workplace, for anticipating human hazards from a substance, and for identifying possible toxic effects based on chemical structure.

As of June 1976, the registry contained 82,908 listings of chemical substances, of which 21,729 are names of different chemicals with qualifying toxic dose information and 61,179 are synonymous names and codes acquired from the published literature, cooperating industries, individuals, and the American Chemical Society. Among these substances are 1913 compounds classed as carcinogens, 300 compounds classed as mutagens, and 1717 compounds classed as teratogens.

Future improvements in the registry will result in the inclusion of more physical descriptors, toxicity reviews, definitions of mixtures, eye and skin irritation effects, chronic and cumulative effects, plant toxins, and, standards prepared by the Environmental Protection Agency, Food and Drug Administration, and Department of Transportation.

IV. Special-Purpose Information Services

The services that have been described thus far have mostly been ones that provide bibliographic data, either lists of references, or references with abstracts, as the output from any query of the system. There are, however, some services that meet different purposes and provide other kinds of output.

A. World Health Organization Activities

As an international organization devoted to all aspects of health, the World Health Organization (WHO) is in the unique position of being able to gather information in many different subject areas from many different geographic areas. It can then coordinate this information, evaluate it, and disseminate it to those who are interested in it. There is in Geneva the International Drug Monitoring Program which includes the WHO Center for International Monitoring of Adverse Reactions to Drugs. In addition, there is an international network that covers psychotropic drugs.

WHO International Reference Centers Network for Psychotropic Drugs

This network has been in operation since 1968, with the mission of facilitating the communication of psychopharmacologic research activities among the world's scientific community. The network consists of an International Reference Center, three Regional Reference Centers (for

Europe, Asia, and Africa), and nineteen Collaborative and National Reference Centers.

The International Reference Center has the responsibility for coordinating the activities of the other centers, and is located at the Psychopharmacology Research Branch of the National Institute of Mental Health in Rockville, Maryland.

The individual centers do not attempt to duplicate services that are available in most nations through libraries or information centers. Thus, they do not function as disseminators of technical papers, bibliographies, or other published materials. Similarly, they are not storehouses of information on psychotropic drugs. Their emphasis is on the substantive component of psychotropic drug information. The centers are actively involved in research themselves and also continuously survey psychotropic drug research in their geographic areas of responsibility. These research activities are reported to the International Reference Center in the United States, where all incoming information is duplicated and immediately disseminated to all the other centers. The other centers then make this information available to interested investigators in the field.

All information exchanged and available through the centers is related to psychotropic drugs used in the treatment of mental illness. Drug abuse and alcoholism are not included within the program. The concern is with new drugs as well as with drugs already in use for which new applications in mental health have been found or claimed. Information included in the exchange among countries relates to research methodologies, research results, analyses of results, as well as indications, contraindications, interactions, and concomitant effects, including toxicology. The program serves to keep the international scientific community alerted to ongoing work in psychopharmacology in any part of the world and enables investigators anywhere to communicate with colleagues of similar research interest.

Several publications of the network encourage and facilitate contact among researchers in psychopharmacology. The first is an *International Directory of Investigators in Psychopharmacology,* which lists thousands of professionals around the world who are actively engaged in or responsible for psychotropic drug research. Indexes to the directory cover geographic areas and subject headings that cover drug names, animal or human subjects, psychiatric symptoms and syndromes, age groups, and research methodologies.

Another important publication is the *Psychopharmacology Bulletin*, which is published in the United States by the Psychopharmacology Research Branch. It serves as the main organ of communication among centers and researchers in the field with emphasis on rapid informal reporting of work that is usually not covered by the usual scientific journals..

The program is administered by WHO in Geneva, but depends on the voluntary exchange of information among centers and the willingness and readiness of each center to disseminate this information to the scientific community in its geographic area of responsibility. Being kept abreast of the latest developments in the field is of equal importance both to those gathering the information and to those receiving it.

All information provided by the centers is free of charge and is available to any investigator in the field. Upon receiving a request for information, a center will provide referral to resource persons or other sources where specific information on a particular psychotropic drug can be obtained. Data on new drugs that are on file at each center are also available at no cost to requesters. Since the emphasis of the program is on the latest research information and not on the published literature, which is often out-dated before it reaches the reader, investigators are often able to make use of this unique resource in the planning and implementation of their drug studies.

B. The CRISP System

The CRISP system (*C*omputer *R*etrieval of *I*nformation on *S*cientific *P*rojects) is a computer-based data system containing information on the scientific and fiscal aspects of research projects supported by the various research grants and contract programs of the National Institutes of Health and other components of the Public Health Service (DHEW).

Research grants awarded by the National Institutes of Health cover all areas of biomedicine. Many of these grants relate to pharmacological and chemotherapeutic research projects. From this system, scientists and administrators of science programs can obtain immediate answers to a wide range of inquiries, such as: How many current research grants relate to cancer chemotherapy with bleomycin? What are the names of investigators studying clinical pharmacology and cancer chemotherapy? How many current NIH projects are using anthramycin or streptonigrin?

The CRISP system was developed and is maintained and operated by the Division of Research Grants of the National Institutes of Health. The computer files consist of a master dictionary of scientific subject headings that are used to describe the projects supported by the Public Health Service; a file of all the subject index terms with their associated grant number, in sequence by index term; a file of all the grants in grant number order; and, a grant identification master file that contains information such as investigator's name, address, project title, and amount of funds awarded. Queries to the CRISP system may be formulated to obtain either all the terms associated with specific projects or all the grants indexed by a specific term or combination of terms, using traditional Boolean language expressions.

C. The PROPHET System

The PROPHET system is a specialized computer resource sponsored by the Division of Research Resources of the National Institutes of Health (1966) for the study of drug action mechanisms and other chemical/biological interrelationships (Raub, 1974). It was developed by the Chemical/Biological Information-Handling (CBIH) Program, whose goal is to assist the biomedical research community to employ modern computer-based information-handling concepts and methods in its efforts to place knowledge about chemical/biological interactions on an improved theoretical base.

The PROPHET system consists of a remotely accessible, time-shared computer facility and multifaceted, ever-evolving computer programs that are oriented toward the information-handling problems of scientists studying chemical/biological interactions. The computer files consist mostly of the researcher's own data. Thus, the computer serves as a tool that laboratory and clinical investigators can use to represent, organize, manipulate, and communicate their research data and other information in the most scientifically meaningful ways. In addition, the computer contains other files, such as the data base of amino acid sequences of the variable regions of immunoglobulin light and heavy chains.

A variety of research projects has been studied during the past year by PROPHET users. These projects include research applications such as: propranolol uptake by the liver; pharmacokinetics of bethanidine; stimulation of pancreatic enzymes by Sincalide, methacholine, and pancreozymin; histamine-sensitive cardiac adenyl cyclase; metabolic interactions of tetrahydrocannabinol and amphetamine; synthesis of antischistosomal chemotherapeutic agents; and, structure–activity relations of angiotensin analogs.

Presently the PROPHET system serves over 100 scientists located at twelve institutions in nine states. The computer is located at the First Data Corporation in Waltham, Massachusetts, and is accessed via telecommunication lines. One of the objectives of the CBIH Program staff is to increase the number of PROPHET user groups over the next few years. The CBIH Review Committee has recommended that the

PROPHET user community should continue to be comprised principally of high-quality investigators working in the area of chemical/biological interaction mechanisms, even though scientists in other areas of biomedical research could benefit from PROPHET's proven features. New users are selected on the basis of research prospectuses that they submit. The prospectus is assessed on the basis of the following criteria: the scientific merit of the research activities described and their relevance to the objectives of the CBIH Program; the likelihood that access to the PROPHET system can facilitate the offeror's research; and, the likelihood that the offeror's uses of the PROPHET system will contribute significantly toward the system's further development.

Although many needs and opportunities for further development of PROPHET exist, PROPHET already is the most nearly comprehensive array of computer tools for the study of chemical/biological interrelationships that has ever been integrated into a single system and made available as a service to the biomedical community.

D. The MYCIN System

Named after the common suffix used for many antibiotic names, MYCIN is an interactive computer program that uses clinical decision criteria acquired from medical experts to advise physicians who request information concerning antimicrobial therapy selection. The system was developed at Stanford University by Shortliffe *et al.* (1973, 1975).

It is often the case with patients who have infectious diseases that therapy must be initiated before complete information on the nature of the infecting organism is available. MYCIN is an attempt to alleviate this situation by gathering clinical and historical criteria that have been identified by experts in infectious diseases and incorporating these criteria into a computer system. The physician using the MYCIN system enters certain data (patient's name, age, sex, etc.) into the computer at his data terminal and then, in turn, is queried by the computer to provide whatever information he has regarding the patient's infection. On the basis of hundreds of decision criteria that have been stored in the computer, MYCIN can give appropriate advice that the physician can consider in diagnosing and treating his patients with bacteremia. New decision criteria are acquired by MYCIN during interactions with experts and these can be used during future consultation sessions. Additional rules for MYCIN are still being identified and formulated, but, once it has been implemented on hospital wards, its clinical effectiveness can be formally evaluated. The methodology of MYCIN also has possible application in other areas of clinical medicine.

E. de Haen Drug Information Services

Paul de Haen, Inc., of New York City, is a firm that has been engaged in providing a variety of drug information services for many years. All the services represent published products, either file cards, report sheets, or computerized indexes, with microfilm editions available in some cases.

The data for the de Haen drug information systems are extracted from more than 400 worldwide biomedical journals. Some of the services are aimed at providing citations to the published literature but most provide detailed annotations and specific data on number of patients, sex, age, dosages, and reactions to the drugs used. Some of the specific de Haen products that are published are *Drug Adverse Reactions, Drug Interactions, Drugs in Research, Drugs in Use, Drugs in Medical Practice (USA), Nonproprietary Name Index,* and, *Diagnostic Trends.*

V. Concluding Remarks

The need for information on drugs is continuous and expanding constantly. It is not just the scientists engaged in drug research who need this information, but many others with varying and widespread interests. Public health officials, toxicologists, environmentalists, regulatory agency officials, government officials at all levels, and patient care physicians all have strong interest in this information. It is not surprising that so much effort has already been expended and continues to be expended in developing the means by which drug information can be gathered, analyzed, evaluated, and disseminated to all the different groups that need it. Computerized systems have been of great value in speeding up this information-handling process. Some of them have been described here in the hope that the users of drug information can benefit from these powerful services.

Acknowledgement

The author is greatly obliged to Dr. Robert J. Schnitzer for his active interest, helpful advice, and constant encouragement in the initiation and completion of this report.

References

Christensen, H. E. (1976a). *In* "Symposium on the Handling of Toxicological Information." Natl. Inst. Health, Bethesda, Maryland (in preparation).

Christensen, H. E. (1976b). "Registry of Toxic Effects of Chemical Substances, 1976 Edition." Natl. Inst. Occup. Safety and Health, Rockville, Maryland. HEW Publ. No. (NIOSH) 76-191.

Cosmides, G. J. (1976). *In* "Symposium on the Handling of Toxicological Information." Natl. Inst. Health, Bethesda, Maryland (in preparation).

Division of Research Resources, National Institutes of Health. (1976). "Fiscal Year 1976 Annual Report," pp. 53–86. Chemical/Biological Information Handling Program, Bethesda, Maryland.

Herxheimer, A. (1974). *Drugs* **8,** 321–329.

Huff, J. E., Gerstner, H. B., Ulrikson, G. U., and Kissman, H. M. (1976). *In* "Symposium on the Handling of Toxicological Information." Natl. Inst. Health, Bethesda, Maryland (in preparation).

Kissman, H. M. (1976). *In* "Symposium on the Handling of Toxicological Information." Natl. Inst. Health, Bethesda, Maryland (in preparation).

Laney, M. J. (1976). *Tox-Tips* **1,** 1.

Miller, K. C., Gerstner, H. B., and Beauchamp, R. O., Jr. (1974). *J. Chem. Doc.* **14,** 32–36.

National Library of Medicine (1975). "Fact Sheet." Toxicology Information Program, Natl. Inst. Health, Bethesda, Maryland.

Oxman, M. A., Kissman, H. M., Burnside, J. M., Edge, J. R., Haberman, C. B., and Wykes, A. A. (1976). *J. Chem. Inf. Comput. Sci.* **16,** 19–21.

President's Science Advisory Committee. (1966). "Handling of Toxicological Information," The White House, Washington, D.C.

Raub, W. F. (1974). *Fed. Proc. Fed. Am. Soc. Exp. Biol.* **33,** 2390–2392.

Shortliffe, E. H., Axline, S. G., Buchanan, B. G., Merigan, T. C., and Cohen, S. N. (1973). *Comput. Biomed. Res.* **6,** 544–560.

Shortliffe, E. H., Davis, R., Axline, S. G., Buchanan, B. G., Green, C. C., and Cohen, S. N. (1975). *Comput. Biomed. Res.* **8,** 303–320.

Weinstein, L. (1976). "Teratology and Congenital Malformations: A Comprehensive Guide to the Literature." IFI/Plenum Data Corporation, New York.

Weinstock, M. (1971). *Encyl. Lib. Inf. Sci.* **5,** 16–40.

Pharmacology and Neurochemistry of Apomorphine*

GAETANO DI CHIARA AND GIAN LUIGI GESSA

Institute of Pharmacology, University of Cagliari
Cagliari, Italy

* Much of the work reported herein was supported by grants from the Consiglio Nazionale delle Richerche, Rome.

I. Introduction

Apomorphine was first employed as a powerful emetic agent. In 1948, Dordoni called attention to apomorphine 's ability to attenuate decerebrate rigidity in dogs and opened the way to its use by Schwab *et al.* (1951) to treat parkinsonian disturbances. These results were confirmed by others, but this line of research was soon interrupted. In the meantime, the research on the mechanism of the emetic effects of apomorphine received a major impulse and led to the discovery by Borison and Wang (1953) of the chemoreceptor trigger zone as the site of apomorphine emesis.

Interest in apomorphine as an antiparkinsonian agent was resumed only after Ernst's studies (1967), which indicated the direct dopaminergic nature of apomorphine effects, and after the introduction of L-dopa* as a specific treatment for Parkinson's disease (Cotzias *et al.*, 1967). In 1970, when Cotzias *et al.*, rediscovered the antiparkinsonian effect of apomorphine, almost 20 years had elasped since Schwab's first report. At that time apomorphine had already acquired its place as a specific tool for the study of dopamine function in the nervous system. Now, to say that apomorphine research has contributed to our present knowledge of dopamine function might be, indeed, an understatement.

II. Chemical Pharmacology of Apomorphine

Apomorphine can be obtained by the acid-catalyzed rearrangement of morphine (Matthiessen and Wright, 1869; Small *et al.*, 1940) and by total synthesis (Neumeyer *et al.*, 1973a).

* List of Abbreviations: ACh, acetylcholine; AMP, adenosine 5′-monophosphate; AP, area postrema; COMT, catechol-*O*-methyltransferase; CTZ; chemoreceptor trigger zone; DBH, dopamine-β-hydroxylase; DA, dopamine; L-dopa, 3,4-dihydroxyphenylalanine; DOPAC, 3,4-dihydroxyphenylacetic acid; GH, growth hormone; 5-HIAA, 5-hydroxyindolacetic acid; 5-HT, 5-hydroxytryptamine (serotonin); HVA, homovanillic acid; LSD, lysergic acid diethylamide; M-7, 5,6-dihydroxy-2-dimethylaminotetrahydronaphthalene; MAO, monoamine oxidase; MOPEG, 3-methoxy-4-hydroxyphenylglycol; α-MT, α-methyltyrosine; NA, norepinephrine; NPA, *N*-*n*-propylnorapomorphine; 6OH-DA, 6-hydroxydopamine; PIF, prolactin-inhibiting factor.

The hydrochloride forms colorless crystals that readily undergo superficial oxidation and assume a greenish tinge. Apomorphine solutions in water are unstable, turning green upon exposure to light and to air oxygen. Oxidation of apomorphine is much slower in acidic media. These properties of apomorphine explain the current addition of ascorbic acid to apomorphine solutions. The oxidation of apomorphine has been studied by Burkman (1963a,b) and by Kaul and Brochmann-Hansen (1961).

A. Structure–Activity Relationships

1. *Apomorphine Pharmacophore*

By simple comparison of apomorphine and DA structural formulas, Ernst (1965) detected their striking resemblance which led him to postulate that apomorphine acts as a dopaminergic agonist. He apparently envisioned the tetrahydronaphtalene and not the isoquinoline moiety as the part of apomorphine responsible for its dopaminomimetic activity. The two moieties correspond to different conformations of DA; in the tetrahydronaphthalene moiety the DA molecule is in the extended transconformation with maximal distance between the amino group and the ring; in the tetrahydroisoquinoline moiety, the DA molecule is, instead, in a folded cis conformation, with reduced distances between the amino group and the ring.

The problem of establishing which of the two moieties is responsible for the DA-like activity of apomorphine is important, since it is directly connected to that of the active conformation of DA. Indeed, the clarification of the first problem has greatly contributed to the solution of the second one.

The problem of the identity of the active conformer of DA was studied by Kier and Truitt (1970) by calculating with a semiempirical quantum-mechanical treatment the preferred conformation of DA. Accordingly, DA would exist in two low-energy gauche conformations, corresponding to an angle of torsion of 60° and of 300°, respectively. In these conformers the aliphatic chain of DA is folded, and the distances between the amino group and the ring are minimal. According to these calculations, a transconformation was not found to be thermodynamically preferred. Kier and Truitt (1970) therefore suggested that apomorphine would interact with its receptor by the tetrahydroisoquinoline moiety and that absence of ring hydroxyl groups would be compatible with DA activity. Both these predictions have been disproved by experiment.

Thus, Pinder *et al.* (1971, 1972) found that aporphine, tetrahydroisoquinoline, and *N*-methyltetrahydroisoquinoline, which contain the pharmacophore proposed by Kier and Truitt (1970), are inactive as central as well as peripheral DA receptor stimulants. In addition, 1,2-dihydroxy-aporphine, which corresponds to a rigid cis conformer of DA, has been found to be inactive as emetic in the dog at doses 10 times higher than apomorphine (Neumeyer *et al.*, 1973b). Methylation of one hydroxy group of apomorphine as in apocodeine (Koch *et al.*, 1968; Lal *et al.*, 1972a); Saari *et al.*, 1974) as well as abolition of the 10,11-catechol configuration as in 10- or 11-hydroxyaporphine, results in loss or large reduction of activity (Neumeyer *et al.*, 1974). Similar results have been obtained *in vitro* by testing the ability of various rigid conformational analogs of DA to stimulate the DA-sensitive adenyl cyclase of rat striatal homogenates (Miller *et al.*, 1974). Interestingly, in this system, dihydroxytetrahydroisoquinoline is fairly active even if less than the rigid trans conformer, aminodihydroxytetrahydronaphthalene.

Recently, Kier and Truitt (1970) conclusions have been disproved also on the basis of theoretical calculations (Bustard and Egan, 1971; Rekker *et al.*, 1972) as well as by direct physical analysis. It has been shown that the interatomic distances between the catechol oxygens and the nitrogen atom of DA in the trans conformation correspond perfectly to that in the apomorphine molecule (Rekker *et al.*, 1972). Direct evidence for the existence of a transconformer has been given by NMR analysis of DA in solution (Bustard and Egan, 1971).

From these results, it is possible to draw the following conclusions: (*1*) the pharmacophore of apomorphine is the tetrahydroaminonaphthalene moiety; (*2*) hydroxylation at the 10- or 11-position of the ring is essential for the activity but a catechol configuration is optimal; and (*3*) DA interacts with its receptor in an unfolded trans conformation.

2. *Methylethers of Apomorphine*

In spite of older reports of emetic activity, later ascribed to contamination by apomorphine, methoxylation at the 10- or 11-position, as in apocodeine and in isoapocodeine, results, according to Koch *et al.* (1968) and to Cannon *et al.* (1972a), in complete loss of the ability to produce gnawing in mice, emesis in dogs, and pecking in pigeons. Apocodeine still produces emesis in pigeons (Koch *et al.*, 1968). However, this response in pigeons does not seem to be a purely dopaminergic one.

In contrast to Koch *et al.* (1968), it has been reported that apocodeine retains some dopaminergic activity in mice and in rats (Saari, *et al.*, 1974; Lal *et al.*, 1972a). A possible explanation for these discrepancies might be the different sensitivity of the tests used for DA activity or that rats and mice (Saari *et al.*, 1974; Lal *et al.*, 1972a), in contrast to dogs and pigeons (Koch *et al.*, 1968), demethylate apocodeine to apomorphine. In fact, apomorphine has been identified in the urine of rats treated with apocodeine (Smith and Cook, 1974). This might also explain the activity of 10,11-methylenedioxyaporphine (Lal *et al.*, 1972a).

On the basis of the inactivity of apocodeine and isoapocodeine, Cannon *et al.* (1972a) concluded that both hydroxy groups of apomorphine are essential for agonist activity. However, this conclusion should be revised in the light of the recent evidence gained with monohydroxyaporphines (Neumeyer *et al.*, 1974).

3. *Modification of the Catechol Configuration of Apomorphine*

The catechol configuration, although optimal for DA agonist activity, might be nonessential for it. This conclusion has been recently drawn from the finding that 11-hydroxyaporphine has some agonistic properties on DA receptors *in vivo* (Neumeyer *et al.*, 1974). *N-n*-Propyl substitution increases the potency of the 10- or 11-hydroxynoraporphine derivatives (Neumeyer *et al.*, 1974).

However, before concluding that the catechol configuration is not a strict requirement for DA receptor activation, it is necessary to exclude that monohydroxyaporphines act *in vivo* through conversion to apomorphine. Since this reaction would require the activity of a P-450-containing, oxygen-dependent, enzyme system, which is absent in brain, a way to settle this question might be to test the ability of the monohydroxylated aporphines to stimulate the striatal adenylcyclase activity. Hydroxylation of the aporphine ring system at positions other than 10 or 11 results in very weak or no activity (Neumeyer *et al.*, 1973a,b; Saari *et al.*, 1973; Lal *et al.*, 1972a).

4. *N-Substituted Apomorphine Derivatives*

Increasing the length of the aliphatic substituent of apomorphine increases lipid solubility and partition into the brain compartment is also expected to increase. On the other hand, modification of the N-substituent might drastically reduce the affinity of apomorphine for the DA receptor. Thus, it can be predicted that DA-mimetic activity *in vivo* might be augmented by increasing the length of the aliphatic N-substituent until the increased brain partition compensates for a decrease in receptor affinity.

According to Koch *et al.* (1968), who have performed the most extensive study on N-substituted aporphines, *N*-demethylated apomorphine (norapomorphine) is 50–100 times less potent than apomorphine; ethyl substitution coincides with maximal activity; and the introduction of an allyl substituent (Hensiak *et al.*, 1965) reduces activity but results in a less toxic compound.

Substitution of an *n*-propyl group increases potency by 14–28% depending on the test used (Koch *et al.*, 1968). By contrast, according to Neumeyer *et al.* (1973a) and to Schoenfeld *et al.* (1975), NPA is 25–35 times more potent than apomorphine. The reason for this discrepancy is obscure and is not accounted for by differences in testing procedures since it occurs also when the same test is used (emesis to threshold doses in the dog).

5. *Dextro-Apomorphine*

The preparation of apomorphine by the acid-catalyzed rearrangement of morphine results in the retention of the configuration at the C6a chiral center leading to the corresponding (−)-isomer. For these reasons the preparation of the optical antipode of apomorphine and its pharmacological evaluation had to wait until apomorphine could be obtained by total synthesis in amounts large enough to permit its resolution. Recently, Neumeyer *et al.* (1970) have worked up a procedure that satisfies these requirements. By applying Neumeyer's synthesis, Saari *et al.* (1973) have obtained (+)-apomorphine. This enantiomer has been found to be inactive as a DA agonist as well as a (−)-apomorphine antagonist (Saari *et al.*, 1973).

The inactivity of (+)-apomorphine as a DA-like drug makes it a valuable tool to differentiate DA-mediated from nonspecific effects of apomorphine.

B. Estimation Procedures

Apomorphine has been measured in biological samples by spectrophotometric (Kaul *et al.*, 1961a) and fluorimetric (Van Tyle and Burkman, 1971; Andén *et al.*, 1973) methods and by fluorescence quenching after chromatographic separation (Smith *et al.*, 1973).

The method of Van Tyle and Burkman (1971) is particularly suited for estimation of apomorphine in tissues, because it is simple and sensitive to as little as 100 ng of apomorphine per sample.

C. Pharmacokinetics

Kaul *et al.* (1961b) and Burkman *et al.* (1974) reported that the biological half-life of apomorphine in mice is 8.5 and 47 minutes, respectively. Such a large discrepancy is not due to differences in experimental data but to the use of the slopes of different portions of the time course in calculating the biological half-life. Thus, Kaul *et al.* (1961b), assuming a one-compartment model of apomorphine distribution, used the slope of the first-order portion (alpha phase) whereas Burkman *et al.* (1974) on the basis of a two-compartment model used the slope of the terminal portion of the time plot (beta phase). Calculation of apomorphine half-life from the alpha phase of the experimental time course obtained by Burkman *et al.* (1974) gives a value of 7.3 minutes which agrees very well with that of 8.5 minutes reported by Kaul *et al.* (1961b).

Norapomorphine and *N*-*n*-propylapomorphine have a biological half-life of 20 and 29 minutes, respectively (Burkman *et al.*, 1974).

After intravenous administration, apomorphine distribution into the brain compartment is rapid, reaching completion in 5 minutes, at which time the brain-to-blood concentration ratio becomes constant. Norapomorphine is distributed less rapidly (50 minutes), whereas *N*-*n*-propylapomorphine equilibrates with brain in less than 1 minute.

The time course of apomorphine in brain is an exponential profile which mirrors that in the blood; the same applies to *N*-*n*-propylapomorphine. Their brain-to-blood ratio is a constant that depends on the partition coefficient. By contrast, the time course of norapomorphine in brain has a parabolic profile, very dissimilar to that in the blood (Burkman *et al.*, 1974). The reason for this is that norapomorphine in blood equilibrates slowly with brain so that the brain-to-blood concentration ratio varies with time, being kinetically related to the continuously changing concentrations of the drug in the blood.

The comparative behavior of N-substituted apomorphine is an excellent example of the fact that brain-to-blood concentration ratios of drugs are not always and simply related to their partition coefficient but, rather, to the kinetics of the drug in the blood.

D. Metabolism

Apomorphine is metabolized by *O*-glucuronidation, *O*-methylation, and, probably, by *N*-demethylation.

"Bound" apomorphine excreted in the urine was reported by Kaul *et al.* (1961b) to account for a major fraction of administered apomorphine. In the rabbit, 71% and, in the rat, 56–64% of administered apomorphine was recovered in the urine in the bound form. Bound apomorphine was described by Kaul *et al.* (1961b) to consist of a 2:1 mixture of two glucuronides. Because they consider the 10-position as the less hindered, Kaul *et al.* (1961b) postulate that the most represented metabolite of apomorphine is the 10-glucuronide.

Administration of *p*-hydroxyacetanilide prolongs apomorphine effects; this might be due to a competitive inhibition of glucuronide conjugation of apomorphine by *p*-hydroxyacetanilide (Missala *et al.*, 1973).

Administration of the microsomal inhibitor SKF-525A, failed to inhibit apomorphine metabolism and glucuronidation. Induction of drug-metabolizing enzymes by administration of phenobarbital or testosterone failed to induce apomorphine metabolism and glucuronidation. Only apomorphine, administered for 3 days once a day, induced its own metabolism, but estradiol, administered in a single dose 4 days earlier, inhibited apomorphine metabolism (Kaul and Conway, 1971).

Apomorphine is methylated *in vitro* when incubated with rat liver soluble fraction in the presence of *S*-adenosylmethionine as methyl donor (White and McKenzie, 1971; Cannon *et al.*, 1972a; McKenzie and White, 1973; Missala *et al.*, 1973). This reaction is carried by the enzyme COMT. The products of the reaction are the 10- and the 11-methoxyapomorphine; 10,11-dimethoxyapomorphine is not observed (Cannon *et al.*, 1972a). This could be evidence in favor of the hypothesis of Kaul *et al.* (1961b) that the less hindered 10-position is preferred for metabolic attack.

O-Methylation of apomorphine has been measured by the formation of labeled products when the drug is incubated with liver homogenates in the presence of *S*-adenosylmethionine-^{14}C (McKenzie and White, 1973). The apparent K_m of the reaction is fairly high: 1.4×10^{-3} *M*. This suggests that the COMT pathway is of minor importance for apomorphine metabolism *in vivo*. On the other hand, the ability of COMT inhibitors to potentiate and to prolong apomorphine effects seems to indicate that *O*-methylation of apomorphine has some role in its *in vivo* disposition (McKenzie and White, 1973). However, this conclusion needs to be substantiated by the study of the effect of COMT inhibitors on the apomorphine half-life *in vivo*.

N-Dealkylation of apomorphine is postulated on the basis of the presence of norapomorphine in the urine of rats treated with 10-methoxyapomorphine (apocodeine) (Smith and Cook, 1974) and by analogy with the *in vitro* metabolism of *N*-alkylated derivatives of nornuciferine, a methylated isomer of norapomorphine (Smith and Sood, 1971).

Apomorphine is excreted as a free base in the acidic urine of the rat, but not in the alkaline urine of the rabbit. This behavior can be explained by ionization of the basic group at acidic pH, preventing tubular reabsorption of apomorphine and its breakdown in the bladder.

III. Emetic Effects of Apomorphine

If a historian were to trace the development of apomorphine systematically, he would probably distinguish an emetic era from a postemetic one. In fact, apomorphine has been known for many years as an emetic agent, the most potent and specific in man. As a result of this, the emetic effect of apomorphine was the first to be subjected to thorough study. Unfortunately, however, as interest in the behavioral actions of apomorphine mounted, research on emesis declined dramatically. Thus, little progress has been made on this subject since the studies of Borison and Wang (1953) in the late forties and in the fifties. Owing to this fact and to the existence of excellent reviews on the subject (Borison and Wang, 1953; Wang, 1965; Borison, 1974), this chapter is restricted to the neurochemical characterization of the emetic receptor and to the theoretical and practical significance of the antiemetic properties of neuroleptics.

A. Intracerebral Site of Action

The monumental work of Borison and Wang on emesis may be summarized by saying that they discovered the existence, in the AP, of a CTZ that constitutes the primary site of action of emetic drugs such as apomorphine, ergot alkaloids, digitalis, glycosides, morphine, and intravenous but not intragastric copper sulfate (Wang and Borison, 1952; Wang and Glaviano, 1954; Borison, 1952; Gaitondé *et al.*, 1965).

The AP is often reported in textbooks as a superficial area located in the floor of the fourth ventricle. This is actually incorrect: anatomically AP is a circumventricular formation, forming a pedestal to the tela choroidea which separates the fourth ventricle from the cisterna magna (Koella and Sutin, 1967; Weindl, 1973). For this reason, on the surface of AP one distinguishes a pial (cisternal) and an ependymal (ventricular) side. Whereas in dogs the ependymal side is the most represented, in rats and rabbits AP is a median mass covered by pia mater.

The capillaries of AP consist of leaky fenestrated endothelium surrounded by a double basement membrane (Rohr, 1966; Andres, 1965; Dempsey, 1968; Brightman and Reese, 1969). This structural feature leads to an important characteristic of AP, namely that it is permeated by vital dyes (Wislocki and King, 1936), drugs (Wilson and Brodie, 1961; Wilson *et al.*, 1962), and proteins (Torack and Finke, 1971) that do not normally cross the blood–brain barrier.

The AP consists of large glial cells (Brizzee and Neal, 1954) and neurons (Cammermayer, 1949; Morest, 1960; Andres, 1965; Shimizu and

Ishii, 1964). In rodents and lagomorphs, some neurons show a catecholamine-type fluorescence intensified by L-dopa administration (Fuxe and Owman, 1965). Serotonin-containing neurons have been also observed after treatment with MAO inhibitors. Catecholamine terminals are described in the AP but are reportedly scarce (Fuxe and Owman, 1965).

Sampling difficulties, due to the paucity of the tissue, has lead to controversy over the presence of biogenic amines in the AP. Early reports on the presence of high concentrations of catecholamines (Vogt, 1954) and serotonin (Amin *et al.*, 1954) in AP have not been confirmed and are ascribed to contamination by nearby tissue (Fuxe and Owman, 1965).

The AP is present in all mammalian species; however, only a few species do vomit. According to early studies by Hatcher and Weiss (1923), solipeds, ruminants, rodents, and birds are incapable of vomiting. More recently, it has been reported that certain avian species (pigeon, herring gull, cowbird) vomit in response to apomorphine (Burkman, 1960; Chaney and Kare, 1966). This might indicate that in these animals which are unable to vomit, the AP is only a rudimentary organ. However, according to Borison and Brizzee (1951), CTZ is not equivalent to AP but only to a small part of it, specifically, the most lateral one, which is devoid of neurons. Contrasting views were later expressed by Brizzee and Neal (1954).

At the moment, CTZ seems to be more a physiological and a pharmacological entity than a morphological one. A correlation between emetic response and morphological characteristics of the AP does not allow any conclusion regarding the morphological substrate of apomorphine-induced emesis.

B. Mechanism of Apomorphine-Induced Emesis

Wang and Borison (1952) demonstrated that CTZ-lesioned dogs were resistant to apomorphine emesis but normally responsive to intragastric copper sulfate. Destruction of the nucleus fasciculi solitarii makes the dog resistant also to the intragastric copper sulfate; stimulation of this nucleus consistently elicits emesis (Wang, 1965). Single-unit recording from the nucleus fasciculi solitarii in the cat has shown an increased firing rate in response to apomorphine administered intravenously or locally applied on the AP; this response to apomorphine was blocked by metoclopramide and by chlorpromazine (Takaori *et al.*, 1968, 1970).

These results enable us to envision apomorphine-induced emesis as due to a primary activation of a receptive zone of the AP (CTZ) which, in turn, stimulates an emetic center located in the area of the nucleus fasciculi solitarii. The emetic center constitutes the neural basis for the act of vomiting itself; it can also be activated by afferent volleys originating in the gastrointestinal mucosa.

Anatomical connections between CTZ and the nucleus fasciculi solitarii are made through axons originating in the AP and through dendrites extending from the nucleus into the AP (Morest, 1960, 1967; Borison and Brizzee, 1951).

C. Nature of Apomorphine Receptors for Emesis

The dog is exquisitely sensitive to the emetic action of apomorphine: 0.01 mg/kg i.v., produces emesis in 85% of the animals; on the contrary, according to Borison and Wang (1953), the cat is about 1000 times less sensitive to apomorphine than dogs. The monkey does not vomit after doses of apomorphine as high as 25 mg/kg i.v. and 100 mg/kg s.c. which induce an overt stereotypic response (Brizzee *et al.*, 1955). In man, 5 mg of apomorphine administered subcutaneously induce emesis in most subjects (Sollmann, 1957).

Apomorphine receptors for emesis are able to function soon after birth, but the dose of apomorphine required for producing emesis is higher than in the adult; during development there is a steady decrease of the emetic dose toward the adult values (Pi and Peng, 1971).

A major discovery in the area of apomorphine-induced emesis was the finding that chlorpromazine markedly protected dogs from this effect while it did not prevent vomiting to oral copper sulfate (Courvoisier *et al.*, 1953). In contrast to chlorpromazine, antihistaminic agents even in large doses did not exert a protective effect (Brand *et al.*, 1954; Glaviano and Wang, 1955). In dogs, chlorpromazine prevented not only the emesis produced by apomorphine but also that induced by ergot alklaoids and, to a lesser extent and less predictably, the emesis induced by morphine (Brand *et al.*, 1954; Glaviano and Wang, 1955). The differential action of chlorpromazine on emesis by apomorphine and by intragastric copper sulfate makes its administration analogous to the ablation of CTZ.

However, an important feature distinguishes chlorpromazine-treated from CTZ-ablated dogs: the former are normally sensitive to the emetic actions of cardiac glycosides and intravenous copper sulfate, whereas the latter are insensitive to these agents too. This indicates that in the CTZ there is a distinct population of emetic receptors that have the property of being blocked by chlorpromazine and by neuroleptic drugs when challenged with apomorphine, ergot alkaloids, and morphine (Brand *et al.*, 1954). Assignment of these receptors to the dopaminergic type is now obvious since a strict correlation exists between the potency of neuroleptics in blocking apomorphine-induced emesis in dogs and their cataleptogenic and antistereotypic activity in rats (Janssen *et al.*, 1965a,b). A positive correlation also exists between the emetic potency of DA receptor agonists in dogs and their ability to induce stereotypy in rodents (Koch *et al.*, 1968). In this respect, it might be recalled that DA itself has emetic properties when administered systemically (Wang, 1965) and that nausea and vomiting is a common side-effect of patients undergoing L-dopa therapy (Cotzias, 1971).

Amphetamine, however, an indirectly acting dopaminomimetic agent, is devoid of emetic properties. This could indicate that in the CTZ, dopaminergic receptors responsible for triggering emesis but not DA nerve terminals are present. Thus, the presence in AP of a DA-sensitive cyclase can be predicted, but has not been reported so far.

The problem of the relationship between the antiemetic and the antistereotypic effects of neuroleptics has been analyzed by Rotrosen *et al.* (1972a) in dogs. According to them, haloperidol is a better blocker of stereotypy than of emesis, whereas the reverse is valid for pimozide. The authors conclude on this basis that the DA receptor for emesis can be differentiated pharmacologically from that for stereotyped behavior. However, a closer scrutiny of the data does not substantiate this conclusion. In fact, if the hypothesis of Rotrosen *et al.* is correct, the ratio between the potency of neuroleptics as blockers of emesis and stereotypy, respectively, should be maintained for each neuroleptic through the time of its action. This is not the case: although at 1 and 3 hours post drug, pimozide blocks emesis more effectively than stereotypy, at 20 hours post drug it resembles haloperidol since it blocks stereotypy more efficiently than emesis. Thus, haloperidol and pimozide appear to differ in the time course of the effect on emesis and on stereotypy rather than in their specificity toward these two effects of apomorphine. This conclusion is substantiated by Janssen *et al.* (1968), who find that the ratio of antiemetic to antistereotypy potency at the peak of action is similar for pimozide and haloperidol. Viewed from this point, the results of Rotrosen *et al.* (1972a) are still interesting since they might indicate that pimozide accumulates on striatal receptors more slowly than does haloperidol. The results of Rotrosen *et al.* (1972a) could be explained as the result of differential partition of the drugs between intra (striatal) and extra (CTZ) blood–brain barrier compartments.

A relation seems to exist between the antiapomorphine action in dogs and the antipsychotic effect of neuroleptics in man (Janssen, 1965a,b, 1967, 1968). Indeed, the antiapomorphine test has become a routine method for screening antipsychotic drugs (Niemegeers, 1971). Even if notable exceptions exist, this relationship cannot be simple chance. In fact, together with the ability of *d*-amphetamine to produce psychotic symptoms (Angrist and Gershon, 1970; Griffith *et al.*, 1970), the correlation between the antidopaminergic and the antipsychotic potency of neuroleptics is the most suggestive evidence for the role of brain dopamine in mental illnesses.

IV. Behavioral Effects of Apomorphine

A. Stereotyped Behavior

Apomorphine, administered to rats by a variety of routes, produces in threshold doses an increase in exploratory activity and discontinuous sniffing. As the dose is increased normal activities such as grooming, social interaction, and feeding are replaced by continuous sniffing, accompanied by small head movements and ptosis. Higher doses of the drug produce the full-blown apomorphine syndrome, characterized by continuous gnawing, biting, and licking while the rat stands in a restricted area of the cage (Ernst, 1967). The continuous, purposeless nature of this behavior justifies the name "stereotyped" which has been applied to it. After very high doses, exophthalmus and convulsions are observed (Janssen *et al.*, 1960).

The dose of apomorphine capable of producing the full-blown stereotyped behavior varies according to the experimental conditions used; since Ernst (1967), most investigators use wire mesh on the cage floor; too fine a grid inhibits gnawing (Lal and Sourkes, 1973) whereas the presence of wooden shavings facilitates it (personal observation).

The latency and the duration of the stereotyped syndrome depends on the dose and the route of administration; it has been reported by Janssen *et al.* (1960) that as little as 0.08 mg/kg of apomorphine administered intravenously elicited stereotyped gnawing in 25% of the rats. After doses higher than 0.31 mg/kg, the rats exhibited exaggerated motor reactions to various stimuli such as noise and light (Janssen *et al.*, 1960).

From data in the literature, it appears that in rats the threshold dose of apomorphine for the induction of a full-blown stereotypy is 0.5 mg/kg s.c. (McKenzie, 1972), 2.0 mg/kg i.p. (Costall and Naylor, 1973a), and 0.31 mg/kg i.v. (Janssen *et al.*, 1960). The higher effectiveness of the subcutaneous compared to the intraperitoneal route is in keeping with the high rate of apomorphine inactivation by liver enzymes.

Increased exploratory behavior and sniffing is the most characteristic response of mice to apomorphine, whereas gnawing is produced only in some strain or after very high doses of the drug (Ther and Schramm, 1962; Frommel, 1965; Pedersen, 1967; Scheel-Krüger, 1970; Maj *et al.*, 1972b).

Stereotyped behavior characterized by gnawing has been described after the administration of apomorphine to rabbits (Harnack, 1874) and guinea pigs (Frommel, 1965; Srimal and Dhawan, 1970; Klawans *et al.*, 1973; Costall *et al.*, 1975b).

Stereotypies in dogs take the form of head bobbing, eye shifting, and incessant running around the cage (Nymark, 1972; Willner *et al.*, 1970).

Side-to-side head movements are observed in cats (Wallach *et al.*, 1972).

In the monkey *(Macaca,* baboon), apomorphine , administered subcutaneously or intravenously in doses of 0.5–1.0 mg/kg, produced restlessness and agitation, aggressiveness, and a form of stereotyped behavior consisting of licking, lip-smacking, and chewing. This behavior lasted for 30–40 minutes after the injection of apomorphine (Brizzee *et al.*, 1955; Peng and Wang, 1962; Shintomi and Yamamura, 1975; Meldrum *et al.*, 1975).

In pigeons (Koster, 1957; Burkman and Nelson, 1957) and in various other species of birds (sparrows, quails, parrots, herring gull, cowbirds) but not in chickens, apomorphine elicits stereotyped pecking (Deshpande *et al.*, 1961; Chaney and Kare, 1966). In pigeons, apomorphine-induced pecking is vigorous and directed to the floor so that it can be easily monitored by a microphone apparatus (Van Tyle and Burkman, 1970).

Stereotyped behavior after apomorphine administration, in spite of its continuous and purposeless character, is influenced to a certain extent by external stimuli. In rats, distracting stimuli, such as loud noises, have an inhibitory influence on the stereotypy produced by intermediate doses of apomorphine: sniffing becomes discontinuous and is directed upward; the same applies to pigeons which stop pecking when suddenly exposed to a bright light or placed in the dark (Dhawan and Saxena, 1960).

Chronic or subchronic administration of apomorphine does not result in modification of the intensity or of the characteristics of the stereotyped response; this applies to the rat as well as to the pigeon (Dresse and Niemegeers, 1961; Lal and Sourkes, 1973; Dhawan and Saxena, 1960; Burkman, 1961). The only observed modification after repeated administration of apomorphine in rats and pigeons is a decreased latency in the onset of the stereotyped behavior (Dresse and Niemegeers, 1961); no explanation for this effect has been suggested.

The stereotyped behavior produced in rodents has been measured by a scoring system (Ernst, 1967). A more objective method of quantitation, consisting of placing the animals in cages with the floor covered by corrugated paper and measuring gnawing by the number of holes made by the animals in the paper, has been devised (Ther and Schramm, 1962). Both techniques have been used to screen drugs for psychotropic activity (Janssen *et al.*, 1965a; Möller-Nielsen *et al.*, 1973).

1. *Neurochemical Mechanism of Stereotyped Behavior*

Ernst (1965, 1967) first indicated that apomorphine produces stereotyped behavior in rats by a direct stimulation of DA receptors located in the neostriatum. The following evidence supports this hypothesis: (1) apomorphine stereotypy is abolished by lesions of the neostriatum (Amsler, 1923); (2) apomorphine and DA elicit stereotyped behavior when placed in the striatum (Ernst and Smelik, 1966); (3) pretreatment with α-methyldopa or α-methyltyrosine, which block the synthesis of brain catecholamines, does not reduce the stereotypies induced by apomorphine in rats, guinea pigs, dogs, and pigeons but prevents those induced by amphetamine (Ernst, 1965); and (4) the DA molecule is present in the apomorphine structure (Ernst, 1965).

Point 3 indicates a fundamental difference between apomorphine and amphetamine and has been considered as evidence that amphetamine acts indirectly by releasing DA whereas apomorphine stimulates DA receptors directly.

Further support for the dopaminergic nature of apomorphine effects is that chlorpromazine and other neuroleptics, which are considered to block central catecholamine receptors, antagonize the stereotyped behavior produced by apomorphine in rats (Janssen *et al.*, 1960), guinea pigs (Srimal and Dhawan, 1970), dogs (Rotrosen *et al.*, 1972a; Nymark, 1972), monkeys (Shintomi and Yamamura, 1975; Meldrum *et al.*, 1975), and pigeons (Deshpande *et al.*, 1961; Burkman, 1961, 1962; Dhawan *et al.*, 1961; Gupta and Dhawan, 1965; Cheng and Long, 1974). Among neuroleptics, the most powerful antagonizers of apomorphine are haloperidol, spiroperidol, and pimozide, which are reported to be pure DA receptor blockers at doses effective in antagonizing the apomorphine syndrome (Janssen *et al.*, 1967, 1968).

Definitive evidence for a direct stimulation by apomorphine of striatal DA receptors comes from the study of apomorphine effects in animals whose striatal DA terminals have been destroyed with 6OH-DA. In intact rats, local application of DA in the caudate of one side produces contralateral turning of the head and of the tail (Ungerstedt *et al.*, 1969). Unilateral lesions of the substantia nigra produce in rats ipsilateral turning shortly after the lesion. By 15 days these asymmetries disappear and the rats' locomotion is apparently normal (Ungerstedt, 1971a).

Systemic administration of apomorphine to rats bearing unilateral nigral lesions produces contralateral turning, indicating a dominance of the lesioned side over the innervated one (Ungerstedt, 1971a). Thus, denervation not only does not abolish apomorphine action but, in fact, potentiates it. These results demonstrate that apomorphine acts directly by stimulating DA receptors and that denervation induces a supersensitivity to its effects. In this model, amphetamine produces ipsilateral turning, indicating that intact DA terminals are essential for the action of amphetamine on the striatum (Ungerstedt, 1971a). These results further stress the basic differences in the mechanism of apomorphine and amphetamine action on DA terminals.

The foregoing findings have been confirmed in mice lesioned by intrastriatal 6OH-DA (von Voigtlander and Moore, 1973a,b; Thronburg and Moore, 1975).

Schoenfeld and Uretsky (1972) reported that pretreatment with 6OH-DA administered intraventricularly facilitates the response of rats to apomorphine, so that the ED_{50} for stimulation is halved.

Curiously, in 6OH-DA-treated rats, apomorphine fails to produce the gnawing syndrome; instead, a combination of increased locomotion and wall-climbing is observed. The repetitive, exaggerated, and uninterrupted character of this modified response to apomorphine indicated its stereotyped nature. This modified response was blocked by low doses of perphenazine. The sensitivity of 6OH-DA-treated rats to apomorphine correlates with the degree of destruction of DA terminals but not of NA terminals (Schoenfeld and Uretsky, 1972).

An increased sensitivity to apomorphine in rats treated with intraventricular 6OH-DA was also found by Jalfre and Haefely (1971). At variance with the findings of Schoenfeld and Uretsky (1972), apomorphine was still able to produce compulsive gnawing in the 6OH-DA-pretreated rats.

Ungerstedt (1971a) found that, in rats with bilateral lesion of the substantia nigra obtained with the local injection of 6OH-DA, apomorphine produced a furious compulsive gnawing far more intense than when the same dose was administered to intact rats.

Recently, Creese and Iversen (1973) found an enhancement of the stereotypy in response to apomorphine in adult rats, to which 6OH-DA had been administered intraventricularly in the neonatal period. In these animals, *d*-amphetamine was no longer able to elicit stereotypy nor locomotor stimulation. These findings were associated with an almost complete destruction of the dopaminergic input to the striatum and to a less complete destruction of the noradrenergic system.

Thus, although there is some disagreement on the characteristics of the stereotypy induced by apomorphine in the 6-OH DA-treated rats, all reports are in agreement on the existence of a supersensitivity to apomorphine.

2. *Pharmacological Interactions*

Various pharmacological treatments are able to modify apomorphine-induced stereotyped behavior.

The effect of reserpine pretreatment on apomorphine-induced stereotypies is controversial. Ther and Shramm (1962), in mice, and Andén *et al.* (1967) and Lal *et al.* (1972a), in rats, reported that reserpine did not affect the action of apomorphine, but Fekete *et al.* (1970) found inhibition in mice. Rotrosen *et al.* (1972b) and Costall and Naylor (1973a) have reexamined this problem and found that reserpine potentiates both the intensity and the duration of the stereotypies produced by apomorphine in rats.

These discrepancies might be due in part to a difference in the time interval between reserpine and apomorphine administration and, in part, to a difference in the method of quantitating stereotypy. Thus, the authors who showed potentiation (Rotrosen *et al.*, 1972b; Costall and Naylor, 1973a) used the scoring system, which allows the measurement of the whole stereotyped syndrome (exploration, sniffing, gnawing, biting), whereas the investigators who showed inhibition (Fekete *et al.*, 1970) used the rating method based on the number of holes gnawed on corrugated paper. In the latter case, decreased motility could have resulted in dissociation between the rating values and the actual gnawing activity.

The mechanism by which reserpine increases apomorphine stereotypy is uncertain. A receptor supersensitivity due to functional denervation produced by reserpine pretreatment might be an explanation, but the fact that the potentiation is evident within 1 hour after reserpine might argue against this mechanism.

The effect of α-MT on the ability of apomorphine to produce gnawing is debated. Although most authors have reported that α-MT pretreatment does not affect the potency of apomorphine in producing stereotyped behavior (Weissman *et al.*, 1966; Ernst, 1967; Jalfre and Haefely, 1971), recently a 40% reduction was obtained after α-MT pretreatment (Srimal and Dhawan, 1970). This effect of α-MT might be related in part to its neurotoxic action since the dose used was the maximal nonlethal dose (Srimal and Dhawan, 1970). In a recent careful study, Costall and Naylor (1973a) have reported potentiation by α-MT pretreatment of apomorphine-stereotypy. The potentiation was almost maximal at 1 hour after α-MT and lasted for at least 48 hours. Interpretation of these findings is difficult and must await confirmation.

Contrasting findings have also been reported in regard to the effects of MAO inhibitors on the stereotyped behavior produced by apomorphine. Thus, Fekete *et al.* (1970), measuring gnawing by the number of holes made on corrugated paper, reported that pretreatment of mice with tranylcypromine or nialamide potentiates the ability of apomorphine to elicit gnawing. On the other hand, Costall and Naylor (1973a) showed that tranylcypromine, in various doses, decreased the potency of apomorphine in eliciting stereotyped behavior in rats. Nialamide, in low doses prolonged, whereas in higher doses protected, from the effects of apomorphine (Costall and Naylor, 1973a). The reason for these discrepancies is unexplained.

Recently, it has been reported that amantadine blocks apomorphine stereotypies (Cox and Tha, 1973). It has been argued that the blockade of apomorphine effects by amantadine is secondary to its weak receptor-agonist properties.

The interaction of narcotic analgesics with apomorphine deserves special consideration because from this interaction much speculation has been derived on the mechanism of narcotic effects on the DA system. Narcotics produce catatonia in the rat (Winter *et al.*, 1954; Poignant *et al.*, 1974a); this effect is correlated to their analgesic potency and is antagonized by nalorphine (Smith *et al.*, 1951). Associated with the catatonic effect of narcotic analgesics and apparently correlated to it is an increase of brain DA synthesis and turnover, which has been measured by various methods (Sasame *et al.*, 1971, 1972; Perez-Cruet *et al.*, 1972; Kuschinsky and Hornykiewicz, 1972; Ahtee and Kaariainen, 1973). Apomorphine effectively antagonizes the catatonia and the increase of DA synthesis induced by narcotics (Sasame *et al.*, 1972; Kuschinsky and Hornykiewicz, 1972; Ahtee and Kaariainen, 1973; Poignant *et al.*, 1974). These findings have been taken as evidence that narcotics block DA receptors in brain and that the increase of DA synthesis is due to a feedback mechanism triggered by DA-receptor blockade (Sasame *et al.*, 1971, 1972; Ahtee and Kaariainen, 1973). This hypothesis, however, has been challenged since no inhibition by morphine has been observed on striatal DA-sensitive adenylate cyclase (Iwatsubo and Clouet, 1975).

The other facet of the interaction between apomorphine and narcotic analgesics involves their ability to influence apomorphine effects. Even if opposite results have been reported (McKenzie and Sadof, 1974; Vedernikov, 1970), most authors agree that morphine and various narcotic analgesics are able to antagonize some apomorphine effects: stereotyped behavior in rats, guinea pigs, and pigeons (Puri *et al.*, 1973; Srimal and Dhawan, 1970; Dhawan *et al.*, 1961) and emesis in dogs (Janssen *et al.*, 1960). This would be further evidence for the proposed blockade of DA receptors by narcotic analgesics.

Recently, another kind of interaction between apomorphine and narcotic analgesics has been reported. Low doses of apomorphine, which are liminal for the induction of stereotyped sniffing, prevent the behavioral stimulation produced by low doses of morphine in rats (Fog, 1970). L-Dopa, in doses that produce sedation, has effects similar to apomorphine (Ayhan and Randrup, 1973). In mice, apomorphine, L-dopa, 2-bromoergocryptine, administered in doses that produce sedation (see Section IV,B), antagonize the hypermotility and the increased DA turnover after morphine (Di Chiara *et al.*, 1977f). These data suggest that morphine hyperactivity in contrast to amphetamine hyperactivity, is related to an increase in impulse flow in DA neurons. From this point of view, morphine hyperactivity resembles that produced by alcohol (Read *et al.*, 1960; Carlsson *et al.*, 1974).

Fenfluramine, an anorectic drug resembling amphetamine in chemical structure, increases the level of HVA in the striatum and reduces motility in rats (Jori *et al.*, 1973). This drug antagonizes apomorphine-induced stereotypy, hypermotility, and hypothermia in rats (Jori *et al.*, 1974a; Grabowska and Michaluk, 1974a). Conversely, apomorphine prevents the increase of striatal HVA produced by fenfluramine (Jori *et al.*, 1974a). These results have been taken to indicate that fenfluramine increases DA turnover in the striatum by blocking DA receptors (Jori *et al.*, 1974a).

A major criticism that applies to most studies on the effects of pharmacological interactions with apomorphine on behavior is that no attempt has been made to ascertain the influence of the various drugs on the distribution and metabolism of apomorphine.

3. *Intracerebral Site of Action*

Amsler (1923) was the first to postulate that the striatum is essential for apomorphine action in rodents; the basis for this statement was the finding that ablation of the striatum abolished the ability of the drug to produce stereotyped behavior. Later Ernst and Smelik (1966) supported this view by showing that apomorphine and dopa could induce stereotypy when implanted in the dorsal part of the caudate nucleus or in the pallidum; negative results were obtained when apomorphine was implanted in the ventral part of the caudate, in the nucleus lateralis septi, in subthalamic structures, and in the substantia nigra (Ernst and Smelik, 1966). In keeping with the findings of Amsler (1923) and of Ernst and Smelik (1966), stereotyped behavior has been obtained after injection of dopamine into the striatum (Fog *et al.*, 1967; Fog and Pakkenberg, 1971; Cools and Van Rossum, 1970).

The effect of electrolytic or mechanical brain lesions on stereotyped behavior has been subjected to a systematic study. The results of these studies are as follows:

1. In contrast with the results of past studies, large lesions of the complex caudate putamen (neostriatum) either increase (Wolfart, 1974) or fail to affect (McKenzie, 1972; Divac, 1972; Costall and Naylor, 1973b) the potency of apomorphine in eliciting stereotypies.
2. Bilateral lesions placed in an area of the lateral hypothalamus that contains the ascending dopaminergic fiber system, lesions of the dopaminergic pathways directed to the mesolimbic areas (Costall and Naylor, 1973b), or lesions of the substantia nigra (Baum *et al.*, 1971; Costall *et al.*, 1972), all abolish or greatly decrease the stereotyped behavior produced by apomorphine.
3. The stereotypy is decreased also by lesions of mesolimbic areas (tuberculum olfactorium, nucleus amygdaloideus centralis and lateralis, nucleus accumbens septi) and of paleostriatal areas (nucleus pallidus) (McKenzie, 1972; Costall and Naylor, 1973b).

Two main conclusions can be drawn from these studies:

1. Mesolimbic and paleostriatal areas would be more important than neostriatal areas for the production of stereotyped behavior by apomorphine. Similar conclusions have been drawn from studies of amphetamine and methylphenidate-induced stereotypy (Costall and Naylor, 1974a,b).
2. Lesions of dopaminergic tracts or nerve cells are as effective as the lesions of the corresponding areas of distribution in abolishing or decreasing apomorphine-induced stereotypy.

This would indicate that apomorphine stereotypy requires the presence of intact dopaminergic terminals. On the basis of these results, we would be forced to revise the long and widely accepted theories on apomorphine action and to postulate that apomorphine produces stereotypy by a presynaptic mechanism. This is, in fact, what Costall *et al.* (1972) suggest with great caution. Even if the latter conclusion is not unreasonable in the context of the experiments performed by Costall *et al.* (1972), it is inconsistent with the large body of evidence supporting the postsynaptic nature of apomorphine stereotypy.

In addition, a most pertinent criticism to the results obtained by physical brain lesions comes from studies utilizing 6OH-DA as a selective means of destroying DA terminals in restricted brain areas. Thus, Price and Fibiger (1974) found in rats that nigral lesions, produced by local 6OH-DA injections, potentiate apomorphine stereotypy but abolish amphetamine stereotypy. These authors suggest that the different results obtained by Costall *et al.* (1972) might be due to unspecificity of the electrolytic lesions. Very recently, Kelly *et al.* (1975) have reported that the injection of 6OH-DA in the nucleus accombens septi potentiates the hypermotility produced by apomorphine but abolishes the amphetamine hypermotility without changing the intensity of the stereotyped behavior produced by both drugs. The injection of 6OH-DA in the caudate nucleus did not affect the locomotor response to the drugs, but it intensified the stereotypy produced by apomorphine and decreased that in response to amphetamine (Kelly *et al.*, 1975).

These results indicate that the locomotor response is localized in the nucleus accumbens septi, and the stereotypy in the caudate.

Lastly, Asher and Agajahian (1974) reported that bilateral 6OH-DA lesions of the DA terminals in the olfactory tubercles and in the nucleus accombens fail to affect amphetamine stereotypy, whereas chemical lesions of the caudate abolished it.

In conclusion, results obtained by destroying DA terminals with 6OH-DA confirm the postsynaptic nature of apomorphine stereotypy and indicate that the nigrostriatal but not the mesolimbic system is the locus of this response. These conclusions are in complete disagreement with studies that employ electrolytic or mechanical lesions. The reason for this discrepancy might be due to (1) incompleteness of the physical lesion, as in the case of the persistence of apomorphine stereotypy after striatal lesions (McKenzie, 1972; Divac, 1972; Costall and Naylor, 1973b) and of amphetamine stereotypy after nigral lesions (Costall *et al.*, 1972); (2) destruction of neuronal systems affecting the behavior or having a facilitatory influence on it, as after lesions of rhinencephalic areas (McKenzie, 1972; Costall and Naylor, 1973b); (3) destruction of nigral non-DA neurons mediating apomorphine-stereotypy (Di Chiara *et al.*, 1977b).

Recently, Costall *et al.* (1975a) have attempted to differentiate both pharmacologically and anatomically two components of stereotypy: sniffing and repetitive head and limb movements (low-intensity component) and biting, gnawing, and licking (high-intensity component). The authors reported that the low-intensity stereotyped behavior occurs with low doses whereas the high-intensity stereotyped behavior is elicited by higher doses of apomorphine; NPA is reported to be weakly potent in producing low-intensity stereotyped behavior. Biting is claimed to be the predominant effect of NPA. Pretreatment with amantadine abolished the high-intensity stereotyped behavior of apomorphine, whereas reserpine or α-MT pretreatment removed the low-intensity one.

After ablation experiments, Costall *et al.* (1975a) concluded that the tuberculum olfactorium and the nucleus accumbens are responsible for the low-intensity stereotyped behavior, whereas the substantia nigra and the central nucleus of the amygdala are the effectors of the high-intensity stereotyped behavior. According to this distinction, it would seem that the current method of scoring the stereotypy would have to be rejected since it is based on the assumption that stereotyped behavior is a continuum in a response of increasing intensity from sniffing to gnawing and biting. On the contrary, the latter interpretation might provide the simplest explanation for the results of Costall *et al.* (1975a). Accordingly, the abolition of biting by amantadine can be due to a reduced response to apomorphine, whereas the abolition of sniffing after reserpine or α-MT pretreatment might simply indicate an increased response with the consequent emergence of gnawing. An analogous explanation can be given for the differential effects of apomorphine as compared to its more potent analog NPA.

Thus, a more detailed dose–response study with low doses of NPA seems to be necessary to conclude that NPA is, indeed, specific for producing the high-intensity components of the stereotyped syndrome.

4. *Drug-Induced Stereotyped Behavior in the Human*

Apomorphine, given in threshold emetic doses, has not been described yet to produce behavioral changes in man resembling the stereotypies observed in the animal. Due to the emetic potency of apomorphine, higher doses of the drug have not been administered. Blockade of the emetic properties of apomorphine would, if specific, open the way to the study of the effects of apomorphine on human behavior. Since apomorphine seems to be the more powerful stimulant of central DA receptors, the study of its effects on human behavior might greatly contribute to the knowledge of the role of DA in human psychology and psychopathology.

On the other hand, stereotyped behavior has been observed in man after administration of high doses of amphetamine and also in "tardive dyskinesia," which develops in patients after long treatment with neuroleptics.

Amphetamine has been described to induce a form of psychosis characterized by paranoid ideation with well-formed delusions, sexual excess, and hallucinations (Connell, 1958; Griffith *et al.*, 1970; Angrist and Gershon, 1970). A recently emphasized symptom of amphetamine psychosis is a stereotyped compulsive behavior (Ellinwood, 1967). Patients analyze details in a repetitive manner; they have a compulsion to take objects apart, to sort, and, sometimes, to put them back together ("punding") (Rylander, 1969). The repetitive and purposeless character of this behavior indicates its stereotyped nature. Moreover, an exquisitely motor stereotypy has also been described in amphetamine psychosis, which is strikingly similar to that induced by apomorphine in animals. Patients pace back and forth and move their mouth from side to side in a stereotyped grimacing fashion. Ellinwood (1967) has reported that the stereotyped behavior appears to be invariably concomitant to the psychosis, since stereotyped behavior does not occur in amphetamine addicts who have not developed psychosis.

Indirect evidence for a dopaminergic mediation of amphetamine psychosis in man derives from the comparison of the relative potency of the *d*- and *l*-isomers of amphetamine in eliciting psychosis in man (Angrist *et al.*, 1971). In this study, the *l*-isomer, in spite of its ineffectiveness in producing central stimulation, showed a potency comparable to the *d*-isomer in the induction of psychosis. Thus, in these studies, *d*- and *l*-amphetamine were much more similar in their ability to elicit psychosis than to produce central stimulation. The *d*- and *l*-forms of amphetamine have similar potency in inhibiting the uptake of DA-^{3}H by brain synaptosomes and in eliciting stereotypy in animals. However, the *d*-isomer is 10 times more potent than the *l*-isomer in inhibiting the uptake of NA-^{3}H and in stimulating motility in animals (Taylor and Snyder, 1970); On this basis, it has been concluded that the psychosis-eliciting properties of amphetamine are correlated to its dopaminergic activity, whereas its behavior stimulating properties depend on the activation of central noradrenergic systems (Angrist *et al.*, 1971).

Tardive dyskinesia develops during prolonged treatment with neuroleptic drugs a few days after reduction in the dosage or after a discontinuation of the drug. It is characterized by involuntary rythmic movements of various appearance and localization but more commonly centered around the mouth (oral dyskinesia or buccolingual-masticatory syndrome). The syndrome consists of chewing movements, rhythmic opening of the mouth and protrusion of the tongue, stereotyped movements of the lips and rumination. The movements are intensified by stress and by the movements of other muscles; they are reduced by the voluntary movement of the affected muscles or during sleep (Ayd, 1967; Crane, 1968, 1973; Klawans, 1973).

Various treatments that decrease the activity of the dopaminergic system ameliorate the syndrome; drugs falling into this category include α-MT, reserpine and α-methyldopa, tetrabenazine, and haloperidol (Gerlach *et al.*, 1974; Kazamatsuri *et al.*, 1972a,b). Worsening of the syndrome is caused by treatments that produce a central dopaminergic stimulation, such as L-dopa alone or in combination with a peripherally acting decarboxylase inhibitor (Klawans and McKendall, 1971). On the basis of these pharmacological results, it is suggested that overstimulation of dopamine receptors could be the cause of tardive dyskinesia.

Chronic treatment of experimental animals with neuroleptics produces an increased sensitivity to various effects of DA-receptor agonists. Schelkunov (1967) showed an increase in the duration of amphetamine and apomorphine stereotypies during chronic treatment with perphenazine. This effect was also present 20–72 hours, as well as 14–19 days, after withdrawal of the drug. These results have been confirmed and extended by various investigators (Tarsy and Baldessarini, 1973, 1974; Christensen and Möller-Nielsen, 1974; Gianustos *et al.*, 1974). Chronic treatment with neuroleptics also results in increased sensitivity to the inhibitory effect of apomorphine on DA turnover and on the firing of caudate neurons (Gianustos *et al.*, 1975; Yarbrough, 1975). These findings could be applied to explain the development of tardive dyskinesia as due to supersensitivity of DA receptors secondary to chronic blockade by DA receptor antagonists (neuroleptics).

B. Motility

Apomorphine produces hypermotility in rats (Maj *et al.*, 1972a, 1973) and in mice (Andén *et al.*, 1973). Decreased motility after very low or very high doses of apomorphine has also been described (Puech *et al.*, 1974).

Presynaptic inhibition of DA synthesis and release has been postulated to be the cause of the sedation and hypomotility produced by the low doses of apomorphine (Carlsson, 1975a; Strömbom, 1976) (see Section VIII,A). Inhibition of locomotor activity due to paroxismal gnawing and biting in a restricted area is probably the cause of the hypomotility occurring when high doses are administered (Creese and Iversen, 1973).

The effect of apomorphine on motility in mice has been correlated to ambient temperature (Maj *et al.*, 1972b). Thus, apomorphine depressed the motility of mice kept at 22°C, whereas it stimulated mice kept at 36°C. However, the lowest dose of apomorphine used in this study (0.05 mg/kg) still caused hypomotility at 36°C.

Neurochemical Mechanisms

The mechanism of apomorphine-induced hypermotility has been recently studied by Maj and his colleagues (1972a, 1973; Grabowska *et al.*, 1973a). Pretreatment with neuroleptics blocked apomorphine-induced hypermotility and stereotypy in rats. Pretreatment with reserpine + α-MT, which inhibit catecholamine storage and synthesis, and with diethyldithiocarbamate, which inhibits NA synthesis, and with diethyldithiocarbamate, which inhibits NA synthesis by blocking dopamine-β-hydroxylase, partly abolished the ability of apomorphine to increase motility but not to induce stereotyped behavior. Since phenoxybenzamine, a blocker of α-adrenergic receptors, is also able to diminish the hypermotility but not the stereotypy produced by apomorphine, it has been postulated that an indirect stimulation of the noradrenergic system plays a role in apomorphine-induced hypermotility.

Since blockade of the catecholamine synthesis with intact stores, as can be produced soon after treatment with α-MT, does not modify the effect of apomorphine but blocks that of amphetamine, Maj *et al.* (1972a) exclude that an amphetamine-like effect on NA terminals is the mechanism by which apomorphine exerts its effect on motility.

An alternative explanation for these findings could be that the activation of the NA system is a feedback response to the stimulation of DA receptors by apomorphine. In fact, there are indications that apomorphine stimulates central NA activity and turnover (Persson and Waldeck, 1970a,b). However, the relevance of central NA activity for the induction of hypermotility by apomorphine remains an open question, since the mechanism by which the pretreatments influence the apomorphine-induced hyperactivity could be unrelated to their effect on the central NA system but simply due to the neurotoxicity of the pretreatments used to inhibit NA synthesis.

Very recently, Kelly *et al.* (1975) have found that selective depletion of DA in the nucleus accombens, after local injection of 6OH-DA in rats pretreated with desmethylimipramine, potentiated the hypermotility produced by apomorphine but abolished that of amphetamine. In addition, Roberts *et al.* (1975) have shown that the depletion of up to 95% of brain NA does not affect the hypermotility induced by *d*-amphetamine. These results, although confirming the critical role played by mesolimbic DA in motility (Pijnenburg and Van Rossum, 1973), tend to exclude the involvement of NA.

An inhibitory influence of 5-HT on apomorphine-induced hypermotility in rats has been recently postulated (see Section VIII,C).

C. Sexual Behavior

The interest in the effects of apomorphine on sexual behavior originates mainly from the consideration that results of such studies might help to understand the role of endogenous DA in the regulation of this behavior.

The results of the experiments with apomorphine support the view that brain DA stimulates copulatory behavior in male animals.

The intraperitoneal injection of 0.5 mg/kg of apomorphine to sexually sluggish male rats was found to increase significantly the percentage of animals displaying mountings, penile intromission, and ejaculations. On the other hand, 5 mg/kg of the compound produced a marked stereotyped behavior, which prevented the occurrence of other goal-directed behaviors, including the copulatory one. The stimulant effect of apomorphine on copulatory behavior was prevented by haloperidol. Moreover, doses of this drug that did not produce other overt behavioral changes, suppressed the spontaneous copulatory behavior of rats with a high basal level of sexual activity (Tagliamonte *et al.*, 1974a,b).

Analogous results were obtained by Malmnäs (1973) in castrated rats treated with suboptimal doses of testosterone. In these animals, intraperitoneal doses of apomorphine ranging from 30 to 100 μg/kg increased the percentage of subjects that displayed mounts and intromissions. These effects were prevented by 100 μg/kg of pimozide, a dose that did not produce other overt behavioral changes.

Finally, apomorphine was found to prevent tetrabenazine-induced suppression of copulatory behavior in male rats (Bütcher *et al.*, 1969). No published data are available on the effect of apomorphine on the copulatory pattern of normal rats, nor on the effect of apomorphine on the copulatory behavior of other animal species.

In female rats, lordosis behavior (sexual receptivity) is dependent on ovarian hormones. Ovariectomy abolishes this behavior, which is restored by the administration of estrogen followed by progesterone. Progesterone administration might be replaced by different treatments that deplete either brain 5-HT (such as *p*-chlorophenylalanine) or brain DA (such as α-MT) or both (such as tetrabenazine or reserpine) (Meyerson, 1964a,b; Meyerson and Lewander, 1970; Ahlenius *et al.*,

1971). These results suggest that both brain 5-HT and DA play an inhibitory role on the lordosis behavior in female rats. Consistently, pimozide, a potent DA-receptor blocker, significantly increased the sexual receptivity of estrogen-treated ovariectomized female rats, whereas ET-495 (a DA-receptor-stimulating agent) lowered estrogen–progesterone-induced receptivity (Everitt *et al.*, 1974).

In contrast with the preceding conclusion are the recent results of Hamburger-Bar and Rigter (1975), showing that the subcutaneous injection of apomorphine in a dose of 0.25 mg/kg facilitated the lordosis behavior of spayed female rats primed with estrogen or estrogen + progesterone. Interestingly, this facilitatory action was demonstrable even 48 hours after apomorphine administration. The effect of apomorphine was dependent on estrogen but was not prevented by adrenalectomy (thus, it was not mediated by adrenal progesterone release). The mechanism of this long-lasting facilitating effect of apomorphine is not clear. The possibility that it is related to some hormonal release might be considered. Indeed, the injection of DA in the third ventricle has been shown to release LH-RH (Kamberi *et al.*, 1971), and this peptide is able to facilitate the lordosis behavior in spayed rats primed with estrogen (Pfaff, 1973; Moss and McCann, 1973).

D. Aggressive Behavior

Apomorphine has been reported to produce "bizzare social behavior" in rats, consisting of "wrestling" postures not accompanied by fighting ("mock fighting") (Van Rossum, 1970). This behavior has been described also after administration of amphetamine (Evetts *et al.*, 1970) or after L-dopa with a peripherally acting decarboxylase inhibitor (Lammers and Van Rossum, 1968).

Apomorphine is also able to induce vigorous fighting in rats (Senault, 1970; McKenzie, 1971). The characteristics of this behavior have been described and its pharmacology and brain localization investigated.

According to Senault (1970), apomorphine, at the optimal dose of 1 mg/kg i.v., produces aggressive behavior in 37% of male Wistar rats housed in couples in metal cages and submitted to the sound of an electric bell.

Strain, age, and sex of the rats are critical for maximal effect since lower percentages of aggressive animals were obtained when Holtzman or Long-Evans females or young rats were used instead of Wistar, male, adult rats. Sensory or painful stimulation (sound or pinching of the tail) exerts a facilitating action on the elicitation of the behavior (Senault, 1970; McKenzie, 1971).

The duration of the aggressive episodes among the rat population has a bimodal distribution. On this basis rats can be divided into two groups: those in which the aggressive episodes have a mean duration of less than 5 minutes and those with a mean duration of more than 50 minutes (Senault, 1970). In the first group ("weak fighters") the aggressive behavior consist mainly of wrestling postures with rare fighting. In the second group ("strong fighters"), the aggressive episodes are violent and result in wounds and sometimes in fatalities.

In the apomorphine-induced aggressive behavior, as in the spontaneous one, a hierarchy is quickly established; if two dominant rats are placed togehter, a hierarchy is reestablished and fighting continues (McKenzie, 1971).

Apomorphine-induced aggressive behavior appears to be sharply distinct from the aggressiveness induced by septal lesions or by bulbectomy and from mouse-killing behavior.

Thus, rats made aggressive by apomorphine do not attack inanimate objects nor a mouse presented to them (Senault, 1970). Aggression instead is strictly directed toward a member of the same species and, most important, follows the same ritual that regulates spontaneous intraspecific aggression. Thus, the assumption of submissive postures by one of the rats has an inhibiting influence on the continuation of the attack by the other rat (McKenzie, 1971). In addition, rearing in isolation or treatment with testosterone increase the ability of apomorphine to produce aggressive behavior (Senault, 1971, 1972).

Apomorphine-induced aggression appears to be a directed, nonstereotyped behavior produced by doses of apomorphine that are able themselves to induce stereotyped gnawing. However, gnawing is not present during the attacks but only in the intervals between them (Senault, 1970). This is an example of the possibility that the stereotyped gnawing produced by apomorphine is abolished by the emergence of another kind of behavior. A similar observation has been made for the stereotyped pecking produced by apomorphine in pigeons: sensory stimuli are able to divert the animals from the stereotyped behavior (Koster, 1957).

1. *Pharmacological Interactions*

Senault (1970, 1974) and McKenzie (1971) have studied the effect of various drugs on the aggressive behavior induced by apomorphine.

Low doses of neuroleptics are able to prevent the induction of aggressive behavior by apomorphine (Senault, 1974). Among a series of six neuroleptics, their ability to block aggression was roughly correlated to their potency as DA-receptor antagonists, as measured by their activity as blockers of amphetamine and apomorphine-induced stereotypies. However, many inconsistencies are evident if one wants to correlate the antistereotypy to the antiaggressive activity of neuroleptics. Thus, haloperidol, although having a potency similar to that of pimozide in blocking apomorphine-induced stereotypies, is 10 times more potent than pimozide in blocking the aggressive behavior induced by apomorphine. Conversely, pimozide, which is 800 times more potent than thioridazine in blocking stereotyped behavior, is, on the other hand, only 8 times more potent than thioridazine in antagonizing the aggressive behavior induced by apomorphine (Senault, 1974). These discrepancies between antistereotypy and antiaggression potency of neuroleptics might be explained by the existence of different DA receptors responsible for the aggressive and the stereotyped behavior.

Another possibility is that the antiaggressive activity of the neuroleptics results from some other action of the neuroleptics that is additive to the blockade of DA receptors. Relevant to this possibility is the ability of phenoxybenzamine, an α-adrenergic-blocking agent, to inhibit completely the induction of aggressive behavior induced by apomorphine (Senault, 1974). This finding is interesting since phenoxybenzamine does not affect the stereotypies produced by apomorphine.

On the basis of these results it might be postulated than an intact central noradrenergic function is essential for apomorphine to induce aggressive behavior (Senault, 1974). The involvment of noradrenergic activity in the aggressive behavior produced by apomorphine is also indicated by the fact that clonidine, a central NA-receptor stimulant, is able in association with apomorphine, to induce aggression in rats that did not become aggressive with apomorphine alone (Senault, 1974).

Reserpine pretreatment did not decrease the ability of apomorphine to induce aggressive behavior in sensitive rats but, instead, made apomorphine capable of producing aggressive behavior in rats that were resistant to apomorphine alone (Senault, 1974; McKenzie, 1971).

Also MAO inhibitors potentiate the action of apomorphine on aggressive behavior. This has been taken as a further demonstration that stimulation of the central NA system plays a permissive role in the elicitation of aggressiveness by apomorphine (Senault, 1974).

2. *Site of Action in Brain*

Senault (1973) has reported that, olfactory bulb ablation and lesions of the anterior part of the striatum facilitate the production of aggressive behavior by apomorphine. Lesions of the amygdala and of the substantia nigra had an inhibitory effect; septal lesions increased the duration of the attacks but did not render aggressive rats that did not respond to apomorphine prior to the lesion (Senault, 1973).

Interestingly, the same lesions affect in a similar way other forms of aggressiveness. Thus, septal and olfactory bulb lesions produce aggressive behavior (Brady and Nauta, 1953; Kumadaki *et al.*, 1967). Conversely, lesions of the amygdala are known to exert a taming effect on spontaneous and induced aggressive behavior (King and Meyer, 1958; Allikmetes and Ditrikh, 1965; Karli, 1955).

Lesions that depress the aggressive behavior produced by apomorphine (amygdala, substantia nigra) have been reported either to decrease or to potentiate the gnawing syndrome (Costall and Naylor, 1973b; Ungerstedt, 1971a). Thus, no correlation exists between the ability of apomorphine to elicit aggressive behavior and to induce stereotyped gnawing.

E. Operant Behavior

The effect of apomorphine on operant behavior is debated. Weissman (1966) showed that apomorphine decreased the rate of responding in 4 out of 5 pigeons previously trained to peck under a differential reinforcement of low-rate schedule of food presentation. Only in 1 pigeon apomorphine administration resulted in very high and constant rates of responding. Low or high rates of responding after apomorphine might simply depend on the chance that the pigeons would direct their stereotyped pecking on the floor or on the key, respectively.

Bütcher (1968) also observed an unpredictable effect of apomorphine on free-operant avoidance in rats. Some animals showed an increase in lever-pressing rate, accompanied by a decrease in shock frequency. The opposite effect was observed in the remaining animals. Apomorphine elicited stereotyped behavior in all the rats tested. Rats that failed to press the lever gnawed primarily on the grid floor, despite the repeated presentation of shock. By contrast, in rats displaying an increased rate of responding, the stereotyped gnawing was directed toward the lever.

At variance with these studies, apomorphine consistently decreased the rate of lever pressing by rats trained on a fixed-interval schedule of water presentation. In addition, apomorphine did not increase response rates in rats treated chronically with reserpine (De Oliveira and Graeff, 1972). By contrast, apomorphine increased the rate of responding in a free-operant avoidance situation, in rats administered tetrabenazine (Bütcher and Andén, 1969).

Recently, two studies report a consistent stimulation of operant behavior by apomorphine. Baxter *et al.* (1974) reported that rats with jugular cannulas, self-administer apomorphine at doses ranging from 0.129 to 1 mg/kg/injection. The acquisition of the self-injection behavior follows a typical learning curve; intervals between injections are timed precisely by the rat and the day-to-day intake is constant; large doses produce lower rates of responding. On this basis, the authors conclude that apomorphine maintains self-injection behavior by a reenforcing action rather than by nonspecific stimulation. Pimozide administration disrupts the regular pattern of apomorphine self-injection and, at higher doses, blocks it. It is an open question if pimozide disrupts the self-injection behavior of apomorphine by blocking the action of apomorphine in brain or by interfering with the neurochemical substrate of operant behavior. Thus, the hypothesis suggested by these results (i.e., "stimulation of brain DA receptors is rewarding") is extremely encouraging, but still to be proven.

Terada and Masur (1973) report that apomorphine and amphetamine stimulate the behavior of rats submitted to a competitive situation to obtain food in a straight runway. The effect of neuroleptics on the stimulation produced by apomorphine is difficult to ascertain because these drugs disrupt the competitive behavior of several rats and fail to block the increase of victories in the remaining animals at doses effective in preventing stereotypies. The response of this behavior to neuroleptics resembles that of the aggressive behavior produced by apomorphine. Taking into consideration the competitive nature of the behavior tested, it is quite possible that apomorphine increases the number of victories because it stimulates aggressiveness and not goal-directed behavior.

F. Self-Stimulation

The effect of apomorphine on self-stimulation behavior has been studied by Broekkamp and Van Rossum (1974) in rats implanted in various brain areas. Apomorphine consistently facilitated self-stimulation in a number of rats but inhibited it in others. The effect of the drug was highly reproducible for individual animals. However, no relationship was found to the brain areas in which the electrode was implanted. Most important, once self-stimulation was initiated, it continued even if the rewarding current was reduced to zero, its duration being dependent solely on the duration of drug action.

In another study, apomorphine was found to produce in rats a facilitation of self-stimulation at low doses and depression at high doses (Wauquier and Niemegeers, 1973). In agreement with these results, apomorphine has been reported first to depress and then to stimulate the response in rats pretreated with α-MT, which by itself depresses self-stimulation; apomorphine administered to normal rats depressed the responding irrespective of the dose (St. Laurent *et al.*, 1973).

Apomorphine decreased self-stimulation at normal current. Doubling of the stimulation current produced greater than normal rates of lever pressing at 0.75 mg/kg, but no increase was observed at 1.5 mg/kg (Liebman and Butcher, 1973).

These results have been taken to indicate that the DA system is critically involved in electrical self-stimulation of the brain and in reward.

In order to explain apomorphine effects on behavior, various workers have suggested that the depressive effect of apomorphine on operant behavior is due to an induction of competing stereotyped behaviors (Weissman, 1966; Bütcher, 1968). Carlsson (1972), on the basis of the finding that apomorphine stimulates exploration, suggests that this view might be only partially correct: at high doses, apomorphine would produce an increased and persistent reactivity to many types of stimuli, making the necessary focus on the goal stimulus less probable; at low doses, the stimulation of exploration produced by apomorphine would facilitate operant behavior.

G. Feeding

The fact that the anorexigenic response to *d*-amphetamine is prevented by α-MT has led to the conclusion that this effect is mediated by the release of endogenous catecholamines (Weissman *et al.*, 1966; Holtzmann and Jewett, 1971; Baez, 1974). However, in recent years it has been suggested that brain DA is the catecholamine mediating the amphetamine effect and not NA, as previously considered. Among the arguments in support of such a hypothesis are the following:

1. Doses of *d*-amphetamine effective in producing anorexia are also effective in stimulating brain DA turnover but not that of NA (Costa and Groppetti, 1970; Costa *et al.*, 1972; Groppetti *et al.*, 1972).
2. The anorexigenic effect of *d*-amphetamine is prevented by pimozide, at doses that selectively block DA receptors (Barzaghi *et al.*, 1973).
3. *d*-Amphetamine is only twice as potent as *l*-amphetamine in inhibiting food intake (Baez, 1974), a ratio of potency similar to the ratio of the potency of the two isomers in blocking DA uptake; *d*-amphetamine instead is 10 times more potent than the *l*-isomer in blocking NA uptake in brain slices (Taylor and Snyder, 1970).

4. Finally, apomorphine has been found to be 3 times as potent as *d*-amphetamine in inhibiting food intake in rats, a species in which apomorphine produces no emetic response (Barzaghi *et al.*, 1973). In fact, in fasted rats, 0.25 mg/kg of apomorphine reduced food intake by 50% during the first hour of access to food. The anorexigenic effect of apomorphine, as well as that of *d*-amphetamine, was prevented by pimozide (0.5 mg/kg), which per se did not affect food intake.

Because of the foregoing considerations, DA has gained the reputation of playing a major role in controlling feeding behavior. This conclusion is in apparent contrast with the results of Ungerstedt, who observed long-lasting aphagia and adipsia after bilateral complete degeneration of the nigrostriatal DA pathway, obtained either by electrocoagulation or by intracerebral injection of 6OH-DA (Ungerstedt, 1971b).

Obviously, the question that arises is, Does DA stimulate food intake or inhibit it? A possible source of confusion in this area is that of equating aphagia with lack of appetite. Indeed, Ungerstedt (1971b) has suggested that aphagia in lesioned rats originated from their inability to initiate any activity including eating: these animals may not be anorectic but might lack the drive or the ability to perform such activity. Consistently, the administration of apomorphine to these animals induced gnawing but did not restore eating behavior.

In conclusion, striatal DA seems to be essential for initiating or maintaining mastication (a repetitive movement), whereas nonstriatal DA (or NA) might have an inhibitory role in appetite control. A more detailed discussion on this matter is beyond the scope of this review.

V. Neuropharmacological Effects of Apomorphine

A. Sympathetic Nervous System

1. *Effects on Sympathetic Responses*

Whitnack *et al.* (1970, 1971) and Whitsett *et al.* (1970a,b) were the first to report, at the same session of the 1970 Federation Meeting, that L-dopa attenuates postganglionic sympathetic nerve function in dogs and cats, thus providing an explanation for the postural hypotension commonly observed in patients undergoing L-dopa therapy.

More recently, DA and DA-receptor agonists, such as apomorphine and M-7 have been shown to be potent inhibitors of reflex or electrically induced responses of the sympathetic nervous system (Long *et al.*, 1975).

In anesthetized dogs and cats, M-7 reduces resting heart rate, inhibits the pressor response and the increased heart rate produced by bilateral carotid occlusion or by stimulation of the central stumps of the vagi or of the sciatic nerve. This drug also blocked both *in vivo* and *in vitro* the positive chronotropic response resulting from electrical stimulation of the postganglionic right cardioaccelerator nerve. Maximal blockade by M-7 was obtained with a frequency of stimulation of 2Hz; responses to higher frequencies were not antagonized. Dopamine had qualitatively similar effects on sympathetic responses, but they were of lower magnitude than after apomorphine or M-7; pretreatment with cocaine was needed to obtain maximal inhibition of sympathetic responses by DA (Long *et al.*, 1975; Ilhan *et al.*, 1975).

The following characteristics of the action of DA and its analogs indicate that it is mediated by specific DA receptors: (1) sympathetic inhibition is obtained at low doses *in vivo* (5 mg/kg of M-7 and 10 mg/kg of apomorphine) and at low concentrations *in vitro* (2×10^{-8} M M-7 produces 50% blockade of atrial chronotropic responses); (2) the potency of M-7 and apomorphine in producing sympathetic blockade closely parallels their emetic activity since for both effects the activity ratio of M-7 and apomorphine is about 10; and (3) DA-receptor blockers (haloperidol, chlorpromazine, bulbocapnine) are potent antagonists of the sympathetic blockade by M-7 and apomorphine and their rank order of potency is the same as for antiemetic activity (Long *et al.*, 1975; Ilhan *et al.*, 1975).

Since cocaine, which prevents DA uptake, potentiates its sympathetic blocking effects, the DA receptors involved in this action seem to be located on the outer side of the membrane of the adrenergic nerve terminal.

In this action, DA agonists closely resemble clonidine, which also inhibits cardioaccelerator responses to low-frequency (2 Hz) but not to high-freauency stimulation (Armstrong and Boura, 1973; Scriabine and Stavorski, 1973).

Effects of DA agonists and clonidine (Starke and Altmann, 1973) on peripheral sympathetic transmission can be related to two separate sets of inhibitory receptors recently identified on presynaptic adrenergic terminals: DA receptors and α-adrenergic recerpors, respectively.

2. *Presynaptic DA Receptors*

The entire field of catecholamine research has undergone a major development with the discovery of a fine, simple, and efficient mechanism by which NA regulates its own release. The biophysical substrate for this regulation is a population of presynaptic α-adrenergic receptors whose stimulation inhibits the release of transmitter (Langer *et al.*, 1971; Farnebo and Hamberger, 1971a; Starke, 1971). The efficiency of this mechanism is such that its blockade by phenoxybenzamine results in a ten- to twenty-fold increase of NA release.

The steps that have lead to this discovery are a paradigmatic example of a basic research on the mechanism of action of a drug (phenoxybenzamine) which resulted in a major advance in the field of neurophysiology (Langer, 1974).

The concept of presynaptic regulation was soon transferred from the peripheral to the central nervous system, seeming perfectly tailored to explain the inhibitory action exerted by NA- and DA-receptor stimulants on impulse flow and transmitter synthesis (see Section VIII,A).

Direct evidence has been given for the existence of presynaptic DA receptors on postganglionic noradrenergic terminals, which exert an inhibitory influence on NA release (Enero and Langer, 1975; McCulloch *et al.*, 1973). These receptors are quite distinct from the α-adrenergic ones. In spite of the high affinity of DA and of apomorphine for them, these receptors do not normally participate in the regulation of NA release because the amounts of DA released from sympathetic terminals are insufficient to stimulate them (Enero and Langer, 1975). Yet, the inhibition of sympathetic chronotropic heart responses by L-dopa, DA, and its agonists can be fully explained in terms of stimulation of presynaptic DA receptors, as characterized by Langer in cat's nictitating membrane and spleen (Langer, 1973).

B. Thermoregulation

Lapin and Samsonova (1968) and Schelkunov (1971) reported that apomorphine elicits hypothermia when administered systemically to mice.

This effect of apomorphine has been confirmed and its mechanism studied (Barnett *et al.*, 1972; Kruk and Brittain, 1972; Kruk, 1972; Fuxe and Sjöqvist, 1972). Dopamine-receptor blocking agents such as spiroperidol, pimozide, and haloperidol, given in doses that do not affect body temperature, are able to antagonize competitively the hypothermia produced by apomorphine. The blockade of the hypothermia is apparently related to the potency of the neuroleptics as blockers of DA receptors and not of adrenergic receptors. Thus, chlorpromazine and thioridazine, which are poor DA-receptor blockers but of similar potency to NA-receptor blockers in comparison to spiroperidol and haloperidol, are 10–20 times less potent than the latter drugs in antagonizing apomorphine-induced hypothermia. Phenoxybenzamine and other α-adrenergic blocking agents have been reported to have no effect on apomorphine-induced hypothermia (Barnett *et al.*, 1972; Fuxe and Sjöqvist, 1972). On this basis, apomorphine-induced hypothermia has been indicated to be secondary to stimulation of DA receptors.

Since hypothermia has also been obtained after intraventricular injection of apomorphine and since pimozide antagonizes this hypothermia, it has been concluded that the hypothermia produced by apomorphine is secondary to the stimulation of central DA receptors (Kruk and Brittain, 1972; Kruk, 1972).

In a more general context, this action of apomorphine has been taken as evidence for a role of DA in thermoregulation. In fact, this view is supported by a large body of evidence gained in several species and under a variety of experimental conditions. Thus, L-dopa, which increases DA levels in brain, causes a fall in core temperature in the mouse (Yehuda and Wurtman, 1972).

In rats, 6OH-DA, administered intraventricularly, produces a fall in core temperature; this hypothermia is prevented by a pretreatment with 6OH-DA plus imipramine, which destroys specifically brain DA terminals without affecting NA terminals (Breese *et al.*, 1972). On this basis, the hypothermia produced by 6OH-DA is interpreted as secondary to a release of DA.

Systemic administration of *d*-amphetamine produces hyperthermia in rats kept at room temperature (20°C) and hypothermia in rats kept in a cold environment (Yehuda and Wurtman, 1972). The amphetamine-induced hyperthermia appears to be due to a peripheral or central NA release; conversely, the hypothermia seems to be the result of a central release of DA. Consistently, pimozide and haloperidol are potent antagonizers of the hypothermia (Yehuda and Wurtman, 1972). In addition, the relative potency of the *d*- and *l*-forms in producing hypothermia are better correlated to the dopaminergic than to the noradrenergic activity. Amphetamine also produces hypothermia when administered intraventricularly to rats kept at room temperature (20°C) (Yehuda and Wurtman, 1972). Tolerance develops in rats to the hypothermic effects of apomorphine, amphetamine, and ET-495 (Chiel *et al.*, 1974).

Involvement of other amines in the hypothermia produced by apomorphine, although postulated, in unclear. Thus, Grabowska *et al.* (1973b) have proposed that the hypothermia is secondary to the activation of 5-HT synthesis by apomorphine. The basis for this hypothesis is that

LSD-25 and pimozide prevent both the hypothermia and the increase in 5-HT synthesis. However, blockade of 5-HT synthesis and lowering of 5-HT levels by *p*-chlorophenylalanine failed to affect the ability of apomorphine to produce hypothermia.

In contrast to its hypothermic effects in rats and mice, intravenous or intraventricular administration of apomorphine to rabbits elicits an increase in body temperature; this hyperthermia is dose-dependent and antagonized by pimozide and haloperidol (Hill and Horita, 1972; Quock *et al.*, 1975). The hyperthermic response to apomorphine is abolished by pretreatment with *p*-chlorophenylalanine; administration of 5-hydroxytryptophan with a decarboxilase inhibitor regenerates the brain 5-HT stores and restores in part the hyperthermic response to apomorphine (Quock and Horita, 1974). On the basis of these results, it has been suggested that apomorphine produces hyperthermia in rabbits by stimulation of DA receptors and by secondary activation of serotoninergic mechanisms in brain (Quock and Horita, 1974).

VI. Cardiovascular Effects of Apomorphine

A. Blood Pressure

In 1942, Holtz and Credner clearly differentiated the cardiovascular effect of DA from that of NA. Dopamine, in contrast to NA, decreased the blood pressure of the guinea pig and rabbit and only in very high doses had a pressor effect in these species. Since then, extensive investigation has been performed on the vasodepressor effects of DA, which led to the discovery of its vasodilatatory action on the renal, celiac, and mesenteric vascular beds (Goldberg, 1972).

At the present time, there are only three papers giving detailed studies on the cardiovascular effects of apomorphine.

Apomorphine causes hypotension in various animal species. Since the first report by Krayer (1926), 45 years elasped before the mechanism of this effect of apomorphine was subjected to study. In 1971, Barnett and Fiore observed that apomorphine lowered blood pressure in the anesthetized cat. Since this effect was antagonized by haloperidol and abolished by spinal transection, they concluded that the hypotensive effect of apomorphine was due to stimulation of DA receptors within the CNS.

An alternative interpretation of these findings (e.g., Grabowska, 1974b) (see in the following) is that apomorphine lowers blood pressure by an action on presynaptic receptors in the peripheral nerve terminals;

however, hypotension takes place only in the presence of a normal sympathetic tone.

Contrasting conclusions were reached by Finch and Hausler (1973) who studied the cardiovascular effect of apomorphine in the anesthetized rat. In urethan but not in pentobarbitone-anesthetized rats, apomorphine, in low doses (0.1 mg/kg) produced a hypotensive effect and, at higher-dose levels (0.5–1 mg/kg), also a marked bradicardia. Since atropine pretreatment or bilateral vagotomy abolished the hypotensive effect of apomorphine, this was considered to be secondary to an increased efferent vagal discharge: recording of vagal activity showed increased frequency and amplitude. In contrast with the results of Barnett and Fiore (1971), neither haloperidol nor spiroperidol antagonized the hypotensive effect of apomorphine. Thus, the hypotensive effect of apomorphine in the rat appears unrelated to stimulation of DA receptors.

However, this conclusion is not supported by the study of Grabowska (1974b) on ether- or urethan-anesthetized rats. In this study, apomorphine produced a dose-dependent hypotension in doses as low as 0.001 mg/kg i.v.; maximal effect was obtained with 1 mg/kg. In contrast with Finch and Hausler (1973), neither vagotomy nor atropine affected the hypotensive response to apomorphine. Haloperidol, pimozide, and spiroperidol antagonized it, the lower doses of apomorphine being antagonized more efficiently than the higher ones. Since decerebration abolished apomorphine action, the author concludes that the hypotension produced by apomorphine is due to stimulation of DA receptors located in the CNS.

The reasons for the discrepancy between Finch and Hausler's (1973) and Grabowska's (1974b) studies are difficult to ascertain. Apart from the contrasting results on the effect of vagotomy and atropine, for which we have no explanation, the most critical difference between the two studies concerns the effect of DA-blocking agents; in fact, depending on the result of this interaction, we would conclude for or against a dopaminergic mediation of apomorphine-induced hypotension.

Failure of Finch and Hausler (1973) to observe blockade of apomorphine effect by haloperidol might be due to the prolonged interval (15 minutes) between haloperidol and apomorphine administrations. In this regard, Goldberg (1972) reports that the blocking effect of haloperidol on DA-induced renal vasodilatation persists for only 2 minutes; maximal antagonism was best demonstrated when haloperidol was injected simultaneously with DA. In addition, it should be noted that Finch and Hausler (1973) obtained significant antagonism by the DA-receptor blocking agents against the 0.01-mg/kg dose of apomorphine, which was the lowest and the first administered in the dose–response curve.

It is evident that more investigations are needed to clarify the nature and the mechanism of the hypotensive effect of apomorphine. Interest in this effect is justified by its possible clinical application in the management of clinical hypertension.

B. Renal Effects

In addition to its effects on blood pressure and not necessarily correlated with it, apomorphine exerts vasodilation on the renal vascular bed of the dog (Goldberg *et al.*, 1968). In producing this effect apomorphine is considerably less effective than DA but as for DA the vasodilation is not blocked by propranolol, a β-adrenergic blocking agent. Although the effect of haloperidol on apomorphine-induced renal vasodilation has not been studied, Goldberg *et al.* (1968) label the apomorphine effect as DA-like.

VII. Endocrine Effects of Apomorphine

Recent evidence indicates that DA controls the release of some pituitary hormones (De Wied and De Jong, 1974).

A. Prolactin Release

Dopamine and apomorphine decrease the release of prolactin from pituitaries incubated *in vitro*. This effect of DA and of apomorphine is blocked by neuroleptics (Birge *et al.*, 1970; MacLeod *et al.*, 1970; MacLeod and Lehmeyer, 1973a,b; Shaar *et al.*, 1973; Smalstig *et al.*, 1974), demonstrating the existence in the pituitary of DA receptors having an inhibitory influence on prolactin release.

Since neuroleptics increase prolactin secretion in animals and in normal individuals, it is postulated that DA effectively controls prolactin secretion *in vivo* by tonically inhibiting its release (Franz, 1973; Sulman, 1970; De Wied, 1967; Kleinberg *et al.*, 1971). However, neuroleptics fail to stimulate prolactin secretion from disconnected (Kleinberg *et al.*, 1971), transplanted (Blackwell *et al.*, 1973), or isolated pituitaries (MacLeod and Lehmeyer, 1973a), indicating that the site of origin or the site of action of the DA that inhibits prolactin secretion is not the pituitary but the brain and probably the hypothalamus.

The necessity of an intact hypothalamohypophyseal connection for the action of neuroleptics might result from the fact that DA exerts its effect on prolactin by releasing hypothalamic factors that reach the hypophysis through the portal system (Kamberi, 1973); alternatively, DA itself stimulates the inhibitory DA receptors of the pituitary by being released from tuberoinfundibular DA neurons into the portal system.

This second hypothesis is certainly the more economic and is not contradicted by the most recent results.

In fact, two kinds of hypothalamic factors affecting prolactin secretion have been postulated: PIF and the prolactin-releasing factor. The former would account for the ability of hypothalamic extracts to inhibit prolactin secretion from isolated pituitaries. Its nature is controversial. However, recent evidence indicates that the prolactin-inhibiting activity of hypothalamic extracts is totally accounted for by the DA and NA that they contain (Takahara *et al.*, 1974; Shaar and Clemens, 1974). In fact, PIF found in these extracts has the same characteristics as catecholamines, namely, it is destroyed by MAO and absorbed by alumina; conversely, PIF is not of peptidic nature, being unaffected by protrease (Shaar and Clemens, 1974).

These results are not in disagreement with the concept that hypothalamic DA, released into the bloodstream of the portal hypophyseal system, directly inhibits prolactin secretion in the hypophysis.

Apomorphine, L-dopa and other DA-receptor stimulants (see Sections X,B and C) decrease serum prolactin in animals (Lu and Meiters, 1972; Euker *et al.*, 1973; Smalstig *et al.*, 1974), in normal individuals of both sexes (Frantz, 1973; Lal *et al.*, 1973a), and in various conditions associated with hyperprolactinemia (secreting pituitary tumors, oral contraceptive medication, postpartum) (Turkington, 1972; Martin *et al.*, 1974). L-Dopa and apomorphine antagonize the increase in plasma prolactin produced by chlorpromazine (Kleinberg *et al.*, 1971; Smalstig *et al.*, 1974). Lal *et al.* (1973a) did not obtain the same results.

Apomorphine and DA, administered intraventricularly, decrease prolactin in the plasma of rats. This action of DA-receptor stimulants is mimicked by dibutyryl cyclic-AMP; its effect is not affected by pimozide, which, however, blocks the effects of DA (Ojeda *et al.*, 1974).

These results might indicate that cyclic-AMP can initiate the same series of biochemical events that are produced by the stimulation of pituitary DA receptors by acting beyond the DA-receptor itself. This corresponds to the notion of cyclic-AMP as the second messenger of dopaminergic transmission (see Section VIII,E).

B. Growth-Hormone Release

Dopamine affects growth-hormone release in a complicated manner. In fact, its effects on growth hormone are not univocal and vary depending on the species, the route of administration, the animal preparation, or the clinical condition studied (Müller, 1976). The secretion of growth hormone appears to be regulated by DA, but by a different mechanism than prolactin secretion. Thus, DA-receptor stimulants, although they increase growth-hormone secretion in normal individuals (Podolski and Leopod, 1973; Lal *et al.*, 1972b, 1973a; Brown *et al.*, 1973), do not affect the release of growth hormone from isolated pituitaries (Mac Leod, 1969; Birge *et al.*, 1970).

These results have been taken to indicate that DA and apomorphine affect growth hormone release indirectly, through an action on the release of hypothalamic factors (decrease of somatostatin or increase of somatotropin release).

Apomorphine appears to be more potent and its effect more consistent and prompt but shorter-lasting than those of L-dopa and CB-154. Chlorpromazine antagonizes apomorphine effects (Lal *et al.*, 1973a). Men have a higher percent increase of growth hormone than do women (Ettigi *et al.*, 1974); parkinsonian patients show a decreased response to apomorphine (Brown *et al.*, 1973).

Recently, it has been found that acromegalic patients respond to apomorphine and to other DA-receptor stimulants with a decrease of serum growth hormone, that is, in a manner opposite to that of the normal subjects (see Section X, B).

VIII. Neurochemical Effects of Apomorphine

A. Effects on the Dopamine System

Apomorphine produces drastic changes in the synthesis and disposition of brain DA. Apomorphine was first shown to reduce the rate of disappearance of DA in brain after blockade of tyrosine hydroxylase with α-MT (Andén *et al.*, 1967). This was taken to indicate that the drug reduces the turnover of brain DA. In agreement with this hypothesis, it was reported that apomorphine decreases the rate of disappearance of labeled DA from brain after intravenous infusion of labeled tyrosine (Nybäck *et al.*, 1970) and reduces the concentrations of striatal DOPAC and HVA (the main metabolites of DA), while slightly increasing DA levels (Roos, 1969; Di Chiara *et al.*, 1974).

Apomorphine was also reported to reduce the rate of conversion of labeled tyrosine to DA (Nybäck *et al.*, 1970) and to decrease the accumulation of brain DOPA after blockade of cerebral decarboxylase (Carlsson, 1974a), indicating an inhibition of brain DA synthesis.

The inhibitory effect of apomorphine on both DA turnover and DA synthesis appears to be mediated by stimulation of brain DA receptors, since it is prevented by the administration of potent neuroleptics such as haloperidol and pimozide, which are considered to be fairly specific DA-receptor antagonists (Andén *et al.*, 1967; Carlsson, 1975a; Lahti *et al.*, 1972; Kehr *et al.*, 1975; Di Chiara *et al.*, 1976); however, the actual mechanism by which apomorphine produces these effects is still a matter of debate. Its clarification is of particular importance as it is related to the general problem of the DA-receptor-mediated mechanisms regulating the synthesis and the turnover of brain DA (Carlsson *et al.*, 1972).

1. *Postsynaptic Negative-Feedback Theory*

Drugs (such as the neuroleptics) which block DA receptors affect brain DA synthesis and turnover in a manner exactly opposite to apomorphine (Carlsson and Lindquist, 1963; Nybäck and Sedvall, 1968; Andén *et al.*, 1970; O'Keefe *et al.*, 1970; Chéramy *et al.*, 1970). A unifying theory for the interpretation of the above result was proposed by the Swedish school of Carlsson (Carlsson *et al.*, 1972; Andén *et al.*, 1967). This theory postulates that the changes of DA synthesis and turnover induced by the drugs are a feedback response to their interaction with postsynaptic DA receptors. Accordingly, stimulation of postsynaptic DA receptors by DA released from striatal terminals activates a strionigral polisynaptic loop, inhibiting dopaminergic neuronal activity. Neuroleptics—by antagonizing DA actions at postsynaptic sites—remove the feedback inhibition, thus stimulating DA neurons; apomorphine, in contrast, reinforces the feedback thus inhibiting dopaminergic activity.

Essential for the negative feedback theory is the concept that the drug-induced changes of DA synthesis and turnover are secondary to changes in the activity (firing) of the DA neurons. In agreement with this hypothesis, it was shown that electrical stimulation of the nigroneostriatal DA neurons results in an *in vivo* activation of DA synthesis and turnover (Roth *et al.*, 1976). In addition, both neuroleptic administration (Chéramy *et al.*, 1970) and electrical stimulation of the nigroneostriatal tract (Roth *et al.*, 1975) result in a stable activation of striatal tyrosine hydroxylase due to an increase in the affinity of the enzyme for its cofactor (Zivkovic and Guidotti, 1974; Zivkovic *et al.*, 1974). Moreover, neuroleptics were shown to activate and apomorphine to depress the firing of nigral units identified as dopaminergic (Bunney *et al.*, 1973a,b; Bunney and Aghajanian, 1976). In further agreement with the postsynaptic feedback hypothesis, it was reported that the effects of neuroleptics on DA synthesis are prevented by a cerebral transection interrupting the connections between the striatum and the substantia nigra (Nybäck and Sedvall, 1971).

On the basis of these results, the negative-feedback theory has gained large acceptance in the literature. However, further studies on the apomorphine-induced changes of dopaminergic activity suggest the existence of other receptor-mediated regulatory mechanisms which could be alternative to the negative-feedback one.

2. *Prejunctional DA Receptors*

a. In Vitro Studies. It was found that apomorphine, in low concentrations, was able to inhibit DA synthesis in striatal slices, a condition where a polysynaptic feedback loop is not operative (Goldstein *et al.*, 1970). This effect of apomorphine could be shown also on synaptosomal preparations of rat caudate, where it was blocked by low concentrations of potent DA-receptor antagonists (neuroleptics) (Christiansen *et al.*, 1974a,b). These observations have been confirmed and further extended (Ebstein *et al.*, 1974; Iversen *et al.*, 1975b; Snyder *et al.*, 1976). However, apomorphine has also been reported to reduce the release of DA from striatal slices subjected to electrical field stimulation (Farnebo and Hamberger, 1971). These results were interpreted by postulating the existence of presynaptic DA receptors located on the membrane of DA terminals and regulating DA synthesis and DA release. Stimulation of these receptors by DA released by nerve impulses or by DA-receptor agonists such as apomorphine would reduce the activity of tyrosine hydroxylase and the further release of DA.

A similar mechanism has been shown to be operative in the peripheral noradrenergic terminals, where noradrenaline and DA inhibit transmitter release by stimulating, respectively, prejunctional adrenergic (α_2) and dopaminergic receptors (Langer, 1973). However, recent results cast some doubt on the hypothesis that apomorphine inhibits DA synthesis in synaptosomes by stimulating prejunctional DA receptors (Iversen *et al.*, 1975b).

First, neuroleptics do not completely reverse the inhibitory effect of apomorphine on DA synthesis in striatal synaptosomes (Iversen *et al.*, 1975b), indicating that this effect is at least in part independent of an action on DA receptors and is possibly related to the ability of apomorphine to exert a direct inhibitory effect on tyrosine hydroxylase by competing with the reduced pteridine cofactor, a property shared by other catechols besides DA (Goldstein *et al.*, 1970). Second, DA, in contrast to apomorphine, appears to inhibit synaptosomal DA synthesis by a direct effect on tyrosine hydroxylase rahter than by an action on prejunctional DA receptors. In fact, blockade of DA reuptake, but not of DA receptors, prevents the inhibitory action of DA on synaptosomal DA synthesis (Iversen *et al.*, 1975 ; Snyder *et al.*, 1976). In contrast to the results obtained in synaptosomes, it has been reported that in striatal slices DA is able to inhibit DA synthesis by a DA-receptor-mediated mechanism (Westfall *et al.*, 1976). No explanation can be provided for these discrepancies. Third, the prejunctional receptors sensitive to apomorphine do not satisfy the criteria for DA-receptor specificity deduced from studies on other types of DA receptors. For example, α- and β-flupentixol differ by a factor of 50 for their potency in antagonizing apomorphine effects on synaptosomal DA synthesis, while they have been found to differ by more than 1000 times for their potency in antagonizing DA-induced stimulation of striatal adenylate cyclase (Iversen *et al.*, 1975b).

b. In Vivo Studies. In spite of the contradictory results obtained *in vitro*, a prejunctional DA-receptor-mediated mechanism is actually the most rational explanation for the ability of apomorphine to depress DA synthesis *in vivo* independently of dopaminergic firing. Thus, apomorphine was able to reduce DA synthesis in the presence of a cerebral transection, interrupting the nigroneostriatal pathway (Kehr *et al.*, 1972). In addition, apomorphine prevented the increase of DA synthesis produced by γ-butyrolactone (Walters and Roth, 1974), which blocks dopaminergic neuronal firing, or by HA-466 (Van Zwieten-Boot and Noach, 1975), an analog of γ-butyrolactone. These effects of apomorphine appear mediated by stimulation of DA receptors since they are prevented by the administration of DA-receptor blockers. On this basis, it has been postulated that cessation of DA release after interruption of impulse flow stimulates DA synthesis as a result of a relief of tyrosine hydroxylase from DA-receptor-mediated prejunctional inhibition (Walters and Roth, 1974).

Since stimulation of prejunctional DA receptors was not expected to influence neuronal activity, the inhibitory effect of apomorphine on dopaminergic firing was explained by the postsynaptic hypothesis. Thus, it was postulated that apomorphine inhibits DA synthesis by two mechanisms, one mediated by stimulation of prejunctional DA receptors, the other by activation of postsynaptic DA receptors (Carlsson, 1975b).

3. *Regulation of DA Neurons by Nigral DA Receptors*

Recently the inhibitory effect of apomorphine on dopaminergic firing has been shown to be dissociable from a postsynaptic feedback mechanism. In fact, it has been shown that apomorphine continues to depress DA firing after interruption of striatonigral connections by a diencephalic transection (Bunney and Aghajanian, 1975) or by a lesion of the crus cerebri (Bunney and Aghajanian, 1976) and acts even when applied microiontophoretically to the soma of nigral DA neurons (Bunney and Aghajanian, 1975). These effects are reversed by microiontophoretic or systemic administration of neuroleptics and are mimicked by microiontophoretic DA (Bunney and Aghajanian, 1975). On the basis of these findings, it has been postulated that apomorphine depresses dopaminergic firing by acting on DA receptors located within the substantia nigra. More recently, it has been reported that intranigral infusion of haloperidol, a potent DA-receptor blocker, results in activation of the firing of nigral units, while amphetamine, a DA-releasing agent, depresses it. On this basis, it has been postulated that the substantia nigra contains a mechanism for self-regulation of DA neurons via DA released onto inhibitory DA receptors (Groves *et al.*, 1975). The structures responsible for DA release have been indicated to be the dendrites of the DA neurons (Geffen *et al.*, 1976; Korf *et al.*, 1976; Björklund and Lindvall, 1975), but a possible contribution of recurring dopaminergic collaterals should also be envisaged (Rinvik and Grofova, 1970; Schwyn and Fox, 1974).

4. *Localization of Nigral DA Receptors*

The localization of the nigral DA receptors mediating the effects of locally administered drugs on DA firing is debated. While some authors favor a presynaptic localization, i.e., on the membrane of the DA cell bodies or dendrites (Bunney and Aghajanian, 1975; Groves *et al.*, 1975), ("auto-receptors") (Carlsson, 1975a), a postsynaptic localization is favored by the recent discovery in the nigra of DA-sensitive adenylate cyclase activity, the enzymatic marker of DA receptors (Phillipson and Horn, 1976; Kebabian *et al.*, 1972; Spano *et al.*, 1976; Premont *et al.*, 1976). This enzyme is resistant to destruction of nigral DA neurons by 6-OH-DA (Kebabian *et al.*, 1972; Spano *et al.*, 1976; Premont *et al.*, 1976) but is abolished by brain hemitransections cranial to the nigra or by coagulations of the globus pallidus or of the strionigral pathway (Spano *et al.*, 1977). These results, while indicating the existence of DA receptors in the substantia nigra localized on neuronal afferences descending from the corpus striatum, suggest a new mechanism for the regulation of dopaminergic neuronal activity (Di Chiara *et al.*, 1977a).

Thus, nigral DA, by activating nigral DA-sensitive adenylate cyclase, would modulate transmitter release from nigral afferent connections, thus influencing the activity of the DA neurons. In particular, nigral DA might inhibit the release onto DA neurons of an excitatory transmitter (e.g., substance P) (Hökfelt *et al.*, 1975; Brownstein *et al.*, 1976) or stimulate that of an inhibitory one (e.g., GABA) (McGeer *et al.*, 1976), thereby mediating a depression of dopaminergic activity. This model explains the stimulation of DA firing produced by neuroleptics as due to blockade of nigral DA-sensitive adenylate cyclase and the inhibition produced by amphetamine as due to activation of the cyclase by DA released within the nigra. This interpretation appears to reconcile the findings of Groves *et al.* (1975) and of Bunney and Aghajanian (1976) on the inhibition of dopaminergic firing by amphetamine. The apparent contrast between these findings derives from the fact that if one assumes with Groves *et al.* (1975) that amphetamine acts by releasing DA onto nigral DA receptors located on DA neurons, it remains unexplained why, as shown by Bunney and Aghajanian (1976), interruption of afferent nigral connections blocks amphetamine effects. Conversely, if one postulates with Bunney and Aghajanian (1976) that amphetamine inhibits dopaminergic firing by releasing DA onto striatal postsynaptic DA receptors, then it is difficult to justify its effectiveness when infused within the substantia nigra, as shown by Groves *et al.* (1975).

Quite recently, definite evidence for a role of this mechanism in the mediation of amphetamine action on DA firing has been provided by the finding of Groves *et al.* (1976) that interruption of afferent nigral connections prevents the inhibition of DA firing by the intranigral infusion of amphetamine.

5. *Effects of Apomorphine on DA Metabolism after Destruction of Postsynaptic DA Receptors*

In contrast to the effect of neuroleptics on DA firing, there is no evidence that the stimulation of DA synthesis by these compounds is due to a mechanism other than postsynaptic feedback. However, recently it has been shown that the complete destruction of striatal DA-sensitive adenylate cyclase activity by intrastriatal injection of kainic acid (McGeer *et al.*, 1976; Di Chiara *et al.*, 1977d) prevents neither the increase of striatal DOPAC produced by systemic administration of haloperidol nor the decrease of striatal DOPAC produced by apomorphine (Di Chiara *et al.*, 1977a). Actually, the treatment with kainic acid results in an increased sensitivity to the effects of haloperidol and of apomorphine on striatal DOPAC. Taking the loss of DA-sensitive adenylate cyclase activity as an index of destruction of postsynaptic DA receptors and the changes of striatal DOPAC as an index of changes in the rate of metabolism of striatal DA, these results indicate that neuroleptics and apomorphine modify striatal DA metabolism by acting on DA receptors different from the striatal postsynaptic ones.

Figure 1 provides a diagrammatic representation of the mechanisms of dopaminergic regulation discussed above.

6. *Behavioral and Clinical Correlactions*

The concept that dopaminergic activity can be influenced independently from an action on postsynaptic DA receptors has provided an explanation for certain behavioral and clinical effects of apomorphine and related drugs.

Apomorphine, administered in low doses, produces hypomotility and sedation in mice (Di Chiara *et al.*, 1976; Strömbom, 1976) and induces sleep in rats (Mereu *et al.*, 1977). This action is produced in rats by doses as low as 10 μg/kg s.c., which are about 10 times lower than the minimal ones which produce behavioral activation in the form of hypermotility and stereotypies.

The depressant effect of apomorphine is due to the activation of DA receptors, since it is antagonized by the administration of DA-receptor blockers (Di Chiara *et al.*, 1976). The DA receptors responsible for these effects are unlikely to be the postsynaptic ones, since they are stimulated by doses of apomorphine which are insufficient to produce behavioral signs of postsynaptic receptor activation such as hypermotility and stereotypy. On the other hand, the inhibitory effects of apomorphine on behavior are correlated both on a dose and on a time basis to a decrease of brain DA synthesis and turnover (Di Chiara *et al.*, 1976; Strömbom, 1976). Moreover, doses of DA-receptor blockers which prevent the sedative response to apomorphine also prevent the inhibitory effects of apomorphine on DA tunover (Di Chiara *et al.*, 1976). On this basis, it has been postulated that the sedative effect of apomorphine is secondary to depression of dopaminergic activity.

The DA receptors responsible for these effects have been suggested to be presynaptic (auto-receptors), but indeed their actual localization remains to be established.

A similar mechanism has been proposed to explain the hypomotility and sedation produced in mice by low doses of bromocriptine, a postulated DA-receptor agonist; also in the case of bromocriptine, these

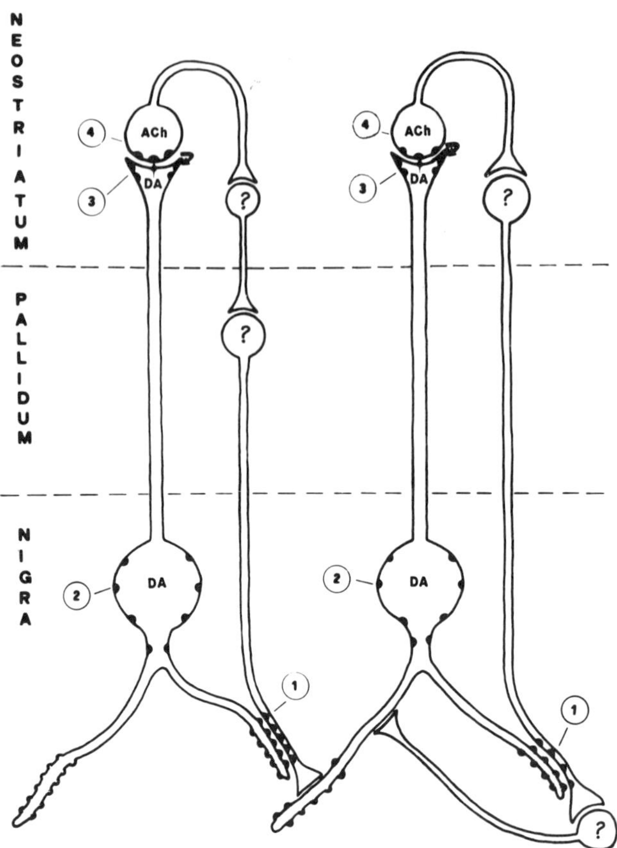

FIG. 1. Diagramatic representation of postulated DA receptors regulating dopaminergic neuronal activity: (1) Nigral postsynaptic DA receptors; (2) nigral presynaptic DA receptors ("auto-receptor"); (3) prejunctional DA receptors ("auto-receptor"); (4) striatal postsynaptic DA receptors.

behavioral effects are associated with a decrease of brain DOPAC and are antagonized by potent DA-receptor blocking agents (Di Chiara *et al.*, 1977b). However, in respect to apomorphine, bromocriptine appears as a more specific and long-lasting stimulant of "regulatory" DA receptors *in vivo*.

By analogy with the results obtained in animals, a depression of dopaminergic activity has been postulated to be the mechanism of certain clinical actions of apomorphine and related drugs. This applies to the ability of subemetic doses of apomorphine (10–25 μg/kg) to produce sedation and somnolence in normal individuals and to worsen parkinsonian symptoms in patients (Corsini *et al.*, 1976). A similar mechanism has also been suggested for the finding that apomorphine ameliorates the motor disturbances of choreic patients, a property shared by bromocriptine (Corsini *et al.*, 1977). In agreement with the hypothesis that these effects are due to stimulation of DA receptors, it has been found that they are blocked by the administration of neuroleptics (Corsini *et al.*, 1977).

Finally, an action on regulatory DA receptors has also been postulated to explain the antimanic action of apomorphine and of ET-495, a postulated DA-receptor agonist (Post *et al.*, 1976).

7. *Inhibition of DA Deamination*

Recent evidence indicates that a direct inhibition of neuronal MAO may contribute to the inhibitory effect of apomorphine on DA turnover (Di Chiara *et al.*, 1974). This concept arises from the following findings:

1. Apomorphine increases the levels of DA and decreases those of DOPAC in brain.
2. Apomorphine prevents, in part, the depletion of DA and the parallel increase of DOPAC and HVA levels produced by reserpine.
3. Apomorphine decreases the accumulation of deaminated metabolites of DA (DOPAC and HVA) in the brain of rats treated with a combination of L-dopa and a peripheral dopa-decarboxylase inhibitor.
4. Apomorphine inhibits competitively DA deamination by mitochondrial fractions of rat brain homogenates.

The major drawback of this theory is the effectiveness of apomorphine as an inhibitor of DA deamination *in vivo* as compared to its low potency as an inhibitor of MAO activity *in vitro*. Until now, this discrepancy has remained unexplained. Two main possibilities can be suggested:

1. Apomorphine concentrates in DA terminals.
2. A DA-specific MAO, very sensitive to the inhibition by apomorphine, deaminates intraneuronal DA; in the homogenate this DA–MAO activity would be masked by the prevailing, nonspecific MAO, insensitive to apomorphine.

8. *Inhibition of DA O-Methylation*

Various investigators have demonstrated *in vitro* the methylation of apomorphine to apocodeine after incubation with purified brain or liver COMT and *S*-adenosyl-L-methionine as the methyl donor (Cannon *et al.*,

1972a; McKenzie and White, 1973). The apparent Km for the reaction is 1.4×10^{-3} *M*. Tropolone and pyrogallol competitively inhibit apomorphine and DA *O*-methylation and potentiate the action of apomorphine *in vivo* (McKenzie and White, 1973; Missala *et al.*, 1973). These data demonstrate indirectly that apomorphine and DA compete for the same site on the enzyme. Thus, apomorphine is expected to be a competitive inhibitor of DA *O*-methylation; since in this case, Ki = Km, apomorphine appears to be a poor inhibitor of COMT. As a consequence of this, *in vivo* inhibition of DA *O*-methylation should take place only at doses higher than 30 mg/kg, which is about 1000 times higher than those which are capable of decreaseing DA synthesis and of affecting behavior.

McKenzie (1974) postulates that apomorphine decreases DA synthesis and turnover by *in vivo* inhibition of COMT. The basis for this view appears to be the finding that a COMT inhibitor, tropolone, also inhibits DA synthesis and turnover and, like apomorphine, antagonizes the increase in DA synthesis produced by chlorpromazine. In addition, according to McKenzie (1974), agroclavine, a DA-receptor agonist, does not inhibit COMT and does not decrease DA synthesis in normal rats. This last finding needs confirmation using a different method of estimation of DA synthesis; since (according to the same author) agroclavine, in spite of its inactivity in decreasing DA synthesis in normal rats, is able to antagonize the increase in DA synthesis produced by chlorpromazine.

Apart from the weakness of such arguments, the basic question that has to be answered before we can make any hypothetical consideration on the significance of COMT inhibition for apomorphine action is if indeed apomorphine inhibits COMT *in vivo*. At the moment, no direct evidence has been given that this is the case.

9. *Inhibition of DA Uptake*

Apomorphine inhibits the uptake of DA and NA by crude synaptosomal preparations of rat striatum and hypothalamus, respectively (Ferris *et al.*, 1975). The constant of inhibition by apomorphine was 1.9×10^{-5} *M* for DA uptake by striatal synaptosomes and 2.0×10^{-5} *M* for NA uptake by hypothalamic synaptosomes. It is unlikley that this apomorphine action contributes to its behavioral and biochemical effects *in vivo*, since apomorphine can produce these effects at brain concentrations about 100 times lower than those necessary for effective blockade of DA or NA uptake.

Does apomorphine accumulate in the DA terminal?

The answer to this question awaits the avilability of labeled apomorphine. The possibility that apomorphine is taken up into the DA terminal by the same membrane pump which concentrates DA is not unlikely, in view of the ability of apomorphine to compete with DA for its uptake. However, the high lipid solubility of apomorphine would probably prevent its concentration into the DA synaptosomes.

B. Effects on the Norepinephrine System

Apomorphine has been shown by Persson and Waldek (1970b) and by Nÿback *et al.* (1970) to decrease NA levels in brain.

Persson and Waldek (1970b) have reported that apomorphine accelerates the rate of NA depletion produced by α-MT. Persson (1970) reported increased formation of NA-^{3}H from tyrosine-^{3}H in the brain of mice treated with apomorphine.

On the basis of these findings, it has been concluded that apomorphine increases NA turnover in brain; this effect has been postulated to be secondary to the DA-receptor stimulation produced by apomorphine. This view is suggested by the finding that pyribedil (ET-495), a DA-receptor agonist, increased the levels of MOPEG, the major NA metabolite in brain (Garattini *et al.*, 1974).

In contrast, Andén *et al.* (1967) reported that apomorphine did not modify the rate of NA depletion after α-MT treatment.

According to Nÿback *et al.* (1970), apomorphine does not modify the synthesis and turnover of NA-^{3}H formed from tyrosine-^{3}H in mouse brain. In addition, apomorphine fails to affect the rate of NA depletion after DBH-inhibition with Fla-63 (Persson and Waldeck, 1970b).

In summary, the reports on the effect of apomorphine on NA neurons are contrasting and difficult to interpret. This is due in part to the difficulties that still afflict the estimation of NA turnover in brain.

C. Effects on the Serotonin System

Apomorphine has been reported to increase the concentration of 5-HT and 5-HIAA in rat brain (Grabowska *et al.*, 1973a; Scheel-Krüger and Hasselager, 1974). After a dose of 5 mg/kg s.c., brain 5-HT and 5-HIAA levels increase steadily and reach a plateau between 45 and 60 minutes following apomorphine; 5-HT levels then return toward normal, but 5-HIAA levels are still significantly elevated 2 hours after apomorphine. In contrast to stereotyped behavior, which remains constant, locomotor activity is maximal at 15 minutes following apomorphine and returns to normal 60 minutes thereafter.

Grabowska *et al.* (1973a) have suggested that stimulation of DA receptors produces hypermotility and also activates the 5-HT system which, in turn, would inhibit motility. Neuroleptics, in doses that prevent hypermotility, also abolish the increase of 5-HT and 5-HIAA levels. Conversely, destruction of raphe nuclei and blockade of 5-HT synthesis by *p*-chlorophenylalanine and *p*-chloroamphetamine potentiate, whereas increase of 5-HT levels by 5-hydroxtryptophan depress apomorphine-induced hypermotility (Grabowska, 1974a; Grabowska and Michaluk, 1974b).

D. Effects on the Acetylcholine System

Apomorphine and DA-receptor agonists produce a reliable and consistent increase of ACh levels in brain areas containing a high concentration of DA terminals (striatum and hypothalamus) but not in mesencephalon, cerebellum, hemispheres, and hippocampus (Sethy and Van Woert, 1973; Consolo *et al.*, 1974; Ladinski *et al.*, 1975; Guyenet *et al.*, 1975). This effect is mediated by an action on DA receptors since neuroleptics prevent it (Ladinski *et al.*, 1975; Guyenet *et al.*, 1975) and denervation by 6OH-DA injection in the substantia nigra results in supersensitivity to the increase of ACh levels (Fibiger and Grewaal, 1974).

Blockade of DA synthesis, although ineffective in preventing the accumulation of ACh by apomorphine and ET-495, blocks the effect of amphetamine (Guyenet *et al.*, 1975). This has been taken as further evidence that the direct action of apomorphine on DA receptors is the cause of its effects on ACh disposition.

Interruption of the nigroneostriatal pathway produces an acute decrease of ACh levels; subsequently, normalization of ACh levels occurs, probably as the result of compensation mechanisms (Rommelspacher and Kuhar, 1975). Neuroleptics that decrease ACh levels do not produce a further decrease of ACh levels that had been lowered by acute denervation (Rommelspacher and Kuhar, 1975). These findings indicate that the effect of neuroleptics on ACh levels is secondary to competition with transmitter DA for its receptor rather than to an anticholinergic effect.

The significance of the changes in ACh levels elicited by DA-receptor agonists and antagonists has been clarified by the finding that drugs which increase ACh levels decrease ACh release and vice versa. Thus, haloperidol stimulates ACh release from the striatum, whereas apomorphine decreases it (Stadler *et al.*, 1973). It is conveivable that the modification of ACh levels by dopaminergic drugs is consequent to a primary action on the firing of ACh neurons. Stimulation of DA receptors by apomorphine, amphetamine, L-dopa, or ET-495 would result in depression of striatal cholinergic firing, decreased ACh release and intraneuronal accumulation of ACh. The reverse would occur after blockade of DA receptors by neuroleptics. Accordingly, ACh turnover is expected to be decreased after apomorphine administration and increased after neuroleptics: this has been found to be the case (Trabucchi *et al.*, 1974; Guyenet *et al.*, 1975). All these results lead to the concept that the dopaminergic input to the striatum exerts an inhibitory action on cholinergic neurons; other evidence indicates that, in turn, cholinergic activation stimulates DA neurons.

A discussion of the anatomical basis and of the practical importance of these concepts, particularly in regard to extrapyramidal disorders, is beyond the scope of this review; for this we refer to published work (Bartholini *et al.*, 1973).

E. Effects on Adenyl Cyclase

A large body of evidence indicates that cyclic-AMP may act as the second messenger of synaptic transmission, mediating the intracellular events that follow the interaction of the neurotransmitter with its receptor (Robison *et al.*, 1967; Kakiuchi and Rall, 1968; Chasin *et al.*, 1971; Seeds and Gilman, 1971; Burkard, 1972; Hoffer *et al.*, 1972; Greengard *et al.*, 1972).

Recently, it has been shown that homogenates of tissues containing DA synapses respond to low concentrations of DA with an increased production of cyclic-AMP. These tissues include bovine superior cervical ganglia (Kebabian and Greengard, 1971), the rat, calf (Brown and Makman, 1972), and rabbit (Bucher and Schorderet, 1974b) retinas, rat basal ganglia (Kebabian *et al.*, 1972), olfactory tubercle, nucleus accumbens (Horn *et al.*, 1974), and the cerebral cortex (von Hugen and Roberts, 1973).

Neuroleptics have been found to be potent competitive inhibitors of the stimulation by DA of the cyclase from various DA-rich regions of the rat brain (Brown and Makman, 1973; Clement-Cormier *et al.*, 1974; Karobath and Leitich, 1974). Alpha-, but not beta-adrenergic-blocking agents are able to inhibit the DA-sensitive cyclase (Brown and Makman, 1972; Kebabian *et al.*, 1972).

Apomorphine mimics the action of DA on homogenates of rabbit retinas (Bucher and Schorderet, 1974b), rat caudate (Kebabian *et al.*, 1972), and on intact rabbit (Bucher and Schorderet, 1974a) and calf retinas (Brown and Makman, 1973). These data show that the pharmacological characteristics of the DA-sensitive cyclase closely resemble those of the DA receptor. Thus, the DA-sensitive cyclase activity represents a unique means of measuring changes in DA-receptor activity and of testing the DA-mimetic or DA-blocking ability of old and new drugs. An extensive study of this kind has been performed by Karobath and Leitich (1974) on DA-receptor antagonists and by Miller *et al.* (1974) on DA-receptor agonists. From these studies, critical information has been gained on the structural requirements of the DA receptor (see Section II,A).

According to Miller *et al.* (1974), apomorphine, added to rat striatal homogenates, has the same affinity as DA for the cyclase but the maximal activity in the presence of apomorphine is less than 50% that obtained in presence of DA. Similar results have been obtained in homogenates of rabbit retina (Bucher and Schorderet, 1974b). By contrast, in intact calf or rabbit retinas the maximal stimulation of cyclase obtained with apomorphine is similar or even higher than that obtained with DA (Brown and Makman, 1973; Bucher and Schorderet, 1974a). The reason for this discrepancy between data obtained with homogenates and with intact tissue is obscure. These results might be explained by postulating that homogenization increases the number of receptors exposed to a polar environment. Under this condition, the number of sites available for interaction would increase for polar agonists, such as DA, and would decrease for nonpolar ones, such as apomorphine. Conversely, in intact tissue, membrane integrity might limit access of polar compounds to receptors, thus resulting in lower activity of DA with respect to apomorphine on the intact retinas of some species.

These considerations might also be applied to explain certain discrepancies between the potency of nonpolar butyrophenones as DA antagonists *in vivo* and *in vitro* (Clement-Cormier *et al.*, 1974; Karobath and Leitich, 1974).

In general, the conclusions drawn from the study of the response of DA-sensitive cyclase from rat striatum to DA-receptor agonists are in close agreement with those drawn from similar studies utilizing different models of DA-receptor activity (see Section II,A). Notable exception is the failure of apomorphine to mimic DA actions on certain neurons of the snail *Helix aspersa* (Woodruff and Walker, 1969; Woodruff, 1971).

Since cyclic-AMP mediates the effects of DA within the CNS, it is predicted that inhibition of cyclic-AMP degradation might potentiate the actions of DA or of DA-receptor agonists. Indeed, apomorphine has been reported to inhibit phosphodiesterase; however, the actual contribution of this action to the effects of apomorphine *in vivo* is unknown (Sheppard and Wiggan, 1971; Nahorski *et al.*, 1973). The recent finding that caffeine, a potent inhibitor of phosphodiesterase potentiates amphetamine and apomorphine-induced stereotyped behavior seems to be perfectly tailored to the proposed role of cyclic-AMP in dopaminergic transmission (Klawans *et al.*, 1974; Fuxe and Ungerstedt, 1974). However, caffeine has been repeatedly reported not to increase cyclic-AMP levels in brain (Sattin, 1971; Rall and Sattin, 1970).

IX. Clinical Effects of Apomorphine

A. Emesis in Man

Apomorphine has a long history as an emetic agent. It has been used clinically to induce vomiting in cases of poisoning by orally ingested toxic substances (Tattersall, 1971), to discourage malingering or hysterical manifestations, and in the aversion therapy of alcoholism, homosexuality, and sexual perversions (Dent, 1953; Rowe, 1967; Quinn and Kerr, 1963; MacConaghy, 1969, 1970).

The usual dose is 0.1 mg/kg s.c.; vomiting ordinarily occurs within a few minutes and is preceded by yawning, nausea, and salivation. However, the concern of the dangers of aspiration of vomited material and disappointing results in aversion therapy has reduced the therapeutic use of apomorphine as an emetic. Nonetheless, the emetic effect of apomorphine is used for screening of antiemetic agents both in animals (see Section III) and in volunteers (Isaacs and Mac Arthur, 1954; Shields *et al.*, 1971).

In dogs, the potency of neuroleptics in blocking the emetic response to apomorphine does not always parallel their potency in blocking the stimulatory effect of DA in the extrapyramidal system nor their clinical efficacy as neuroleptics.

Consistently, Corsini *et al.* (1976) have shown that the emetic effect of apomorphine (5–10 mg, i.m.) in man is prevented by haloperidol (2 mg), metoclopramide (10 mg), and sulpiride (100 mg). However, whereas haloperidol prevents not only emesis but also the therapeutic efficacy of apomorphine in parkinsonism, on the contrary, metoclopramide and sulpiride rather selectively inhibit nausea and vomiting but not apomorphine effectiveness in ameliorating tremor and rigidity in parkinsonian patients. Interestingly, the antiemetic potency of these compounds observed in man did not parallel their antiemetic potency described in dogs (Justin-Besançon and Laville, 1964; Laville and Margarit, 1968).

It would be of interest to correlate the antiemetic potency of neuroleptics in man with their antipsychotic efficacy. This study might clarify whether or not DA receptors responsible for the neuroleptic effect and those at the CTZ are similar.

B. Movement Disorders

Apomorphine has been first shown to be effective in the treatment of tremors in parkinsonian patients by Vernier and Unna (1951) and by Schwab *et al.* (1951) and confirmed by Struppler and von Uexküll (1953). This effect has been rediscovered after nearly 20 years by Cotzias *et al.* (1970) and by Braham *et al.* (1970) and confirmed by many other authors (Cataigne *et al.*, 1971; Cotzias *et al.*, 1972; Corsini *et al.*, 1976).

Indeed, subemetic doses of apomorphine produce rapid improvement of the parkinsonian symptomatology, specially of the tremors (Strian *et al.*, 1972). Moreover, apomorphine enhances the therapeutical effect of L-dopa (Düby *et al.*, 1972; Cotzias *et al.*, 1972; Strian *et al.*, 1972) and decreases the occurrence of dyskinesias induced by this compound (Düby *et al.*, 1972). However, apomorphine itself has been shown to induce involuntary abnormal movements in parkinsonian patients (Cotzias *et al.*, 1970, 1972; Düby *et al.*, 1972).

Unfortunately, apomorphine is of no practical use in the treatment of Parkinson's disease because its beneficial effect is of short duration (about 1 hour) and accompanied by side-effects such as nausea, vomiting, dizziness, hypotension, and bradycardia.

Large oral doses of apomorphine either alone or in combination with L-dopa or L-dopa and a peripheral decarboxylase inhibitor have been administered with positive results, but some patients developed uremia; they recovered, however, after interruption of the treatment (Strian *et al.*, 1972; Cotzias *et al.*, 1972).

Apomorphine (5 mg, i.m.) has been found to suppress promptly the early dyskinetic-dystonic symptoms induced by neuroleptics in schizophrenic patients (Gessa *et al.*, 1972). In these patients apomorphine produced neither vomiting nor other adverse effects. Interestingly, apomorphine did not worsen the schizophrenic symptomatology (see below).

Apomorphine has been shown to improve Sydenham's chorea (Feldman *et al.*, 1954) and not to aggravate (Lal *et al.*, 1973e) or to improve (Tolosa and Sparber, 1974) the abnormal involuntary movements in Huntington's chorea. Moreover, it should be mentioned that in contrast to the majority of observations showing that L-dopa (Chase, 1973) worsens the abnormal involuntary movements of Huntington's chorea, it has been reported that L-dopa produces dramatic improvement in Sydenham's chorea (Spissu *et al.*, 1975) (see Section VIII,A,6).

To explain these conflicting results it might be useful to recall that apomorphine seems to have an action on presynaptic DA receptors that leads to inhibition of DA synthesis and neuronal firing and that small doses of L-dopa also inhibit the firing in DA neurons, decrease motor activity in rodents (see Section VIII,A), and might worsen parkinsonian symptoms in man (Corsini *et al.*, 1976). Therefore it is possible that subemetic doses of apomorphine or small doses of *l*-dopa improve choreic movements by decreasing dopaminergic activity instead of stimulating DA postsynaptic receptors. Indeed, the known sedative effect of apomorphine in man might find a similar "presynaptic" explanation.

C. Psychomotor Effects

The sedative properties of apomorphine have been used in the past in the treatment of excitement accompanying different neuropsychiatric disorders (Feldman *et al.*, 1945) and in the treatment of delirium tremens (Tompkins, 1899).

Various studies have shown that amphetamine, *l*-dopa and methylphenidate precipitate manic episodes and intensify psychotic symptoms in schizophrenic patients (Davis and Janowsky, 1973; Angrist *et al.*, 1973).

Moreover, amphetamine and *l*-dopa can induce psychoses in nonschizophrenics that are indistinguishable from naturally occurring schizophrenia (Connell, 1958; Angrist and Gershon, 1970; Griffith *et al.*, 1970).

These observation are consistent with the hypothesis that an increased dopaminergic activity has a role in the pathogenesis of schizophrenia (Snyder, 1973).

However, in contrast with the foregoing premises, the administration of apomorphine in subemetic doses to schizophrenic patients has caused no exacerbation of the psychopathology, except in 1 case described by Strian *et al.* (1972). The lack of psychotomimetic action of apomorphine might be owing to the fact that the emetic potency of apomorphine is higher than its psychotogenic potency or that subemetic doses of apomorphine are stimulating for presynaptic but not for postsynaptic DA receptors, including those responsible for the psychotomimetic effect.

Consistent with a stimulation of presynaptic DA receptors is the finding that apomorphine caused deep sedation and sleep and worsened the neurological symptoms in parkinsonian patients pretreated with haloperidol (Corsini *et al.*, 1976).

X. Other Dopamine Receptor Agonists

A comprehensive review of nonapomorphine DA-receptor agonists would probably outweigh that on apomorphine itself. However, it is difficult not to even mention in a review on apomorphine the newer DA-receptor agonists, recently introduced in therapy and research. Among them, ET-495 and CB-154 are probably the most interesting.

A. ET-495

The ET-495 (pyribedil; 1-(2″-pyrimidyl)-4-piperonylpiperazine), in doses higher than 0.5 mg/kg has been shown to produce turning contralateral to the lesion in rats and mice with unilateral 6OH-DA-induced degeneration of the nigroneostriatal pathway (Corrodi *et al.*, 1971, 1972). It produces stereotyped sniffing and stimulates locomotion in rats and mice at doses higher than 5–10 mg/kg. These effects of ET-495 are long-lasting, their duration depending on the dose: the effect on turning behavior in rats lasts 1–2 hours after 0.5 mg/kg, 5–10 hours after 5–25 mg/kg, and up to 48 hours after 150 mg/kg (Corrodi *et al.*, 1972). Like apomorphine, ET-495, decreases the rate of depletion of DA but increases that of NA from the brain of rats pretreated with α-MT (Corrodi *et al.*, 1972). This suggests that ET-495 decreases impulse flow in DA neurons while increasing that in NA neurons. Consistent with its action *in vivo* on DA neurons is the ability of ET-495 to inhibit tyrosine hydroxylase activity in striatal slices (Goldstein *et al.*, 1973) and to decrease the levels of HVA in brain (Jori *et al.*, 1974b); ET-495 also increases the levels of brain MOPEG, a metabolite of NA (Garattini *et al.*, 1974; Jenner and Mardsen, 1975).

In contrast to apomorphine, ET-495 does not affect the field stimulation-induced release of DA from neostriatal slices *in vitro* (Corrodi *et al.*, 1972). It does not stimulate *in vitro* the adenyl cyclase activity of striatal homogenates (Miller and Iversen, 1974). Thus, ET-495 appears to be inactive *in vitro* as a DA-receptor stimulant. This fact, as well as the inactivity of ET-495 after intraneostriatal administration (Fuxe *et al.*, 1972), has led to the suggestion that its *in vivo* activity is due to a metabolite. In fact, a catechol metabolite (S-584) has been isolated from hydrolyzed rat urine (Jenner *et al.*, 1973). This metabolite, administered intraperitoneally, produces hypermotility (Creese, 1974), turning behavior in rats (Poignant *et al.*, 1974b) and is active in producing stereotyped behavior after intrastriatal administration (Costall and Naylor, 1974c). The S-584 is also able to decrease HVA *in vivo* (Jori *et al.*, 1974b) and to stimulate *in vitro* the rat striatal adenyl cyclase (Miller and Iversen, 1974).

The catechol metabolite of ET-495 explains the DA-mimetic effect of ET-495 *in vivo* and its long duration.

B. CB-154

The CB-154 (2-bromoergocryptine) produces long-lasting stimulation of DA receptors as measured by contralateral turning behavior in rats lesioned unilaterally with 6OH-DA (Corrodi *et al.*, 1973; Fuxe *et al.*, 1974). In fairly high doses, CB-154 also produces stereotyped sniffing (Fuxe *et al.*, 1974). Threshold doses in rats are reported to be around 0.25–0.5 mg/kg i.p. Pretreatment with pimozide antagonizes the stimulation of turning by CB-154 (Fuxe *et al.*, 1974).

These effects of CB-154 justify its trial in parkinsonian patients (Calne *et al.*, 1974a,b).

In animals and in man, CB-154 inhibits the secretion of thyrotropin (Miyai *et al.*, 1974) and of prolactin (Flückinger and Wagner, 1968; Billeter and Flückinger, 1971; Stähelin *et al.*, 1971; Karg *et al.*, 1972; Flückinger *et al.*, 1972; Del Pozo *et al.*, 1972). These effects are postulated to be due to a stimulation of DA receptors in the pituitary, since they are blocked by neuroleptics (MacLeod and Lehmeyer, 1973b) and can be obtained in pituitary cell cultures (Pasteels *et al.*, 1971) and also after transplantation of pituitaries into mammary glands (Hoshino, 1973) or in the case of hypothalamohypophyseal disconnection (Besser *et al.*, 1972). In humans, CB-154 increases serum gonadotropin levels (Seki and Seki, 1974; Tolis *et al.*, 1973; Seki *et al.*, 1974).

Whereas in normal individuals it stimulates, in acromegalic patients CB-154 depresses the secretion of growth hormone (Chiodini *et al.*, 1974; Liuzzi *et al.*, 1974; Camanni *et al.*, 1975). The differential effect of CB-154 in normal and acromegalic subjects has been suggested to be due to a different locus of action of the drug for each condition (Müller, 1976). In the normal subjects, its effect would be due to the prevalence of hypothalamic DA-receptor stimulation which results in increased growth-hormone secretion. In the acromegalic patients, prevalence of dopaminergic stimulation of the hypophysis would produce inhibition of growth-hormone secretion.

These effects of CB-154 are employed in therapy to suppress lactation in galactorhea syndromes (Varga *et al.*, 1972, 1973; Del Pozo *et al.*, 1974; Lütterbeck *et al.*, 1971) and in acromegaly (Chiodini *et al.*, 1975). Recent evidence indicates that CB-154 produces an inhibition of impulse flow in brain DA neurons (Fuxe *et al.*, 1974). This action of CB-154 has been indicated to be independent from postsynaptic receptor activity but, instead, secondary to stimulation of presynaptic DA receptors (Di Chiara *et al.*, 1977e). In fact, CB-154 decreases DOPAC levels in brain in doses as low as 0.1 mg/kg s.c. and, after a dose of 2.5 mg/kg, for as long as 4 hours. The decrease of brain DOPAC levels after CB-154 is parallel both on a dose and on a time basis to the appearance of sedation, which is considered to be the behavioral correlate of decreased DA activity. As the dose is increased to 50 mg/kg s.c., CB-154, after 1 hour or more, is able to produce hypermotility in mice which is still present 24 hours after administration.

These results have been taken to indicate that CB-154 is a fairly specific and long-lasting stimulant of presynaptic DA receptors.

C. Ergot Alkaloids

The CB-154 is emetic in man (Calne *et al.*, 1974b) and it shares this action with natural ergot alklaoids (Wang, 1965). This effect has been reported to be blocked by neuroleptics (Brand *et al.*, 1954; Glaviano and Wang, 1955) and for this reason might be regarded as evidence that ergot alkaloids have DA-receptor-stimulating properties. In fact, there is evidence that the ergotoxine fraction of the ergot drugs has DA-mimetic activity (Johnson *et al.*, 1973). Ergometrine (Woodruff *et al.*, 1974) and ergocornine (Fuxe *et al.*, 1974) produce contralateral turning and stereotyped behavior in 6OH-DA-lesioned rats. Ergocornine decreases impulse flow in DA neurons (Fuxe *et al.*, 1974). Ergometrine produces hypermotility when injected into the nucleus accumbens (Pijnenburg *et al.*, 1973). Ergot alkaloids are long known to exert endocrine effects similar to those of CB-154 by stimulating DA receptors located in the hypophysis (Floss *et al.*, 1973).

As DA-receptor-stimulating agents, also LSD-25 and agroclavine (Stone, 1973) have to be taken into consideration; both are nonpeptide ergot derivatives and this can be taken as evidence that the DA-mimetic effects of ergot alkaloids are due to the lysergic moiety, where a *trans*-DA configuration can be recognized in the benzene ring linked through carbons 5 and 10 to a *N*-methyl group.

LSD-25 produces contralateral turning and, in high doses, stereotyped behavior in rats (Pieri and Pieri, 1974). It stimulates striatal and retinal adenyl cyclase *in vitro* and this effect is blocked by neuroleptics. Moreover, LSD-25 decreases DA turnover *in vivo*, and this effect is considered to be secondary to DA-receptor stimulation (Spano *et al.*, 1975; Da Prada *et al.*, 1975).

D. Other DA Receptor Agonists

A series of dihydroxyaminotetralines has been prepared by Cannon *et al.* (1972) as analogs and congeners of fragments of the apomorphine molecule. These compounds display emetic effects in dogs, as well as stereotypies in mice and pigeons (Cannon *et al.*, 1972x).

In a series of *N*-dialkyl-substituted aminotetralines the *N*-dipropyl derivatives have displayed the highest potency in producing stereotypy; by contrast, *N*-diethyl substitution appears to be optimal for emetic effects (McDermed *et al.*, 1975).

O-Diacetylation and *N*-methyl substitution of DA results in compounds active *in vivo* in antagonizing oxotremorine-induced tremor and reserpine-induced sedation and ptosis (Borgman *et al.*, 1973). However, these tests are not specific for direct DA-receptor stimulants since they can also be positive after the administration of amphetamine-like drugs.

To list all the compounds that have been reported to possess DA-receptor-stimulating effects is beyond the scope of the present review.

References

Ahlenius, S., Eriksson, H., Larsson, K., Modigh, K., and Södersten, P. (1971). *Psychopharmacologia* **20,** 383.

Ahtee, L., and Kaariainen, I. (1973). *Eur. J. Pharmacol.* **22,** 206.

Allikmetes, L. Kh., and Ditrikh, M. E. (1965). *Fed. Proc., Fed. Am. Soc. Exp. Biol.* **24,** 1000.

Amin, A. H., Crawford, T. B. B., and Gaddum, J. H. (1954). *J. Physiol. (London)* **126,** 596.

Amsler, C. (1923). *Naunyn-Schmiedebergs Arch. Exp. Pathol. Pharmakol.* **97,** 1.

Andén, N. E., Rubenson, A., Fuxe, K., and Hökfelt, T. (1967). *J. Pharm. Pharmacol.* **19,** 627.

Andén, N. E., Butcher, S. G., Corrodi, H., Fuxe, K., and Ungerstedt, U. (1970). *Eur. J. Pharmacol.* **11,** 303.

Andén, N. E., Strömbom, U., and Svensson, T. H. (1973). *Psychopharmacologia* **29,** 289.

Andres, K. H. (1965). *Z. Zellforsch. Mikrosk. Anat.* **68,** 445.

Angrist, B., and Gershon, S. (1970). *Biol. Psychiatry* **2,** 95.

Angrist, B., Shopsin, B., and Gershon, S. (1971). *Nature (London)* **234,** 152.

Angrist, B., Sathananthan, G. S., and Gershon, S. (1973). *Psychopharmacologia* **31,** 1.

Armstrong, J. M., and Boura, A. L. (1973). *Br. J. Pharmacol.* **47,** 850.

Asher, I. M., and Aghajanian, G. K. (1974). *Brain Res.* **82,** 1.

Ayd, F. J., Jr. (1967). *Med. Sci.* **18,** 32.

Ayhan, J. H., and Randrup, A. (1973). *Arch. Int. Pharmacodyn. Ther.* **204,** 283.

Baez, L. A. (1974). *Psychopharmacologia* **35,** 91.

Barnett, A., and Fiore, J. W. (1971). *Eur. J. Pharmacol.* **14,** 206.

Barnett, A., Goldstein, J., and Taber, R. I. (1972). *Arch. Int. Pharmacodyn. Ther.* **198,** 242.

Bartholini, G., Stadler, H., and Lloyd, K. C. (1973). *Adv. Neurol.* **3,** 233.

Barzaghi, F., Groppetti, A., Mantegazza, P., and Muller, E. E. (1973). *J. Pharm. Pharmacol.* **25,** 911.

Baum, E., Etevenon, P., Piarroux, M. C., Simon, P., and Boissier, J. R. (1971). *J. Pharmacol.* **2,** 423.

Baxter, B. L., Gluckman, M. I., Stein, L., and Scerni, R. A. (1974). *Pharmacol. Biochem. Behav.* **2,** 387.

Besser, G. M., Parke, L., Edwards, C. R. W., Forsyth, I. A., and McNeilly, A. S. (1972). *Br. Med. J.* **3,** 669.

Billeter, E., and Flückinger, E. (1971). *Experientia* **27,** 464.
Birge, C. A., Jacobs, L. S., Hammer, C. T., and Daughaday, W. H. (1970). *Endocrinology* **86,** 120.
Björklund, A., and Lindvall, O. (1975). *Brain Res.* **83,** 531.
Blackwell, R., Vale, W., River, C., and Guillemin, R. (1973). *Proc. Soc. Exp. Biol. Med.* **142,** 68.
Borgman, R. J., McPhillips, J. J., Stitzel, R. E., and Goodman, I. J. (1973). *J. Med. Chem.* **16,** 630.
Borison, H. L. (1952). *J. Pharmacol. Exp. Thr.* **104,** 396.
Borison, H. L. (1974). *Life Sci.* **14,** 1807.
Borison, H. L., and Brizzee, K. R. (1951). *Proc. Soc. Exp. Biol. Med.* **77,** 38.
Borison, H. L., and Wang, S. C. (1953). *Pharmacol. Rev.* **5,** 193.
Boyd, A. E., Lebovitz, H. E., and Pfeiffer, J. B. (1970). *N. Engl. J. Med.* **283,** 1425.
Brady, J. V., and Nauta, W. J. H. (1953). *J. Comp. Physiol. Psychol.* **46,** 339.
Braham, J., and Sarova-Pinhas, I. (1973). *Lancet* **2,** 432.
Braham, J., Sarova-Pinhas, I., and Goldhammer, Y. (1970). *Br. Med. J.* **3,** 768.
Brand, E. D., Harris, T. D., Borison, H. L., and Goodman, L. S. (1954). *J. Pharmacol. Exp. Ther.* **110,** 86.
Breese, G. R., Moore, R., and Howard, J. (1972). *J. Pharmacol. Exp. Ther.* **180,** 591.
Brightman, M. W., and Reese, T. S. (1969). *J. Cell Biol.* **40,** 648.
Brizzee, K. R., and Neal, L. M. (1954). *J. Comp. Neurol.* **100,** 41.
Brizzee, K. R., Neal, L. M., and Williams, P. M. (1955). *Am. J. Physiol.* **180,** 659.
Broekkamp, B., and Van Rossum, J. M. (1974). *Psychopharmacologia* **34,** 71.
Brown, J. H., and Makman, M. H. (1972). *Proc. Natl. Acad. Sci. U.S.A.* **69,** 539.
Brown, J. H., and Makman, M. H. (1973). *J. Neurochem.* **21,** 477.
Brown, W. A., Van Woert, M. H., and Ambani, L. M. (1973). *J. Clin. Endocrinol. Metab.* **37,** 463.
Brownstein, M. J., Mroz, E. A., Kizer, J. S., Palkovits, M. P., and Leeman, S. E. (1976). *Brain Res.* **116,** 299.
Bucher, M. B., and Schorderet, M. (1974a). *Biochem. Pharmacol.* **23,** 3079.
Bucher, M. B., and Schorderet, M. (1974b). *Experientia* **30,** 694.
Bunney, B. S., and Aghajanian, G. K. (1975). *In* "Pre- and Post-Synaptic Receptors" (E. Usdin and W. E. Bunney, Jr., eds.), p. 89. Dekker, New York.
Bunney, B. S., and Aghajanian, G. K. (1976). *Science* **192,** 391.
Bunney, B. S., Aghajanian, G. K., and Roth, R. M. (1973a). *Nature (London), New Biol.* **245,** 123.
Bunney, B. S., Walters, G. R., Roth, R. H., and Aghajanian, G. K. (1973b). *J. Pharmacol. Exp. Ther.* **185,** 560.
Burkard, W. P. (1972). *J. Neurochem.* **19,** 2615.
Burkman, A. M. (1960). *J. Am. Pharm. Assoc., Sci. Ed.* **49,** 558.
Burkman, A. M. (1961). *J. Pharm. Sci.* **50,** 156.
Burkman, A. M. (1962). *Arch. Int. Pharmacodyn. Ther.* **137,** 396.
Burkman, A. M. (1963a). *J. Pharm. Pharmacol.* **15,** 461.
Burkman, A. M. (1963b). *J. Pharm. Sci.* **54,** 325.
Burkman, A. M., and Nelson, J. W. (1957). *J. Am. Pharm. Assoc.* **46,** 140.
Burkman, A. M., Notari, R. E., and Van Tyle, W. K. (1974). *J. Pharm. Pharmacol.* **26,** 493.
Bustard, T. M., and Egan, R. S. (1971). *Tetrahedron* **27,** 4457.
Bütcher, L. L. (1968). *Eur. J. Pharmacol.* **3,** 163.
Bütcher, L. L., and Andén, N. E. (1969). *Eur. J. Pharmacol.* **6,** 255.

Bütcher, L. L., Butcher, S. G., and Larsson, K. (1969). *Eur. J. Pharmacol.* **7,** 283.
Calne, D. B., Teychenne, P. F., Claveria, L. E., Eastman, R., Greenacre, J. K., and Petrie, A. (1974a). *Br. Med. J.* **5,** 422.
Calne, D. B., Leigh, P. N., Teychenne, P. F., Bamji, A. N., and Greenacre, J. K. (1974b). *Lancet* **3,** 1355.
Camanni, F., Massara, F., Belforte, L., and Molinatti, G. M. (1975). *J. Clin. Endocrinol. Metab.* **40,** 363.
Cammermeyer, J. (1949). *J. Comp. Neurol.* **90,** 121.
Cannon, J. G., Smith, R. V., Modiri, A., Sood, S. P., Borgman, R. J., Aleem, M. A., and Long, J. P. (1972a). *J. Med. Chem.* **15,** 273.
Cannon, J. G., Kim, J. C., Aleem, M. A., and Long, J. P. (1972b). *J. Med. Chem.* **15,** 348.
Carlsson, A. (1975a). *In* "Pre- and Post-Synaptic Receptors" (E. Usdin and W. E. Bunney, Jr. eds.), p. 49. Dekker, New York.
Carlsson, A. (1975b). *In* "Chemical Tools in Catecholamine Research" (O. Almgren, A. Carlsson, and J. Engel, eds.), Vol. II, p. 219. North-Holland Publ., Amsterdam.
Carlsson, A., and Lindquist, M. (1963). *Acta Pharmacol. Toxicol.* **20,** 140.
Carlsson, A., Kehr, W., Lindqvist, M., Magnusson, T., and Atack, C. V. (1972). *Pharmacol. Rev.* **24,** 371.
Carlsson, A., Engel, J., Strömbom, U., Svensson, T. H., and Waldeck, B. (1974). *Naunyn-Schmiedberg's Arch. Pharmacol.* **283,** 117.
Carlsson, S. G. (1972). *Physiol. Behav.* **9,** 127.
Castaigne, P., Laplane, D., and Dordain, G. (1971). *Res. Commun. Chem. Pathol. Pharmacol.* **2,** 154.
Chaney, S. G., and Kare, M. R. (1966). *J. Am. Vet. Med. Assoc.* **149,** 938.
Chase, T. (1973). *Adv. Neurol.* **1,** 533.
Chasin, M., Rivkin, I., Mamrak, F., Samaniego, S. C., and Hess, S. M. (1971). *J. Biol. Chem.* **246,** 3037.
Cheng, H. C., and Long, J. P. (1974). *Eur. J. Pharmacol.* **26,** 313.
Chéramy, A., Besson, M. J., and Glowinski, J. (1970). *Eur. J. Pharmacol.* **10,** 206.
Chiel, H., Yehuda, S., and Wurtman, R. J. (1974). *Life Sci.* **14,** 483.
Chiodini, P. G., Liuzzi, A., Botalla, L., Cremascoli, G., and Silvestrini, F. (1974). *J. Clin. Endocrinol. Metab.* **38,** 200.
Chiodini, P. G., Liuzzi, A., Botalla, L., Opizzi, G., Muller, E. E., and Silverstrini, F. (1975). *J. Clin. Endocrinol. Metab.* **40,** 705.
Christensen, A. V., and Möller-Nielsen, I. (1974). *Psychopharmacologia* **34,** 119.
Christiansen, J., and Squires, R. F. (1974a). *J. Pharm. Pharmacol.* **26,** 367.
Christiansen, J., and Squires, R. F. (1974b). *J. Pharm. Pharmacol.* **26,** 742.
Clement-Cormier, Y. C., Kebabian, J. W., Petzold, G., and Greengard, P. (1974). *Proc. Natl. Acad. Sci. U.S.A.* **71,** 1113.
Connell, P. H. (1958). "Amphetamine Psychosis," Maudsley Monogr. No. 5. Oxford Univ. Press, London and New York.
Consolo, S., Ladinski, H., and Garattini, S. (1974). *J. Pharm. Pharmacol.* **26,** 275.
Cools, A. R., and Van Rossum, M. J. (1970). *Arch. Int. Pharmacodyn. Ther.* **187,** 163.
Corrodi, H., Fuxe, K., and Ungerstedt, U. (1971). *J. Pharm. Pharmacol.* **23,** 989.
Corrodi, H., Farnebo, L. O., Fuxe, K., Hamberger, B., and Ungerstedt, U. (1972). *Eur. J. Pharmacol.* **20,** 195.
Corrodi, H., Fuxe, K., Hökfelt, T., Lidbrink, P., and Ungerstedt, U. (1973). *J. Pharm. Pharmacol.* **25,** 409.
Corsini, G. U., Del Zompo, M., Cianchetti, C., Mangoni, A., and Gessa, G. L. (1976). *Psychopharmacologia* **47,** 169.

Corsini, G. U., Del Zompo, M., Onali, P. L., Mangoni, A., and Gessa, G. L. (1977). *Life Sci.* **20,** 1613.
Costa, E. , and Groppetti, A. (1970). *In* "Amphetamine and Related Compounds" (E. Costa and S. Garattini, eds.), p. 231. Raven, New York.
Costa, E., Groppetti, A., and Naimzada, M. K. (1972). *Br. J. Pharmacol.* **44,** 742.
Costall, B., and Naylor, R. J. (1973a). *Eur. J. Pharmacol.* **21,** 350.
Costall, B., and Naylor, R. J. (1973b). *Eur. J. Pharmacol.* **24,** 8.
Costall, B., and Naylor, R. J. (1974a). *Eur. J. Pharmacol.* **25,** 237.
Costall, B., and Naylor, R. J. (1974b). *J. Pharm. Pharmacol.* **26,** 30.
Costall, B., and Naylor, R. J. (1974c). *Naunyn-Schmiedeberg's Arch. Pharmacol.* **285,** 71.
Costall, B., Naylor, R. J., and Olley, J. E. (1972). *Eur. J. Pharmacol.* **18,** 95.
Costall, B., Naylor, R. J., and Neumeyer, J. L. (1975a). *Eur. J. Pharmacol.* **31,** 1.
Costall, B., Naylor, R. J., and Pinder, R. M. (1975b). *Eur. J. Pharmacol.* **31,** 94.
Cotzias, G. C. (1971). *J. Am. Med. Assoc.* **218,** 1903.
Cotzias, G. C. , Van Woeret, M. M., and Schipper, L. M. (1967). *N. Engl. J. Med.* **276,** 374.
Cotzias, G. C., Papavasiliou, P. S., Fehling, C., Kaufman, B., and Mena, I. (1970). *N. Engl. J. Med.* **282,** 31.
Cotzias, G. C., Lawrence, W. H., Papavasiliou, P. S., Duby, S. E., Ginos, J. Z., and Mena, I. (1972). *Trans. Am. Neurol. Assoc.* **97,** 156.
Courvoisier, S., Fournel, J., Ducrot, R., Kolsky, M., and Noetschet, P. (1953). *Arch. Int. Pharmacodyn. Ther.* **92,** 305.
Cox, B., and Tha, S. J. (1973). *Eur. J. Pharmacol.* **24,** 96.
Crane, G. E. (1968). *Am. J. Psychiatry* **124,** 40.
Crane, G. E. (1973). *Br. J. Psychiatry* **122,** 395.
Creese, I. (1974). *Eur. J. Pharmacol.* **28,** 55.
Creese, I., and Iversen, S. D. (1973). *Brain Res.* **55,** 369.
Da Prada, M., Saner, A., Burkard, W. P., Bartholini, G., and Pletscher, A. (1975). *Brain Res.* **94,** 67.
Davis, J. M., and Janowsky, D. S. (1973). *In* "Frontiers in Catecholamine Research" (S. H. Snyder and E. Usdin, eds.), p. 977. Pergamon, Oxford.
Del Pozo, E., Brun del Re, E., Varga, L., and Friesen, H. (1972). *J. Clin. Endocrinol. Metab.* **35,** 768.
Del Pozo, E., Varga, L., Wiss, N., Tolis, G., Firese, N., Wenner, R., Vetter, L., and Uetxiler, A. (1974). *J. Clin. Endocrinol. Metab.* **39,** 18.
Dempsey, E. W. (1968). *Exp. Neurol.* **22,** 568.
Dent, J. Y. (1953). *Br. J. Addict.* **50,** 43.
De Oliverira, L., and Graeff, F. G. (1972). *Eur. J. Pharmacol.* **18,** 159.
Deshpande, R., Sharma, M. I., Kherdikar, P. R., and Grewal, R. S. (1961). *Br. J. Pharmacol. Chemother.* **17,** 7.
De Wied, D. (1967). *Pharmacol. Rev.* **19,** 251.
De Wied, D., and De Jong, W. (1974). *Annu. Rev. Pharmacol.* **14,** 389.
Dhawan, B. N., and Saxena, P. N. (1960). *Br. J. Pharmacol.* **15,** 285.
Dhawan, B. N., Saxena, P. N., and Gupta, G. P. (1961). *Br. J. Pharmacol.* **16,** 137.
Di Chiara, G., Balakleevsky, A., Porceddu, M. L., Tagliamonte, A., and Gessa, G. L. (1974). *J. Neurochem.* **23,** 1105.
Di Chiara, G., Porceddu, M. L., Vargiu, L., Argiolas, A., and Gessa, G. L. (1976). *Nature (London)* **264,** 564.
Di Chiara, G., Mereu, G. P., Vargiu, L., Porceddu, M. L., Mulas, A., Trabucchi, M., and Spano, P. F. (1977a). *Adv. Biochem. Psychopharmacol.* **16,** 477.

Di Chiara, G., Olianas, M., Del Fiacco, M., Spano, P. F., and Tagliamonte, A. (1977b). *Nature (London)* **268,** 743.

Di Chiara, G., Porceddu, M. L., Fratta, W., and Gessa, G. L. (1977c). *Nature (London)* **267,** 270.

Di Chiara, G., Porceddu, M. L., Spano, P. F., and Gessa, G. L. (1977d). *Brain Res.* **130,** 374.

Di Chiara, G., Porceddu, M. L., Vargiu, L., Stefanini, E., and Gessa, G. L. (1977e). *Naunyn-Schmiedeberg's Arch. Pharmacol.* **300,** 239.

Di Chiara, G., Vargiu, L., Porceddu, M. L., Longoni, R., Mulas, A., and Gessa, G. L. (1977f). *Adv. Biochem. Psychopharmacol.* **16,** 571.

Divac, I. (1972). *Psychopharmacologia* **27,** 171.

Dordoni, F. (1948). *Boll. Soc. Ital. Biol. Sper.* **24,** 228.

Dresse, A., and Niemergees, C. (1961). *C. R. Seances Soc. Biol. Ses. Fil.* **155,** 1713.

Düby, S. E., Cotzias, G. C., Papavasiliou, P. S., and Lawrence, W. H. (1972). *Arch. Neurol. (Chicago)* **27,** 474.

Ebstein, B., Roberge, C., Tabachnič, J., and Goldstein, M. (1974). *J. Pharm. Pharmacol.* **26,** 975.

Ellinwood, E. H., Jr. (1967). *J. Nerv. Ment. Dis.* **144,** 273.

Enero, M. A., and Langer, S. Z. (1975). *Naunyn-Schmiedeberg's Arch. Pharmacol.* **289,** 179.

Ernst, A. M. (1965). *Psychopharmacologia* **7,** 391.

Ernst, A. M. (1967). *Psychopharmacologia* **10,** 316.

Ernst, A. M., and Semlik, P. G. (1966). *Experientia* **22,** 837.

Ettigi, P., Lal, S., Martin, J. B., and Friesen, H. G. (1974). *Proc. Can. Psychiatr. Assoc., 24th Meet.* p. 25.

Euker, J. S., Shaar, C. J., and Riegle, G. D. (1973). *Fed. Proc., Fed. Am. Soc. Exp. Biol.* **32,** 307.

Everitt, B. J., Fuxe, K., and Hökfelt, T. (1974). *Eur. J. Pharmacol.* **29,** 187.

Evetts, K. D., Uretsky, N. J., Iversen, L. L., and Iversen, S. D. (1970). *Nature (London)* **225,** 961.

Farnebo, L. O., and Hamberger, B. (1971a). *Br. J. Pharmacol.* **43,** 97.

Farnebo, L. O., and Hamberger, B. (1971b). *Acta Physiol. Scand.* **371,** 35.

Fekete, M., Kurti, A. M., and Pribusz, I. (1970). *J. Pharm. Pharmacol.* **22,** 377.

Feldman, F., Susselman, S., and Barrera, S. E. (1945). *Am. J. Psychiatry* **102,** 403.

Ferris, R.M., Tang, F. L., and Russel, A. V. (1975). *Biochem. Pharmacol.* **24,** 1523.

Fibiger, H. C., and Grewaal, D. S. (1974). *Life Sci.* **15,** 57.

Finch, L., and Hausler, G. (1973). *Eur. J. Pharmacol.* **21,** 264.

Floss, H. G., Cassady, J. M., and Robbers, J. E. (1973). *J. Pharm. Sci.* **62,** 699.

Flückiger, R., and Wagner, H. R. (1968). *Experientia* **24,** 1130.

Flückiger, E., Lütterbeck, P. M., Wagner, H. R., and Billeter, E. (1972). *Experientia* **28,** 924.

Fog, R. (1970). *Psychopharmacologia* **16,** 305.

Fog, R., and Pakkenberg, H. (1971). *Exp. Neurol.* **31,** 75.

Fog, R., Randrup, A., and Pakkenberg, H. (1967). *Psychopharmacologia* **11,** 179.

Frantz, A. G. (1973). *Prog. Brain Res.* **39,** 311.

Frommel, I. (1965). *Arch. Int. Pharmacodyn. Ther.* **154,** 231.

Fuxe, K. , and Owman, C. (1965). *J. Comp. Neurol.* **125,** 337.

Fuxe, K., and Sjöqvist, F. (1972). *J. Pharm. Pharmacol.* **24,** 702.

Fuxe, K. and Ungerstedt, U. (1974). *Med. Biol.* **52,** 48.

Fuxe, K., Corrodi, H., Farnebo, L. O., Hamberger, H., and Ungerstedt, U. (1972). *Proc. Int. Symp. Trivastal, 1972,* p. 37.

Fuxe, K., Corrodi, H., Hökfelt, T., Lidbrink, P., and Ungerstedt, U. (1974). *Med. Biol.* **52,** 121.

Gaitondé, B. B., McCarthy, L. E., and Borison, H. L. (1965). *J. Pharmacol. Exp. Ther.* **147,** 409.

Garattini, S., Bareggi, S. R., Marc, V., Calderini, G., and Morselli, P. L. (1974). *Eur. J. Pharmacol.* **28,** 214.

Geffen, L. B., Jessell, T. M., Cuello, A. C., and Iversen, L. L. (1976). *Nature (London)* **260,** 258.

Gerlach, J., Reisby, N., and Randrup, A. (1974). *Psychopharmacologia* **34,** 21.

Gessa, R., Tagliamonte, A., and Gessa, G. L. (1972). *Lancet* **2,** 981.

Gianutsos, G., Drawbaugh, R. B., Hynes, M. D., and Lal, H. (1974). *Life Sci.* **14,** 887.

Gianutsos, G., Hynes, M. D., and Lal, H. (1975). *Biochem. Pharmacol.* **24,** 581.

Glaviano, V. V., and Wang, S. C. (1955). *J. Pharmacol. Exp. Ther.* **114,** 358.

Goldberg, L. I. (1972). *Pharmacol. Rev.* **24,** 1.

Goldberg, L. I., Sonneville, P. F., and McNay, J. L. (1968). *J. Pharmacol Exp. Ther.* **163,** 188.

Goldstein, M., Freedman, L. S., and Backstrom, T. (1970). *J. Pharm. Pharmacol.* **22,** 715.

Goldstein, M., Anagnoste, B., and Shirron, C. (1973). *J. Pharm. Pharmacol.* **25,** 348.

Grabowska, M. (1974a). *Psychopharmacologia* **39,** 315.

Grabowska, M. (1974b). *Pol. J. Pharmacol. Pharm.* **26,** 305.

Grabowska, M., and Michaluk, J. (1974a). *J. Pharm. Pharmacol.* **26,** 549.

Grabowska, M., and Michaluk, J. (1974b). *Pharmacol., Biochem. Behav.* **2,** 263.

Grabowska, M., Antkiewicz, L., Maj, J., and Michaluk, J. (1973a). *Pol. J. Pharmacol. Pharm.* **25,** 29.

Grabowska, M., Michaluk, J., and Antkiewicz, L. (1973b). *Eur. J. Pharmacol.* **23,** 82.

Greengard, P., McAfee, D. A., and Kebabian, J. W. (1972). *Adv. Cyclic Nucleotide Res.* **1,** 373.

Griffith, J. J., Cavanaugh, J., and Oates, J. (1970). *In* "Psychotomimetic Drugs" (D. H. Efron, ed.), p. 287. Raven, New York.

Groppetti, A., Misher, A., Naimzada, M., Revuelta, A., and Costa, E. (1972). *J. Pharmacol. Exp. Ther.* **182,** 464.

Groves, P. M., Wilson, C. J., Young, S. J., and Rebec, G. V. (1975). *Science* **190,** 522.

Groves, P. M., Young, S. J., and Wilson, C. J. (1976). *Neuropharmacology* **15,** 755.

Gupta, G. P., and Dhawan, B. N. (1965). *Psychopharmacologia* **8,** 120.

Guyenet, P. G., Agid, Y., Javoy, F., Beaujouan, J. C., Rossier, J., and Glowinski, J. (1975). *Brain Res.* **84,** 227.

Hamburger-Bar, R., and Rigter, H. (1975). *Eur. J. Pharmacol.* **32,** 357.

Harnack, E. (1874). *Arch. Exp. Pathol. Pharmakol.* **2,** 254.

Hatcher, R. A., and Weiss, S. (1923). *J. Pharmacol. Exp. Ther.* **22,** 139.

Hensiak, J. F., Cannon, J. G., and Burkman, A. M. (1965). *J. Med. Chem.* **8,** 557.

Hill, H. F., and Horita, A. (1972). *J. Pharm. Pharmacol.* **24,** 490.

Hoffer, B. J., Siggins, G. R., Olivier, A. P., and Bloom, F. E. (1972). *Adv. Cyclic Nucleotide Res.* **1,** 411.

Hökfelt, T., Kellerth, J. O., Nilsson, G., and Pernow, B. (1975). *Science* **190,** 889.

Holtz, P., and Credner, K. (1942). *Naunyn-Schmiedebergs Arch. Exp. Pathol. Pharmakil.* **200,** 356.

Holtzmann, W. G., and Jewett, R. E. (1971). *Psychopharmacologia* **22,** 151.

Horn, A. S., Cuello, A. C., and Miller, R. J. (1974). *J. Neurochem.* **22,** 265.

Hoshino, K. (1973). *Experientia* **29,** 882.

Ilhan, M., Long, J. P., and Cannon, J. G. (1975). *Eur. J. Pharmacol.* **33,** 13.

Isaacs, B., and MacArthur, J. G. (1954). *Lancet* **2,** 570.

Iversen, L. L., Horn, A. S., and Miller, R. J. (1975a). *In* "Pre- and Post-Synaptic Receptors" (Usdin and W. E. Bunney, Jr., eds.), p. 207. Dekker, New York.

Iversen, L. L., Rogawski, M. A., and Miller, R. J. (1975b). *Mol. Pharmacol.* **12,** 251.

Iwatsubo, K., and Clouet, D. H. (1975). *Biochem. Pharmacol.* **24,** 1499.

Jalfre, M., and Haefely, W. (1971). *In* "6-Hydroxydopamine and Catecholamine Neurons" (T. Malmfors and H. Thoenen, eds.), p. 333. North-Holland Publ., Amsterdam.

Janowsky, D. S., and Davis, J. M. (1974). *In* "Neuropsychopharmacology of Monoamines and their Regulatory Enxymes" (E. Usdin, ed.), p. 317. Raven, New York.

Janssen, P. A., Niemegeers, C. J. C., and Jageneau, A. H. M. (1960). *Arzneim.-Forsch.* **10,** 1003.

Janssen, P. A., Niemegeers, C. J. E., and Schellekens, K. H. L. (1965a). *Arzneim-Forsch.* **15,** 104.

Janssen, P. A., Niemegeers, C. J. E., and Schellekens, K. H. L. (1965b). *Arzneim.-Forsch.* **15,** 1196.

Janssen, P. A., Niemegeers, C. J. E., Schellekens, K. H. L., and Lenaerts, F. M. (1967). *Arzneim.-Forsch.* **17,** 841.

Janssen, P. A., Niemegeers, C. J. E., Schellekens, K. H. L., Dresse, A., Lenaerts, F. M., Pinchard, A., Schaper, W. K. A., Nuete, J. M., and Verbruggen, F. J. (1968). *Arzneim.-Forsch.* **18,** 261.

Jenner, P., and Marsden, C. D. (1975). *Eur. J. Pharmacol.* **33,** 211.

Jenner, P., Taylor, A. R., and Campbell, D. B. (1973). *J. Pharm. Pharmacol.* **25,** 749.

Johnson, A. M., Vigouret, J. M., and Loew, D. M. (1973). *Experientia* **29,** 763.

Jori, A. , Dolfini, E., Tognoni, G., and Garattini, S. (1973). *J. Pharm. Pharmacol.* **25,** 315.

Jori, A., Cecchetti, G., Ghezzi, D., and Samanin, R. (1974a). *Eur. J. Pharmacol.* **26,** 179.

Jori, A., Cecchetti, G., Dolfini, E., Monti, E., and Garattini, S. (1974b). *Eur. J. Pharmacol.* **27,** 245.

Justin-Bescançon, L., and Laville, G. (1964). *C. R. Seances Soc. Biol. Ses Fil.* **158,** 723.

Kakiuchi, S., and Rall, T. W. (1968). *Mol. Pharmacol.* **4,** 367.

Kamberi, I. A. (1973). *Prog. Brain Res.* **39,** 261.

Kamberi, I. A., Mical, R. S., and Porter, J. C. (1971). *Endocrinology* **88,** 1003.

Karg, H., Schams, D., and Reinhardt, V. (1972). *Experientia* **28,** 574.

Karli, P. (1955). *C. R. Seances Soc. Biol. Ses Fil.* **149,** 2227.

Karobath, M., and Leitich, H. (1974). *Proc. Natl. Acad. Sci. U.S.A.* **71,** 2915.

Kaul, P. N., and Brochmann-Hanssen, E. (1961). *J. Pharm. Sci.* **50,** 266.

Kaul, P. N., and Conway, M. W. (1971). *J. Pharm. Sci.* **60,** 93.

Kaul, P. N. , Brochmann-Hanssen, E., and Way, E. L. (1961a). *J. Pharm. Sci.* ; 244.

Kaul, P. N., Brochmann-Hanssen, E., and Way, E. L. (1961b). *J. Pharm. Sci.* **50,** 840.

Kazamatsuri, H., Chien, C., and Cole, J. O. (1972a). *Arch. Gen. Psychiatry* **27,** 95.

Kazamatsuri, H., Chien, C., and Cole, J. O. (1972b). *Arch. Gen. Psychiatry* **27,** 100.

Kebabian, J. W., and Greengard, P. (1971). *Science* **174,** 1346.

Kebabian, J. W., and Saavedra, J. M. (1976). *Science* **193,** 683.

Kebabian, J. W., Petzold, G. L., and Greengard, P. (1972). *Proc. Natl. Acad. Sci. U.S.A.* **69,** 2145.

Kehr, W., Carmsson, A., Lindqvist, M., Magnusson, T., and Atack, C. V. (1972). *J. Pharm. Pharmacol.* **24,** 744.

Kehr, W., Carlsson, A., and Lindqvist, M. (1975). *Adv. Neurol.* **9,** 185.
Kelly, P. H., Seviour, P. W., and Iversen, S. D. (1975). *Brain Res.* **94,** 507.
Kier, I. B., and Truitt, E. B., Jr. (1970). *J. Pharmacol. Exp. Ther.* **174,** 94.
King, F. A., and Meyer, P. M. (1958). *Science* **128,** 655.
Klawans, H. L. (1973). *Am. J. Psychiatry* **130,** 82.
Klawans, H. L., and McKendall, R. P. (1971). *J. Neurol. Sci.* **14,** 189.
Klawans, H. L. , Goetz, C., and Weiner, W. J. (1973). *J. Neural Trans.* **34,** 187.
Klawans, H. L., Moses, H., and Beaulieu, D. M. (1974). *Life Sci.* **14,** 1493.
Kleinberg, D. L., Noel, G. L., and Frantz, A. G. (1971). *J. Clin. Endocrinol. Metab.* **33,** 873.
Koch, M. V., Cannon, J. G., and Burkman, A. M. (1968). *J. Med. Chem.* **11,** 977.
Koella, W. P., and Sutin, J. (1967). *Int. Rev. Neurobiol.* **10,** 31.
Korf, J., Zieleman, T. M., Cuello, A. C., and Iversen, L. L. (1976). *Nature (London)* **260,** 257.
Koster, R. (1957). *J. Pharmacol. Exp. Ther.* **119,** 406.
Krayer, O. (1926). *Naunyn-Schmiedebergs Arch. Exp. Pathol. Pharmakol.* **111,** 60.
Kruk, Z. L. (1972). *Life Sci.* **11,** Part I, 845.
Kruk, Z. L., and Brittain, R. T. (1972). *J. Pharm. Pharmacol.* **24,** 835.
Kumadaki, N., Hitomi, M., and Kumada, S. (1967). *Jpn. J. Pharmacol.* **17,** 659.
Kuschinsky, K., and Hornykiewicz, O. (1972). *Eur. J. Pharmacol.* **19,** 119.
Ladinsky, H., Consolo, S., Bianchi, S., Samanin, R., and Ghezzi, D. (1975). *Brain Res.* **84,** 221.
Lahti, R. A., McAllister, B., and Wozniak, J. (1972). *Life Sci.* **11,** 605.
Lal, S. , and Sourkes, T. L. (1973). *Arch. Int. Pharmacodyn. Ther.* **202,** 171.
Lal, S., Sourkes, T. L., Missala, K., and Belendiuk, G. (1972a). *Eur. J. Pharmacol.* **20,** 71.
Lal, S., de la Vega, C. E., Sourkes, T. L., and Friesen, H. G. (1972b). *Lancet* **2,** 661.
Lal, S., de la Vega, C. E., Sourkes, T. L., and Friesen, H. G. (1973a). *J. Clin. Endocrinol. Metab.* **37,** 719.
Lal, S., Martin, J. B., and Friesen, H. G. (1973b). *Clin. Res.* **21,** 1025.
Lal, S., de la Vega, C. E., Garelis, E., and Sourkes, T. L. (1973c). *Psychiatr., Neurol., Neurochir.* **76,** 113.
Lammers, A. J. J. C., and Van Rossum, J. M. (1968). *Eur. J. Pharmacol.* **5,** 103.
Langer, S. Z. (1973). *In* "Frontiers in Catecholamine Research" (E. Usdin and S. Snyder, eds.), p. 543. Pergamon, Oxford.
Langer, S. Z. (1974). *Biochem. Pharmacol.* **23,** 1793.
Langer, S. Z., Adler, F., Enero, M. A., and Stefano, F. J. E. (1971). *Int. Congr. Physiol. Sci. [Proc.], 25th, 1971,* p. 335.
Lapin, I. P., and Samsonova, M. L. (1968). *Farmakol. Toksikol. (Moscow)* **31,** 563.
Laville, C., and Margarit, J. (1964). *Pathol. Biol.* **12,** 726.
Liebman, J. M., and Butcher, L. L. (1973). *Naunyn-Schmiedeberg's Arch. Pharmacol.* **277,** 305.
Liuzzi, A., Chiodini, P. G., Botalla, L., Cremascoli, G., Müller, E. E., and Silvestrini, F. (1974). *J. Clin. Endocrinol. Metab.* **38,** 910.
Long, J. P., Heintz, S., Cannon, J. G., and Kim, J. (1975). *J. Pharmacol. Exp. Ther.* **192,** 336.
Lu, K. H., and Meites, J. (1972). *Endocrinology* **91,** 868.
Lütterbeck, P. M., Pryot, J. S., Varga, L., and Wenner, R. (1971). *Br. Med. J.* **3,** 228.
MacConaghy, N. (1969). *Br. J. Psychiatry* **115,** 723.

MacConaghy, N. (1970). *Br. J. Psychiatry* **117,** 555.
McCulloch, M. W., Rand, M. J., and Story, D. F. (1973). *Br. J. Pharmacol.* **49,** 141.
McDermed, J. D., McKenzie, G. M., and Phillips, A. P. (1975). *J. Med. Chem.* **18,** 000.
McGeer, E. G., Innanen, V. T., and McGeer, P. L. (1976). *Brain Res.* **118,** 356.
McKenzie, G. M. (1971). *Brain Res.* **34,** 323.
McKenzie, G. M. (1972). *Psychopharmacologia* **23,** 121.
McKenzie, G. M. (1974). *In* "Neuropsychopharmacology of Monoamines and their Regulatory Enzymes" (E. Usdin, ed.), p. 339. Raven, New York.
McKenzie, G. M., and Sadof, M. (1974). *J. Pharm. Pharmacol.* **26,** 281.
McKenzie, G. M., and White, H. L. (1973). *Biochem. Pharmacol.* **22,** 2329.
MacLeod, R. M. (1969). *Endocrinology* **85,** 916.
MacLeod, R. M., and Lehmeyer, J. E. (1973a). *Fed. Proc., Fed. Am. Soc. Exp. Biol.* **32,** 307. (Abstr.).
MacLeod, R. M., and Lehmeyer, J. E. (1973b). *Endocrinology, Suppl.* **92,** A-50.
MacLeod, R. M., Fontham, E. H., and Lehmeyer, J. E. (1970). *Neuroendocrinology* **6,** 283.
Maj, J. , Grabowska, M., and Gajda, L. (1972a). *Eur. J. Pharmacol.* **17,** 208.
Maj, J., Grabowska, M., Gajda, L., and Michaluk, J. (1972b). *Diss. Pharm. Pharmacol.* **24,** 4.
Maj, J., Sowinska, H., Baran, L., and Kapturkiewicz, Z. (1972c). *Diss. Pharm. Pharmacol.* **24,** 365.
Maj, J., Sowinska, H., and Baran, L. (1973). *Life Sci.* **12,** Part 1, 511.
Malmnäs, C. O. (1973). *Acta Physiol. Scand., Suppl.* **395.**
Martin, J. B., Lal, S., Tolis, G., and Friesen, H. G. (1974). *J. Clin. Endocrinol. Metab.* **39,** 180.
Matthiessen, A., and Wright, C. R. A. (1869). *Proc. R. Soc., Ser. B* **17,** 455.
Meldrum, B., Anlezark, G., and Trimble, M. (1975). *Eur. J. Pharmacol.* **32,** 203.
Mereu, G. P., Scarnati, E., Paglietti, E., Chessa, P., Di Chiara, G., and Gessa, G. L. (1977). *Neuropharmacology* (in press).
Meyerson,m B. J. (1964a). *Acta Physiol. Scand.* **63,** Suppl. 241.
Meyerson, B. J. (1964b). *Psychopharmacologia* **6,** 210.
Meyerson, B. J., and Lewander, T. (1970). *Life Sci.* **9,** 661.
Miller, R. J., and Iversen, L. L. (1974). *Naunyn-Schmiedeberg's Arch. Pharmacol.* **282,** 213.
Miller, R. J., Horn, A., Iversen, L. L., and Pinder, R. (1974). *Nature (London)* **250,** 238.
Mims, R. B., Smit, C. L., Modebe, O. M., and Bethune, J. E. (1973). *J. Clin. Endocrinol. Metab.* **37,** 660.
Missala, K., Lal, S., and Sourkes, T. L. (1973). *Eur. J. Pharmacol.* **22,** 54.
Miyai, K., Onishi, T., Osokawa, M., Ishibashi, K., and Kumahara, Y. (1974). *J. Clin. Endocrinol. Metab.* **39,** 391.
Morest, D. K. (1960). *Am. J. Anat.* **107,** 291.
Morest, D. K. (1966). *J. Comp. Neurol.* **130,** 277.
Moss, R. L., and McCann, S. M. (1973). *Science* **182,** 177.
Möller, Nielsen, I., Pedersen, V., Nymark, M., Franck, K. F., Boeck, V., Fjalland, B., and Cristensen, A. V. (1973). *Acta Pharmacol. Toxicol.* **33,** 353.
Müller, E. E., (1976). *Proc. Int. Congr. Pharmacol., 6th, 1975* Vol. 3, p. 131.
Naharski, S., Rogers, K. J., and Binns, J. (1973). *J. Pharm. Pharmacol.* **25,** 912.
Neff, N. H., and Costa, E. (1968). *J. Pharmacol. Exp. Ther.* **160,** 40.
Neill, D. B., Graut, L. D., and Grossman, S. P. (1972). *Physiol. Behav.* **9,** 655.

Neumeyer, J. L., Neustadt, B. R., and Weinhardt, K. K. (1970). *J. Pharm. Sci.* **59,** 1850.
Neumeyer, J. L. , Neustadt, B. R., Weinhardt, K. K., Boyce, C. B., Rosemberg, F. J., and Teiger, D. G. (1973a). *J. Med. Chem.* **16,** 1223.
Neumeyer, J. L., McCarthy, M., Battista, S. P., Rosemberg, F. J., and Teiger, D. G. (1973b). *J. Med. Chem.* **16,** 1228.
Neumeyer, J. L., Granchelli, F. F., Fuxe, K., Ungerstedt, U., and Corrodi, H. (1974). *J. Med. Chem.* **16,** 1228.
Niemegeers, C. J. E. (1971). *Pharmacology* **6,** 353.
Nybäck, H., and Sedvall, G. (1968). *J. Pharmacol. Exp. Ther.* **162,** 294.
Nybäck, H., and Sedvall, G. (1971). *J. Pharm. Pharmacol.* **23,** 322.
Nybäck, H., Schubert, J., and Sedvall, G. (1970). *J. Pharm. Pharmacol.* **22,** 622.
Nymark, M. (1972). *Psychopharmacologia* **26,** 361.
Ojeda, S. R., Harms, P. G., and McCann, S. M. (1974). *Endocrinology* **95,** 1694.
O'Keeffe, R., Sharman, D. F., and Vogt, M. (1970). *Br. J. Pharmacol.* **38,** 287.
Pasteels, J. L., Danguy, A. Frerotte, M., and Ectors, F. (1971). *Ann. Endocrinol.* **32,** 188.
Pedersen, V. (1967). *Acta Pharmacol. Toxicol..* **25,** Suppl. **4,** 63.
Peng, M. T., and Wang, S. C. (1962). *Proc. Soc. Exp. Biol. Med.* **110,** 211.
Perez-Cruet, J., Di Chiara, G., and Gessa, G. L. (1972). *Experientia* **28,** 926.
Persson, T. (1970). *Acta Pharmacol. Toxicol.* **28,** 378.
Persson, T., and Waldeck, B. (1970a). *Acta Physiol. Scand.* **78,** 142.
Persson, T., and Waldeck, B. (1970b). *Eur. J. Pharmacol.* **11,** 315.
Pfaff, D. W. (1973). *Science* **182,** 1148.
Phillipson, O. T., and Horn, A. S. (1976). *Nature (London)* **261,** 418.
Pi, W. P., and Peng, M. T. (1971). *Proc. Soc. Exp. Biol. Med.* **136,** 802.
Pieri, L., and Pieri, M. (1974). *J. Pharmacol.* **5,** 77.
Pijnenburg, A. J. J., and Van Rossum, J. M. (1973). *J. Pharm. Pharmacol.* **25,** 1003.
Pijnenburg, A. J. J., Woodruff, G. N., and Van Rossum, J. M. (1973). *Brain Res.* **59,** 289.
Pinder, R. M., Buxton, D. A., and Green, D. M. (1971). *J. Pharm. Pharmacol.* **23,** 995.
Pinder, R. M., Buxton, D. A., and Woodruff, G. N. (1972). *J. Pharm. Pharmacol.* **24,** 903.
Podolsky, S., and Leopold, N. A. (1973). *Prog. Brain Res.* **39,** 225.
Poignant, J. C., Gressier, H., and Malecot, E. (1974a). *Eur. J. Pharmacol.* **29,** 195.
Poignant, J. C., Lejeune, F., Malecot, E., Petitjean, M., Regnier, G., and Canevari, R. (1974b). *Experientia* **30,** 70.
Post, R. M., Gerner, R. H., Carman, J. S., and Bunney, W. E., Jr. (1976). *Lancet* **00,** 203.
Premont, J., Thierry, A. M., Tassin, J. P., Glowinski, J., Blanc, G., and Bockaert, J. (1976). *FEBS Lett.* **68,** 99.
Price, M. T. C., and Fibiger, H. C. (1974). *Eur. J. Pharmacol.* **29,** 249.
Puech, A. J., Simon P., Chermat, R., and Boissier, J. R. (1974). *J. Pharmacol. (Paris)* **5,** 224.
Puri, S. K., Reddy, C., and Lal, H. (1973). *Res. Commun. Chem. Pathol. Pharmacol.* **5,** 389.
Quinn, J. T., and Kerr, W. S. (1963). *J. Ir. Med. Assoc.* **53,** 50.
Quock, R. M., and Horita, A. (1974). *Science* **183,** 539.
Quock, R. M., Carino, M. A., and Horita, A. (1975). *Life Sci.* **16,** 525.
Rall, T., and Sattin, A. (1970). *In* "Role of Cyclic AMP in Cell Function" (P. Greengard and E. Costa, eds.), p. 113. Raven, New York.
Read, G. W., Cutting, W., and Furst, A. (1960). *Psychopharmacol. (Berl.)* **1,** 346.
Rekker, R. F., Engel, D. J. C., and Nys, G. G. (1972). *J. Pharm. Pharmacol.* **24,** 589.
Rinvik, E., and Grofova, I. (1970). *Exp. Brain Res.* **11,** 229.
Roberts, D. C. S., Zis, A. P., and Fibiger, H. C. (1975). *Brain Res.* **93,** 441.

Robison, G. A., Butcher, R. W., and Sutherland, E. W. (1967). *Ann. N.Y. Acad. Sci.* **139,** 703.

Rohr, V. U. (1966). *Z. Zellforsch. Mikrosk. Anat.* **73,** 246.

Rommelspacher, H., and Kuhar, M. J. (1975). *Life Sci.* **16,** 71.

Roos, B. E. (1969). *J. Pharm. Pharmacol.* **21,** 263.

Roth, R. H., Walters, J. R., Murrin, L. C., and Morgenroth, V. H. (1975). *In* "Pre- and Post-Synaptic Receptors" (E. Usdin and W. E. Bunney, eds.), p. 5. Dekker, New York.

Roth, R. H., Murrin, L. C., and Walters, J. R. (1976). *Eur. J. Pharmacol.* **36,** 163.

Rotrosen, J., Wallach, M. B., Angrist, B., and Gershon, S. (1972a). *Psychopharmacologia* **26,** 185.

Rotrosen, J., Angrist, B. M., Wallach, M. B., and Gershon, S. (1972b). *Eur. J. Pharmacol.* **20,** 133.

Rowe, W. S. (1967). *Med. J. Aust.* **2,** 637.

Rylander, G. (1969). *In* "Abuse of Central Stimulants" (F. Sjöqvist and M. Motte, eds.), p. 251. Raven, New York.

Saari, W. S., King, S. W., and Lotti, V. J. (1973). *J. Med. Chem.* **16,** 171.

Saari, W. S., King, S. W., Lotti, V. J., and Scriabine, A. (1974). *J. Med. Chem.* **17,** 1087.

Sasame, H. A., Perez-Cruet, J., Di Chiara, G., Tagliamonte, A., Tagliamonte, P., and Gessa, G. L. (1971). *Riv. Farmacol. Ter.* **11,** 99.

Sasame, H. A., Perez-Cruet, J., Di Chiara, G., Tagliamonte, A., Tagliamonte, P., and Gessa, G. L. (1972). *J. Neurochem.* **19,** 1953.

Sattin, A. (1971). *J. Neurochem.* **18,** 1087.

Scheel-Krüger, J. (1970). *Acta Pharmacol. Toxicol.* **28,** 1.

Scheel-Krüger, J., and Hasselager, E. (1974). *Psychopharmacologia* **36,** 189.

Schelkunov, E. L. (1967). *Nature (London)***214,** 1210.

Schelkunov, E. L. (1971). *In* "Problems of the Pharmacology of Psychotropic," p. 98. Riga.

Schoenfeld, R. I., and Uretsky, N. J. (1972). *Eur. J. Pharmacol.* **19,** 115.

Schoenfeld, R. I., Neumeyer, J. L., Dafeldecker, W., and Roffler-Tarlov, S. (1975). *Eur. J. Pharmacol.* **30,** 63.

Schwab, R. S., Amador, L. V., and Lettvin, J. Y. (1951). *Trans. Am. Neurol. Assoc.* **76,** 251.

Schwyn, R. C., and Tox, C. A. (1974). *J. Hirnforsch.* **15,** 95.

Scriabine, A., and Stavorski, J. M. (1973). *Eur. J. Pharmacol.* **24,** 101.

Seeds, N. W., and Gilman, A. G. (1971). *Science* **174,** 292.

Seki, K., and Seki, M. (1974). *J. Clin. Endocrinol. Metab.* **38,** 508.

Seki, K., Seki, M., and Okumura, T. (1974). *J. Clin. Endocrinol. Metab.* **39,** 206.

Senault, B. (1970). *Psychopharmacologia* **18,** 271.

Senault, B. (1971). *Psychopharmacologia* **20,** 389.

Senault, B. (1972). *Psychopharmacologia* **24,** 476.

Senault, B. (1973). *Psychopharmacologia* **28,** 13.

Senault, B. (1974). *Psychopharmacologia* **34,** 143.

Sethy, V. H., and Van Woert, M. H. (1973). *Neuropharmacology* **12,** 27.

Shaar, C. J., and Clemens, J. A. (1974). *Endocrinology* **95,** 1202.

Shaar, C. J., Smalsig, E. B., and Clemens, J. A. (1973). *Pharmacologist* **15,** 256.

Sheppard, H., and Wiggan, G. (1971). *Biochem. Pharmacol.* **20,** 2128.

Shields, K. G., Ballinger, C. M., and Hathaway, B. N. (1971). *Anesth. Analg.* **50,** 1017.

Shimizu, N., and Ishii, S. (1964). *Z. Zellforsch. Mikrosk. Anat.* **64,** 462.

Shintomi, K., and Yamamura, M. (1975). *Eur. J. Pharmacol.* **31,** 273.

Small, U., Faris, B. F., and Mallonee, J. E. (1940). *J. Org. Chem.* **5,** 334.

Smalstig, E. B., Sawyer, B. D., and Clemens, J. A. (1974). *Endocrinology* **95,** 123.
Smith, C. C., Lehman, E. G., and Gilfillan, J. L. (1951). *Fed. Proc., Fed. Am. Soc. Exp. Biol.* **10,** 335.
Smith, R. V., and Cook, M. R. (1974). *J. Pharm. Sci.* **63,** 161.
Smith, R. V., and Sood, S. P. (1971). *J. Pharm. Sci.* **60,** 1654.
Smith, R. V., Cook, M. R., and Stockinski, A. W. (1973). *J. Chromatogr.* **87,** 294.
Snyder, S. H. (1973). *Am. J. Psychiatry* **130,** 61.
Snyder, T. E., Patrick, R. L., and Barchas, J. D. (1976). *Proc. Int. Congr. Pharmacol., 6th, 1975* Abstract No. 193.
Sollmann, A. (1957). *In* "A Manual of Pharmacology and its Application to Therapeutics and Toxicology," 8th ed., p. 000. Saunders, Philadelphia, Pennsylvania.
Spano, P. F., Kumakura, K., Tonon, G., Govoni, S., and Trabucchi, M. (1975). *Brain Res.* **9,** 164.
Spano, P. F., Di Chiara, G., Tonon, G., and Trabucchi, M. (1976). *J. Neurochem.* **27,** 1565.
Spano, P. F., Trabucchi, M., and Di Chiara, G. (1977). *Science* **196,** 1343.
Spissu, A., Corsini, G. U., Mangoni, A., and Gessa, G. L. (1975). *Psychopharmacologia* **44,** 311.
Srimal, R. C., and Dhawan, B. N. (1970). *Psychopharmacologia* **18,** 99.
Stadler, H., Lloyd, K. G., Gadea-Ciria, M., and Bartholini, G. (1973). *Brain Res.* **55,** 476.
Stähelin, H., Burckhardt-Vischer, B., and Flückiger, E. (1971). *Experientia* **27,** 915.
Starke, K. (1971). *Naturwissenschaften* **58,** 420.
Starke, K., and Altmann, K. P. (1973). *Neuropharmacology* **12,** 339.
St. Laurent, J., Leclerc, R. R., Mitchell, M. L., and Miliaressis, T. E. (1973). *Pharmacol., Biochem. Behav.* **1,** 581.
Stone, T. W. (1973). *Arch. Int. Pharmacodyn. Ther.* **202,** 62.
Strian, F., Micheler, E., and Benkert, O. (1972). *Pharmakopsychiatrie Neuro-Psychopharmakol.* **5,** 198.
Strömbom, U. (1976). *Naunyn-Schmiedeberg's Arch. Pharmacol.* **262,** 167.
Struppler, A., and von Uexküll, T. (1953). *Z. Klin. Med.* **152,** 46.
Sulman, F. G. (1970). *In* "Hypothalamic Control of Lactation" (F. G. Sulman, ed.), p. 1. Springer-Verlag, Berlin and New York.
Tagliamonte, A., Fratta, W., Del Fiacco, M., and Gessa, G. L. (1974a). *Pharmacol. Biochem. Behav.* **2,** 257.
Tagliamonte, A., Fratta, W., and Gessa, G. L. (1974b). *Experientia* **30,** 381.
Takahara, J., Arimura, A., and Schally, A. V. (1974). *Endocrinology* **95,** 462.
Talaori, S., Tsakai, Y., Matsuoka, J., Sasa, M., Fukuda, N., and Shimmamoto, K. (1968). *Int. J. Neuropharmacol.* **7,** 115.
Takaori, S., Fukuda, N., and Amano, Y. (1970). *Jpn. J. Pharmacol.* **20,** 424.
Tarsy, D., and Baldessarini, R. J. (1973). *Nature (London), New Biol.* **245,** 262.
Tarsy, D., and Baldessarini, R. J. (1974). *Neuropharmacology* **13,** 927.
Tattersall, R. M. (1971). *Practitioner* **206,** 111.
Taylor, K. M., and Snyder, S. H. (1970). *Science* **168,** 1487.
Terada, C. W., and Masur, J. (1973). *Eur. J. Pharmacol.* **24,** 375.
Ther, L., and Schramm, H. (1962). *Arch. Int. Pharmacodyn. Ther.* **138,** 302.
Thornburg, J. E., and Moore, K. E. (1974). *Neuropharmacology* **13,** 189.
Thornburg, J. E., and Moore, K. E. (1975). *J. Pharmacol. Exp. Ther.* **192,** 42.
Tolis, G., Del Pozo, E., and Goldstein, M. S. (1972). *Endocrinology, Suppl.* **92,** A-50.
Tolosa, E. S., and Sparber, S. B. (1974). *Life Sci.* **15,** 1371.
Tompkins, J. E. (1899). *Med. Rec.* **55,** 56.

Torack, R. M., and Finke, E. H. (1971). *Z. Zellforsch. Mikrosk. Anat.* **118,** 85.
Trabucchi, M., Cheney, D., Racagni, G., and Costa, E. (1974). *Nature (London)* **249,** 664.
Turkington, R. W. (1972). *J. Clin. Endocrinol. Metab.* **34,** 306.
Ungerstedt, U. (1971a). *Acta Physiol. Scand., Suppl.* **367,** 69.
Ungerstedt, U. (1971b). *Acta Physiol. Scand., Suppl.* **367,** 95.
Ungerstedt, U., Bütcher, L. L., Butcher, S. G., Andén, N. E., and Fuxe, K. (1969). *Brain Res.* **14,** 461.
Van Rossum, J. M. (1970). *Int. Rev. Neurobiol.* **12,** 307.
Van Tyle, W. K., and Burkman, A. M. (1970). *J. Pharm. Sci.* **59,** 1757.
Van Tyle, W. K., and Burkman, A. M. (1971). *J. Pharm. Sci.* **60,** 1736.
Van Zwieten-Boot, B. J., and Noach, E. L. (1975). *Eur. J. Pharmacol.* **33,** 247.
Varga, L., Lütterbeck, P. M., Pryot, J. S., Wenner, R., and Erb, H. (1972). *Br. Med. J.* **2,** 743.
Varga, L., Wenner, R., and Del Pozo, E. (1973). *Am. J. Obstet. Gynecol.* **117,** 75.
Vedernikov Yu. P. (1970). *Psychopharmacologia* **17,** 283.
Vernier, V. G., and Unna, K. R. (1951). *J. Pharmacol. Exp. Ther.* **103,** 365.
Villeneuve, A., and Böszörményi, Z. (1970). *Lancet* **1,** 353.
Vogt, M. (1954). *J. Physiol. (London)* **123,** 451.
Von Hungen, H., and Roberts, S. (1973). *Eur. J. Pharmacol.* **36,** 391.
von Voigtlander, P. F., and Moore, K. E. (1973a). *Neuropharmacology* **12,** 451.
von Voigtlander, P. F., and Moore, K. E. (1973b). *J. Pharmacol. Exp. Ther.* **184,** 542.
Wallach, M. B., Angrist, B., and Gershon, S. (1972). *Eur. J. Pharmacol.* **18,** 22.
Walters, J. R., and Roth, R. H. (1974). *J. Pharmacol. Exp. Ther.* **191,** 82.
Wang, S. C. (1965). *Physiol. Pharmacol.* **2,** 255.
Wang, S. C., and Borison, H. L. (1952). *Gastroenterology* **22,** 1.
Wang, S. C., and Glaviano, V. V. (1954). *J. Pharmacol. Exp. Ther.* **111,** 329.
Wauquier, A., and Niemegeers, C. J. E. (1973). *Psychopharmacologia* **30,** 163.
Weindl, A. (1973). *In* "Frontiers in Neuroendocrinology" (W. F. Ganong and L. Martini, eds.), p. 3. Oxford Univ. Press, London and New York.
Weissman, A. (1966). *Arch. Int. Pharmacodyn. Ther.* **160,** 330.
Weissmann, A., Koe, B. K., and Tenen, S. S. (1966). *J. Pharmacol. Exp. Ther.* **151,** 339.
Westfall, T. C., Besson, M.-J., Giorguieff, M.-F., and Glowinski, J. (1976). *Naunyn-Schmiedeberg's Arch. Pharmacol.* **292,** 279.
White, H. L., and McKenzie, G. M. (1971). *Pharmacologist* **13,** 313.
Whitnack, E., Leff, A., and Gaffney, T. E. (1970). *Fed. Proc., Fed. Am. Soc. Exp. Biol.* **29,** 742.
Whitnack, E., Leff, A., Mohammed, S., and Gaffney, T. E. (1971). *J. Pharmacol. Exp. Ther.* **177,** 409.
Whitsett, T. L., Halushka, P. V., Ryan, H., and Goldberg, L. I.(1970a). *Fed. Proc., Fed. Am. Soc. Exp. Biol.* **29,** 742. (abstr.).
Whitsett, T. L., Halushka, P. V., and Goldberg, L. I. (1970b). *Cir. Res.* **27,** 561.
Willner, J. H., Samach, M., Angrist, B. M., Wallach, M. B., and Gershon, S. (1970). *Commun. Behav. Biol.* **5,** 135.
Wilson, C. W. M., and Brodie, B. (1961). *J. Pharmacol. Exp. Ther.* **133,** 332.
Wilson, C. W. M., Murray, A. W., and Titus, E. (1962). *J. Pharmacol. Exp. Ther.* **135,** 11.
Winter, C. A., Orahovats, P. D., Flataker, L., Lehman, E. G., and Lehman, J. T. (1954). *J. Pharmacol. Exp. Ther.* **111,** 152.
Wislocki, G. B., and King, L. S. (1936). *Am. J. Anat.* **58,** 421.
Wolfarth, S. (1974). *Pharmacol., Biochem. Behav.* **2,** 181.
Woodruff, G. N. (1971). *Compt. Gen. Pharmacol.* **2,** 439.

Woodruff, G. N., and Walker, R. J. (1969). *Int. J. Neuropharmacol.* **8,** 279.
Woodruff, G. N., Elkhawad, A. O., and Crossman, A. R. (1974). *J. Pharm. Pharmacol.* **26,** 456.
Yarbrough, G. G. (1975). *Eur. J. Pharmacol.* **31,** 367.
Yehuda, S., and Wurtman, R. J. (1972). *Nature (London)* **240,** 477.
Zivkovič, B., and Guidotti, A. (1974). *Brain Res.* **79,** 505.
Zivkovič, B., Guidotti, A., and Costa, E. (1974). *Mol. Pharmacol.* **10,** 727.

Note Added in Proof

Since this review was completed, several important articles have appeared on the ability of DA-receptor agonists and antagonists to bind stereospecifically and with high affinity to membranes of brain dopaminergic areas. These studies show that apomorphine competes with DA for this binding and provides a direct measurement of its ability to interact with DA receptors.

References for Note Added in Proof

Burt, D. R., Enna, S. J., Creese, L., Snyder, S. H. (1975) *Proc. Natl. Acad. Sci. U.S.A.* **72,** 4655.
Seeman, P., Chau-Wong, M., Tedesco, J., Wong K. (1975). *Proc. Natl. Acad. Sci. U.S.A.* **72,** 4376.
Seeman, P., Lee, T., Chau-Wong, M., Tedesco, J., Wong, K. (1976). *Proc. Natl. Acad. Sci.* U.S.A. **73,** 4354.

Structural Requirements for Tetracycline Activity

J. R. BROWN AND D. S. IRELAND*

Department of Pharmacy
University of Manchester
Manchester, England

I. Introduction

Although the tetracyclines are broad-spectrum antibiotics with low host toxicity, their usage has diminished in recent years. They are no longer first-line drugs for the treatment of staphylococcal, streptococcal, or pneumococcal infections but are currently considered as second-line antibiotics (Finland, 1974). They are reserved mainly for specific indications such as the treatment of respiratory infections, mixed infections, acne vulgaris, rickettsial infections, and some sensitive gram-negative infections. Their usage is restricted in this manner because more specific antibiotics have become available. The broad-spectrum penicillins, for example, have displaced them from their role as first choice, oral, broad-

* Present address: Fazakerley Hospital, Liverpool, England.

spectrum antibiotics since the tetracyclines have some disadvantages not shared by the penicillin group of drugs. Currently, therefore, ampicillin and its congeners are the broad-spectrum orally active antibiotics of choice in most cases. A major drawback of the tetracyclines is that they are deposited in calcified tissue resulting in staining and even impairment of the structure of bone and teeth. They are thereby unsuitable for use in infants and children up to 12 years of age and also during pregnancy as they are able to cross the placenta. Furthermore, the older members of the group are not completely absorbed orally, and unabsorbed drug inhibits the normal flora of the intestine. The newer tetracyclines, notably doxycycline, are completely absorbed, however, and so do not have such a marked effect on the gut flora. Thus one undesirable characteristic of the tetracyclines has been eliminated. A final drawback of this group of antibiotics is that, due to overusage, a high degree of resistance has developed, particularly in the hospital environment, and so other antibiotics are naturally preferred unless the tetracyclines are specifically indicated. Nevertheless, the tetracyclines do have many meritorious properties, in particular their breadth of spectrum, their lack of cross-resistance with the penicillins and cephalosporins, and their low host toxicity. Whereas the penicillins and even the cephalosporins give rise to an allergic response in a relatively high proportion of patients, this does not occur with the tetracyclines, although there is a low incidence of phototoxicity.

Even though the tetracyclines are at present of secondary importance to the penicillins and cephalosporins, they are still a most necessary group of drugs because it is imperative to have at hand orally active, alternative, broad-spectrum antibiotics that are not structurally related to the broad-spectrum penicillins. This is of growing importance as there is a continuing emergence of organisms that are resistant to ampicillin and the cephalosporins. A reappraisal of the structural requirements for activity within the tetracycline group of antibiotics is, therefore, appropriate. This is particularly the case since much of the work on the mode of action and selectivity of action of tetracyclines corroborates the evidence from semisynthesis, which has led to the identification of those features that are essential for tetracycline activity. Also the risk of incidence of tetracycline-resistant infections may now have lessened due to the decreased use of tetracycline in medicine, especially hospitals, and due to the justifiable restriction from use as feed additives in animal husbandry.

This review seeks to delineate the structural requirements for tetracycline activity. No attempt will be made to review completely the overwhelming amount of literature regarding the tetracyclines, which has accumulated since the first isolation of chlortetracycline in 1947. Instead, this review will be restricted to the identification of those features that are responsible for the antibacterial effect and for optimal distribution within the body. In considering the action of an antibiotic, it is not sufficient to study just one aspect, for example the antibacterial activity or structure–activity relationships (using the structural analog, or quantum-mechanical or Hansch approaches), or the mechanism and selectivity of action, or the disposition within the body. All these effects must be correlated. Fortunately, the tetracyclines have been investigated very thoroughly and so each of these areas can be discussed, thereby allowing an appreciation of the features that would be embodied in the "ideal" tetracycline drug.

II. Structure–Activity Relationships

A. Biosynthetic Tetracyclines

Chlortetracycline [Fig. 1(I)], the first member of the tetracycline group to be discovered, was first isolated by Duggar in 1947 from *Streptomyces aureofaciens* during a systematic screening of microorganisms for antimicrobial products (Duggar, 1948) and was followed by the isolation of oxytetracycline [Fig. 1(II)] from *Streptomyces rimosus* (Finlay *et al.*, 1950). Tetracycline [Fig. 1(III)], the parent member of the group, was initially prepared by reductive hydrogenolysis of chlortetracycline

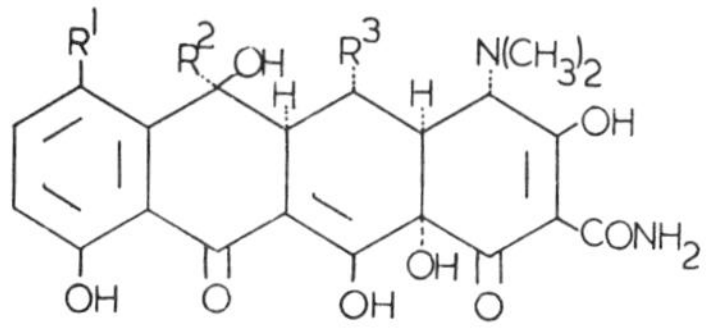

	R^1	R^2	R^3
Chlortetracycline (I)	Cl	CH_3	H
Oxytetracycline (II)	H	CH_3	OH
Tetracycline (III)	H	CH_3	H
Bromotetracycline (IV)	Br	CH_3	H
Demethyltetracycline (V)	H	H	H
Demethylchlortetracycline (VI)	Cl	H	H

FIG. 1. Biosynthetic tetracyclines.

(Boothe *et al.,* 1953; Conover *et al.,* 1953) and subsequently by fermentation (Minieri *et al.,* 1953; Doerschuk *et al.,* 1956). These three antibiotics possess essentially equivalent antibacterial activities. Early attempts to produce improved tetracyclines involved modification of the fermentation conditions, for example the initial isolation of tetracycline was from *S. aureofaciens* (the chlortetracycline-producing organism) grown in a chloride-free medium. Another example is the isolation of bromotetracycline [Fig. 1(IV)] from the same organism grown in the presence of high levels of bromide (Sensi *et al.,* 1955). It proved more difficult to modify the biosynthetic pathway, however, than was the case with the penicillins since tetracyclines are biosynthesized by the acetate pathway (Snell *et al.,* 1956; Miller *et al.*, 1956; Gatenbeck, 1961) and this, by its very nature, is not amenable to modification by addition of alternative precursors.

Although it was not possible to produce a wide range of new tetracyclines by addition of alternative precursors, blocked mutant organisms could be induced. By using these organisms and the "blocked" intermediates, the biosynthetic pathway to the tetracyclines was elucidated. This work was carried out mainly by McCormick and has been the subject of extensive reviews (McCormick, 1965, 1967; Turley and Snell, 1966; Mitscher, 1968; Money and Scott, 1968). The first identifiable product in the pathway is 6-methylpretetramid (McCormick *et al.*, 1963) which then undergoes successive metabolic

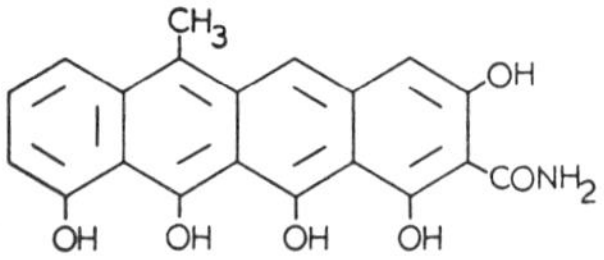

CH_3 OH $CONH_2$ OH OH OH OH

(VII)

reactions to yield the natural antibiotics. All the carbon atoms of 6-methylpretetramid come from acetate except the 6-methyl group which is donated by *S*-adenosylmethionine (Miller *et al.*, 1956). It might be expected, therefore, that deletion of this methyl donation stage would not affect the overall pathway, and, indeed, mutant strains of *S. aureofaciens* that produce 6-demethyltetracyclines (McCormick *et al.*, 1957b) have been isolated. Two of these, 6-demethyltetracycline [Fig. 1(V)] and 6-demethylchlortetracycline [Fig. 1(VI)] have been used quite extensively in medicine. They show comparable antibacterial activity to the natural tetracyclines. This proves that structural variation within the tetracycline molecule is possible without loss of activity at the 6-position as well as at the 5-position (oxytetracycline) and the 7-

position (chlortetracycline). A great deal more information on the effect of structural variation on antibacterial activity has been gleaned from study of semisynthetic derivatives, and this will be considered next.

B. Semisynthetic Tetracyclines

Chemical modification of a fermentation-derived antibiotic is termed *semisynthesis*; it is essentially a process of partial synthesis using the antibiotic as the starting point. Many semisynthetic tetracyclines have been prepared in an attempt to produce a drug with improved activity. This approach has been far more successful than attempts to develop a new biosynthetic tetracycline and has led to the introduction of semisynthetic tetracyclines such as lymecycline [Fig. 2(VIII)], doxycycline [Fig. 2(IX)], and minocycline [Fig. 2(X)]. A consideration of semisynthetic derivatives is pertinent since there are data available on the activity of a large number of structural analogs of the natural tetracyclines against a wide range of bacteria *in vitro* and also *in vivo* (Blackwood and English, 1977). This information will prove useful in determining the basic structural requirements for antibacterial activity and for elucidating the effect of structural variation on tetracycline activity. Previous reviews have been given by Boothe (1962), Barrett (1963), Blackwood and English (1970), Hlavka and Boothe (1973), and Dürckheimer (1975). In the present review, we attempt to identify the features required for activity and to explain the changes in antibacterial activity effected by changes in structure.

The tetracyclines contain two distinct π-electron systems: the phenoldiketone moiety and the tricarbonylmethane moiety (Fig. 3); these are independent due to the presence of the interposed 12*a*-hydroxy group (Fig. 3 gives the numbering of the tetracycline system). Both of these chromophoric groups must be retained intact otherwise activity is lost. Loss of activity, therefore, results from cleavage of one of the rings (Blackwood *et al.*, 1963) or from aromatization of the A or C ring (Green and Boothe, 1960) or from modification of the phenoldiketone moiety by 11*a*-substitution (Stephens *et al.*, 1963) or by deletion of the 12*a*-hydroxy group (Blackwood and English, 1970). It is, therefore, inferred that a compound must contain these groups otherwise it will not possess tetracycline-like activity. A further general requirement of a tetracycline analog is that the oxygenation pattern of the natural tetracyclines is retained (Korst *et al.*, 1968). This would be expected from a consideration of current knowledge on the mode of action of the tetracyclines, which will be discussed later.

Structure–activity relationships of the semisynthetic tetracyclines are

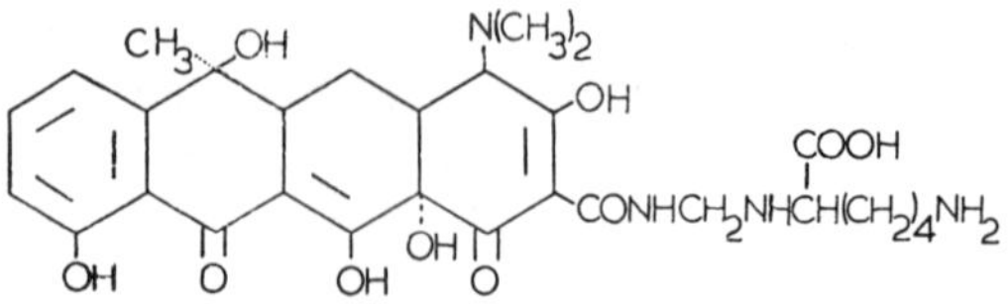

Lymecycline (VIII)

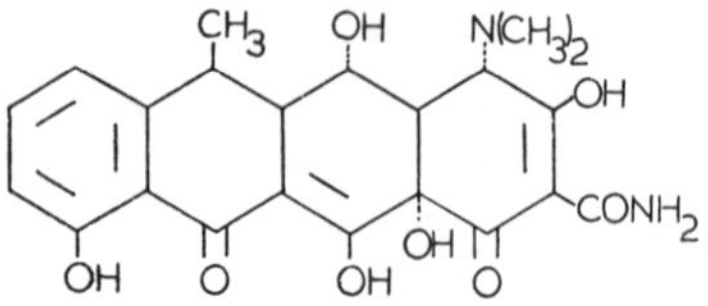

Doxycycline (IX)

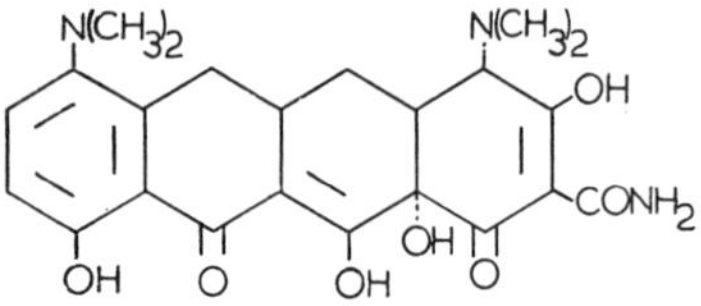

Minocycline (X)

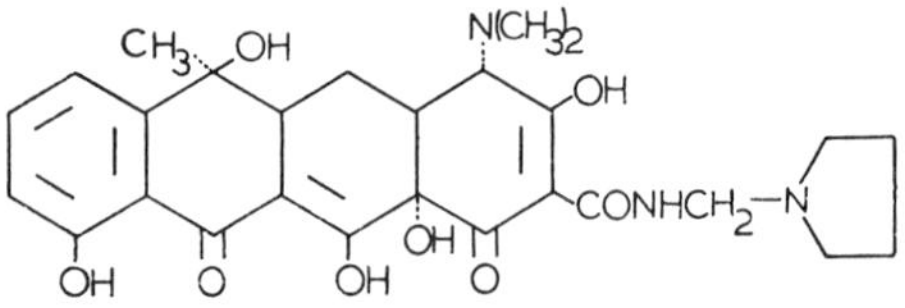

Rolitetracycline (XI)

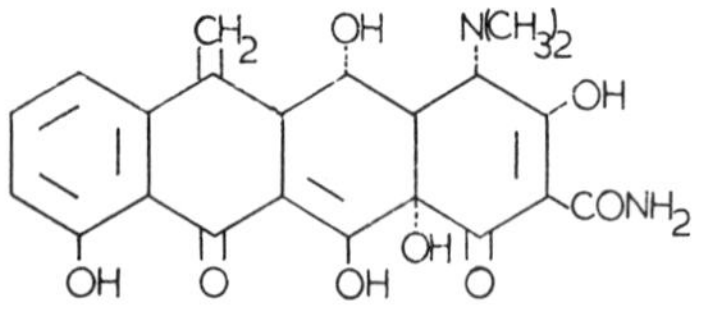

Methacycline (XII)

FIG. 2. Semisynthetic tetracylines.

most conveniently discussed by considering each position of the hydronaphthacene ring skeleton in turn. Dürckheimer (1975) has stressed that when considering these relationships only a qualitative assessment of activity can be derived since the organisms and conditions may have varied when assessing the antibacterial activity of different semisynthetic tetracycline analogs. The results do not indicate clinical usefulness

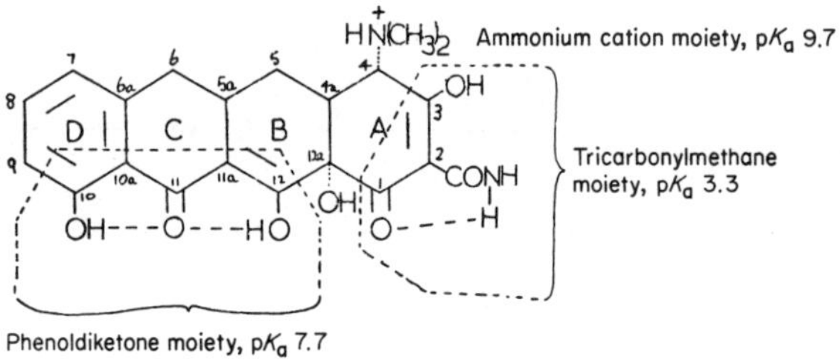

FIG. 3. The tetracycline ring system. The pK_a values quoted are for tetracycline itself; the values will vary for different members of the tetracycline group of antibiotics. (From Stephens *et al.*, 1956; Leeson *et al.*, 1963.)

but rather whether a particular chemical modification reduces, increases, or does not affect some antibacterial effect. This approach is used in interpreting the results of these studies in this review. Table I lists antibacterial activities of tetracycline analogs relative to tetracycline. These values have been culled from data presented by Blackwood and English (1970) and Hlavka and Boothe (1973); the table is complementary to the following discussion on semisynthetic tetracyclines.

1. *C1–3*

Since the tricarbonylmethane group must be present intact for retention of tetracycline activity there must be a keto group at positions 1 and 3, and a carbonyl substituent at position 2. Thus the analog with a nitrile group at position 2 is inactive (Stephens *et al.*, 1963). Although active derivatives at this position have been prepared, for example rolitetracycline [Fig. 2(XI)] (Gottstein *et al.*, 1959), these are labile and are only active *in vivo* after hydrolysis to the parent carbonyl compound. Nevertheless, 2-acetyl-2-decarboxamidotetracycline retains some activity as do several derivatives substituted on the carboxamide nitrogen (Miller and Hochstein, 1962). This demonstrates that it is solely the carbonyl group rather than the total amide function that is the requirement for maintenance of activity. Compounds such as rolitetracycline do have a marginal advantage over tetracycline in parenteral use as they are more water-soluble, although it should be realized that rolitetracycline, for example, will hydrolyze in solution to an equilibrium mixture of rolitetracycline and tetracycline (Hughes *et al.*, 1974).

2. *C4*

The dimethylamino function at the 4 position is essential for retention of antibacterial activity *in vivo* since deletion of this group leads to a

TABLE I

In Vitro ACTIVITIES RELATIVE TO TETRACYCLINE

Drug	Relative activity[a]
Tetracycline (III)	100
Chlortetracycline (I)	130–200
Oxytetracycline (II)	80
6-Demethylchlortetracycline (VI)	150
2-Nitrile analog of tetracycline	Inactive
Rolitetracycline (XI)	100
2-Acetyl-2-decarboxamidotetracycline	7
4-Dedimethylaminotetracycline	17
4-Epitetracycline	2
4-Oxime of tetracycline	Inactive
4-Hydrazone of tetracycline	0.4
5*a*,11*a*-Dehydrochlortetracycline	Inactive
5*a*,11*a*-Dehydro-6-epichlortetracycline	150
5*a*-Epitetracycline	Inactive
5*a*-Epi-6-epitetracycline	40
Anhydrotetracycline	30[b]
Isotetracycline	Inactive
Methacycline (6-methylene-6-demethyl-6-deoxytetracycline) (XII)	150
Doxycycline (α-6-deoxyoxytetracycline) (IX)	110
(β-6-Deoxyoxytetracycline)	50
6-Demethyl-6-deoxytetracycline	160
7-Nitro-6-demethyl-6-deoxytetracycline	640
7-Chloro-6-demethyl-6-deoxytetracycline	300
Minocycline (7-dimethylamino-6-demethyl-6-deoxytetracycline) (X)	200
7-Hydroxy-6-demethyl-6-deoxytetracycline	23
9-Nitro-6-demethyl-6-deoxytetracycline	12
9-Chloro-6-demethyl-6-deoxytetracycline	12
9-Amino-6-demethyl-6-deoxytetracycline	160
7-Amino-6-demethyl-6-deoxytetracycline	40
11*a*-Chloro-6-demethyl-6-deoxytetracycline	3
12*a*-Deoxy-6-demethyl-6-deoxytetracycline	Inactive
4*a*,12*a*-Anhydrotetracycline	0.4

[a] Approximate activity against *S. aureus* (Blackwood and English, 1970; Hlavka and Boothe, 1973); tetracycline = 100.

[b] Activity claimed to be due to a mode of action not typical of other tetracyclines (Koschel *et al.*, 1966).

reduction in *in vivo* activity and in *in vitro* activity against gram-negative organisms (McCormick *et al.*, 1957, 1960). A change in activity of this nature is indicative of a change in distribution characteristics. Since the pK_a of the dimethylamino group is 9.7, it would be expected that over 99% of the drug is ionized at physiological pH. This is not the only consideration, however, as there are three ionizable groups in the tetracycline molecule (Fig. 3) and at physiological pH the tetracycline is in the zwitterionic form. It is this form which has been shown to be the most lipophilic form of the tetracyclines (Colaizzi and Klink, 1969), explaining the requirement for the *N*-dimethylamino group for optimum distribution within the body and for *in vivo* activity. The relatively lipophilic nature of the zwitterion could be due to formation of an "internal salt" in which the positively charged dimethylammonium group interacts with the negatively charged tricarbonylmethane moiety. This gives an effective neutralization of charge, leading to the formation of a relatively lipid-soluble ion pair (Colaizzi and Klink, 1969; Tute, 1975). However, recent X-ray crystallographic studies show that there can be no major interaction between the positive and negative charges (Stezowski, 1976). As an alternative it has been suggested that it is the neutral molecule that is the partitioning species due to its higher lipophilicity, despite the fact that it is present only as an extremely low fraction of the total drug (Purich *et al.*, 1973; Terada and Inagi, 1975; Prewo and Stezowski, 1977). Whatever process is involved, the fact remains that greatest partitioning between an aqueous and a nonaqueous phase occurs between pH's of 5.0 to 6.5 (Colaizzi and Klink, 1969).

In conclusion, the substitution pattern on ring A must be retained totally for optimum tetracycline activity. The stereochemistry at the 4 position is also important since the analogs epimeric at this position have a greatly reduced activity (Kende *et al.*, 1961). The dimethylamino group is optimal because substitution with alternative alkyl functions shows that activity decreases as size of the alkyl group increases (Esse *et al.*, 1964). Derivatives such as the oxime, methiodide, and hydrazone have also been prepared but show little antibacterial activity (Boothe *et al.*, 1958; Blackwood and Stephens, 1964).

3. *C5*

Modification at the 5 position is possible with no loss of activity as evidenced by the activity of oxytetracycline which is 5-hydroxytetracycline. Furthermore, the acetyl (Barrett, 1963), alkoxy (Schach von Wittenau *et al.*, 1963), acyloxy, and formyloxy derivatives (Bernardi *et al.*, 1974) all retain antibacterial activity suggesting that the 5 position can be substituted with no detrimental effect to antibacterial activity.

4. *C5a*

There is some confusion over the effect of dehydrogenation of the 5*a*, 11*a* bond and the effect of changing the configuration at the 5*a* position.

5a,11a-Dehydrotetracyclines were first isolated as intermediates in the biosynthesis of tetracyclines and were found to have insignificant activity (McCormick *et al.*, 1958). By contrast, semisynthetic analogs that have the unnatural configuration at C6 show antibacterial activity both *in vivo* and *in vitro* (Martell *et al.*, 1967). It has been suggested that tautomerism occurs and that the 5,*5a*-dehydro derivative is the active entity (Blackwood and English, 1970). Similarly, epimerization at the *5a* position generally results in loss of activity, the exception again being the analog that has the unnatural configuration at the 6 position (Blackwood and English, 1970). There is no obvious explanation for these anomalies, although, since it is the 6-hydroxy group that confers instability on the molecule, it would be informative to investigate the relative stabilities of all these compounds.

5. *C6*

The isolation of the 6-demethyltetracyclines (described earlier) which have equivalent antibacterial activity to their 6-methyl analogs demonstrated that favorable modification at the 6 position is possible. The presence of the 6-methyl group is, therefore, not essential for activity. In fact the 6-demethyl compounds have a greater stability toward base and slightly enhanced clinical properties since blood levels are sustained longer than for their 6-methyl analogs. Deletion of the 6-hydroxy group by catalytic hydrogenation also has no detrimental effect on activity (McCormick *et al.*, 1960). Indeed, it is the 6-hydroxy function that is involved in both the acidic and basic degradation of the tetracyclines yielding the anhydrotetracyclines and isotetracyclines, respectively (Stephens *et al.*, 1954; Waller *et al.*, 1952; Clive, 1968; Schlecht and Frank, 1975).

The degradation reactions for tetracycline are shown in Fig. 4; although other tetracyclines possessing the 6-hydroxy group are acid- and alkali-labile, the nature of the reaction and the products can vary. Since anhydrotetracyclines have reduced activity (McCormick *et al.*, 1960) and the isotetracyclines are inactive (Boothe, 1962), deletion of the 6-hydroxy group is highly desirable. Further, because 6-deoxytetracyclines are stable they can be used as the starting point for the preparation of other derivatives, for example the 6-methylenetetracyclines (Blackwood *et al.*, 1963) which show excellent antibacterial activity and stability. One of these compounds, methacycline [Fig. 2(XII)], is used clinically. These 6-methylenetetracyclines can be used as intermediates for the preparation of other C6-modified tetracyclines, the most important of which is doxycycline [Fig. 2(IX)] (6-deoxytetracycline)

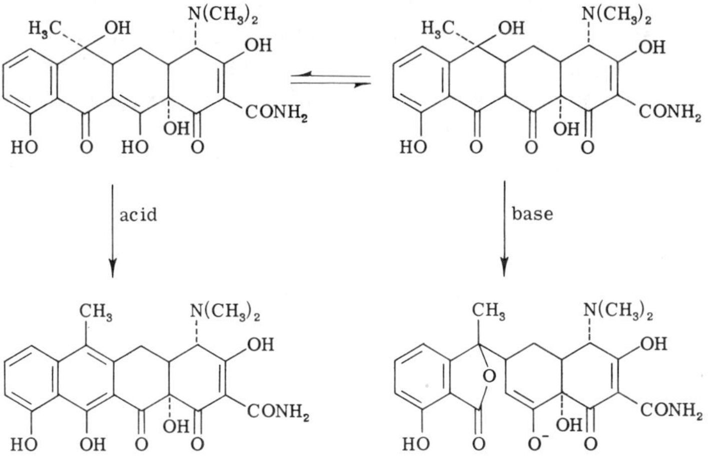

FIG. 4. Acid- and base-catalyzed degradation of tetracycline.

which is now widely established in clinical practice. It shows equivalent antibacterial activity to tetracycline but is much more stable. It should be noted that in doxycycline there has been an inversion to the unnatural α-configuration at the 6 position (Schach von Wittenau *et al.*, 1962); the β-deoxytetracycline has a marginally lower antibacterial activity. Complete replacement of C6 and its substituents by a sulfur atom leads to a retention of activity as would be expected (Rogalski *et al.*, 1976).

6. *Substitution on the D Ring*

Since the 6-deoxytetracyclines are acid-stable, acid-catalyzed substitution reactions can be carried out, whereas this was not possible with the analogous 6-hydroxy compounds. Analogs substituted at the 7 and 9 positions have, therefore, been prepared by electrophilic substitution reactions (Hlavka *et al.*, 1962; Petisi *et al.*, 1962). Many of these compounds possess good *in vivo* activity and the most important compound is 7-dimethylamino-6-demethyl-6-deoxytetracycline, minocycline [Fig. 2(X)] which shows increased activity against many organisms and is also active against many tetracycline-resistant bacteria (Martell and Boothe, 1967; Redin, 1966; Steigbigel *et al.*, 1968).

Several attempts have been made to correlate antibacterial activity with substitution in the D ring either by the Free–Wilson approach (Free and Wilson, 1964; Purcell *et al.*, 1973) or by correlation with physicochemical parameters. No direct correlation was found between antibacterial activity *in vitro* and π value, a measure of the lipophilic nature of the molecule (Collett *et al.*, 1970), but there is a stronger correlation between activity and electronic structure (Cammarata *et al.*, 1970; Peradejordi *et al.*, 1971). Results from semisynthesis indicate that, in general, electron-withdrawing groups at C7 (for example, chloro and nitro) enhance *in vitro* activity and, conversely, electron-donating groups decrease activity. The enhanced activity of 6-methylenetetracyclines (for example, methacycline) can also be explained by this type of electronic effect.

There are, however, some exceptions to this generalization, for example, the 7-dimethylamino derivative, minocycline, would be expected to have lower activity than the parent compound since it has an electron-donating group; in fact, it has increased activity. It has been suggested that the dimethylamino group, which is unionized at physiological pH, becomes protonated in the biophase due to a region of lower pH, thus conferring electron-withdrawing rather than electron-donating properties (Blackwood and English, 1970). Minocycline, however, is considerably more lipophilic than the other tetracyclines and it is more likely that the anomaly regarding this compound is due to differences in uptake of this more lipophilic compound into bacterial cells. It must be borne in mind that *in vitro* tests for antibacterial activity will reflect both the uptake of the drug into the cell as well as the activity at the receptor site. It is known that minocycline is active against tetracycline-resistant organisms (Redin, 1966), and, since tetracycline resistance is due to impairment of the active uptake of tetracyclines into the cell, it can be inferred that uptake of minocycline may not be typical of other tetracyclines. The apparent increase in activity may be, therefore, due to increased penetration into the cell. Evidence in support of this hypothesis is that the 7-hydroxy analog, in which the 7-hydroxy group is also electron-donating, and which is not more lipophilic than the parent compound, shows the expected decrease in activity (Hlavka and Boothe, 1973).

Considering substitution at the 9 position, the activities do not parallel the activities of tetracyclines analogously substituted at the 7 position even though the electronic contributions should be similar. Thus, 9-nitro, 9-methyl, and 9-chloro compounds show depressed activity relative to the corresponding 7-analogs (Hlavka *et al.*, 1962; Bernardi *et al.*, 1975). This could be a result of these groups interfering with the interaction of the 10-hydroxy group with some receptor site either by hydrogen bonding or sterically. Further evidence for a steric factor is the fact that 9-amino-6-demethyl-6-deoxytetracycline shows enhanced activity over the 7-substituted analog, whereas the 9-dimethylamino compound shows depressed activity. All these factors hamper quantitative correlations of structure with activity; nevertheless, correlations of activity with σ^2 (the square of the Hammett factor) or with the related E_R parameter (resonance substituent constant; a measure of the ability to stabilize free radicals by delocalization) or with ΔE_i (perturbation energy; a measure of the interaction of the drug with the receptor) are quoted (Cammarata *et al.*, 1970; Peradejordi *et al.*, 1971), although in the first two cases data for only four compounds were correlated. It should be noted that these correlations have been for *in vitro* antibacterial activity and, therefore, are not a direct guide to *in vivo* activity where factors such as absorption, metabolism, and excretion must modify the relative activities. Distribution within the body will be dependent on the lipophilic nature of the molecule, and this is discussed later when considering pharmacokinetics of the tetracyclines.

Significant information on the structural requirements for tetracycline activity was obtained by Peradejordi *et al.* (1971) from a quantum-mechanical approach to structure–activity relationships. It was shown that the π-electron donor ability of the phenoldiketone moiety is of paramount importance. This is significant since the tetracyclines are thought to act via chelation with magnesium ions (Last, 1969) and the phenoldiketone moiety is a possible site for magnesium chelation. Any substitution on or adjacent to the D ring that increases the charge on the oxygens at positions 10, 11, or 12 or on carbon-6 or delocalizes this charge serves to increase *in vitro* antibacterial activity. It was concluded that the phenoldiketone moiety is involved in the magnesium chelation reaction.

7. *11a*

It is no surprise to find that substitution at the 11*a* position leads to a loss of activity (Blackwood *et al.*, 1963) since substitution at this position would disrupt the vital phenoldiketone moiety.

8. *12a*

The lack of activity of 12*a*-deoxytetracyclines and 4*a*,12*a*-anhydrotetracyclines has been indicated earlier in connection with the requirement for the chromophoric groups to be retained intact. The stereochemistry is also important since the 12*a* epimers have decreased activity compared to the "natural" analogs (Schach von Wittenau *et al.*, 1965).

9. *Overall Requirements for Antibacterial Activity*

From the evidence assembled in the foregoing, it can be seen that any "active" tetracycline derivative must contain the planar phenoldiketone moiety and the tricarbonylmethane group of ring A. These groups must be separated by the 12*a*-hydroxy group, although, in fact, they are not completely isolated from each other as there is extensive hydrogen bonding in the molecule (Rigler *et al.*, 1965; Clive, 1968). This can be seen by consideration of one of the resonant forms (Fig. 5). The configuration at the C4*a*, C5*a*, and C12*a* centers will determine the overall conformation of the molecule, and there is a requirement that they are in the natural configuration (Conover *et al.*, 1962). The presence of the 4-dimethylamino group is essential for the formation of the zwitterion and, therefore, for optimum distribution. This group must also be in the natural configuration. By contrast, modifications at positions 5 and 6 and on the D ring are possible without loss of antibacterial activity provided there is no steric interaction or hydrogen bonding with the oxygen on carbon 10. Substituents that increase the electron-donating ability of the phenoldiketone moiety enhance activity.

These conclusions are consistent with the findings from studies on the synthesis of tetracyclines (reviewed by Barrett, 1963; Money and Scott, 1968; Hlavka and Boothe, 1973; Dürckheimer, 1975); for example, Korst *et al.* (1968) found that 6-methyl-6-deoxytetracycline is the simplest

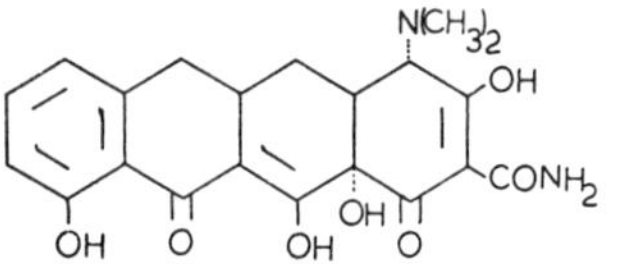

$N(CH_3)_2$, OH, $CONH_2$, OH, O, OH, OH, O

(XIII)

compound that embodies all the features necessary for *in vivo* activity. The 4-dedimethylamino analog is the simplest structure with *in vitro* activity (Blackwood and English, 1970). From the evaluation of semisynthetic tetracyclines, a picture of the active tetracycline unit has emerged. It will be informative to consider current knowledge on the mode of action of the tetracyclines to analyze why these features are required.

III. Structural Features Essential for Activity

A. Molecular Action

Information gleaned from the effects of structural modifications of tetracyclines gives a picture of the overall requirements for tetracycline activity in the compounds analyzed against the test system (usually *in vitro* bacterial growth). This is, however, a composite picture; it may not give a true reflection of the features required for the action of the drug at

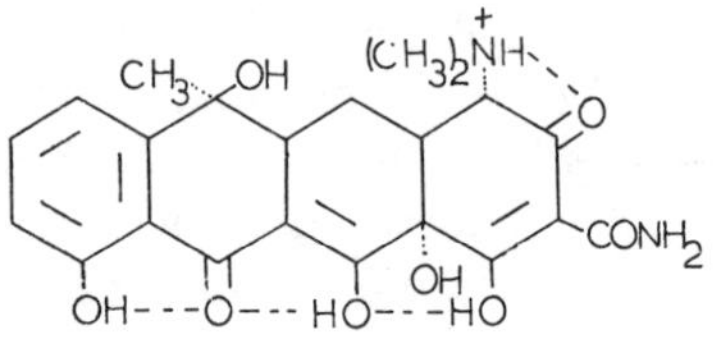

FIG. 5. Hydrogen bonding in tetracyclines.

the molecular level. Analysis of recent work on the mode of action of tetracyclines should serve to identify these latter requirements. The tetracyclines inhibit many cellular processes, and it is now widely accepted that inhibition of protein synthesis is the primary mode of action (for reviews, see Laskin, 1967; Weisblum and Davies, 1968; Pestka, 1971; Kaji, 1973).

Protein synthesis is immediately and totally inhibited after treatment of sensitive organisms with tetracyclines (Gale and Folkes, 1953; Connamacher and Mandel, 1964; Hash *et al.*, 1964; Franklin, 1964), the tetracyclines binding to the bacterial 30 S ribosomal subunit (Connamacher and Mandel, 1965). The amount bound to the 30 S subunit is greater than that bound to the 50 S subunit (Day, 1966; Maxwell, 1968), and the tetracyclines do not inhibit the binding of chloramphenicol (Vasquez, 1965) or lincomycin (Weisblum and Davies, 1968) to ribosomes; both of these drugs are known to bind to the 50 S subunit of the ribosome. This confirms, therefore, that the tetracyclines bind to the 30 S subunit. The binding involves magnesium ions since binding is reduced at low magnesium concentrations (Bodley and Zieve, 1969). The site of binding has now been identified as the acceptor site (Suarez and Nathans, 1965; Sarkar and Thach, 1968), this being the site that accepts the incoming tRNA derivative of the appropriate amino acid. The mechanism by which tetracyclines inhibit binding of aminoacyl–tRNA to the 30 S subunit probably involves binding to the ribosome via chelation with magnesium ions (Last, 1969). Indeed, magnesium chelates of tetracyclines show a greater fluorescence than tetracycline itself and this is further enhanced on binding to *Escherichia coli* ribosomes. This fluorescence enhancement has been attributed to binding to the ribosomes via magnesium chelation (White and Cantor, 1971). Since this type of interaction is likely to be nonspecific, it has been suggested that the selective action at the acceptor site may simply reflect a higher binding of magnesium ions to RNA phosphate at this site (White and Cantor, 1971). Ratios of 1 mole of tetracycline to 1 mole of ribosome were used in this study, and the results will, therefore, reflect the strongest binding site for tetracycline. By inference this would be the site at which they exert the inhibitory effect, but this, of course, may not be true. In addition to the strong binding, there is a weak binding in which up to 300 molecules of tetracycline bind per ribosome (Maxwell, 1968). An attempt has been made to identify which of these interactions is significant in tetracycline action by estimating the number of available sites on *E. coli* ribosomes using fluorescence techniques (Fey *et al.*, 1973). The results indicate that, on average, 1 molecule is bound in a strong interaction with each 50 S subunit and 3 are bound to the 30 S subunit followed by up to 100 molecules in a weak interaction. It was suggested that the strong binding is not the inhibitory interaction, but rather that a weak binding to the 30 or 50 S subunit is the reaction leading to the antibacterial effect. The evidence also showed that a magnesium chelate bridge mediates the action of the tetracyclines. In contrast, the role of magnesium has recently been questioned (Tritton, 1977), and further work is needed.

The evidence to date does not conclusively identify the interaction that is responsible for the inhibitory effect on bacterial protein synthesis. It appears at present that magnesium chelation is involved, and it is surmised that the tetracyclines bind to phosphate residues of the RNA via this chelation. Chelation with magnesium, therefore, may be fundamental to the action of tetracyclines. Consequently, a knowledge of the actual chelation sites on the molecule and of the possible conformations in solution is imperative in identifying the structural features required for tetracycline activity. Before considering chelation, the solution conformation of the tetracyclines needs defining.

Early work on the conformation of tetracyclines involved the use of X-ray crystallography (Hirowaka *et al.*, 1959; Takeuchi and Buerger, 1960; Donohue *et al.*, 1963; Cid-Dresdner, 1965; Kamiya *et al.*, 1971) and NMR spectroscopy (Schach von Wittenau and Blackwood, 1966), neither of which gives a true reflection of the molecule at therapeutic concentrations under physiological conditions. In the most recent X-ray crystallographic studies, the conformations and hydrogen bonding interactions of the nonionized and zwitterionic forms have been defined (Stezowski, 1976; Prewo and Stezowski, 1977; Stezowski, 1977). More appropriately, circular dichroism also has been used and the conformation investigated under physiological conditions (Mitscher *et al.*, 1968, 1969, 1972). It was found that the BCD phenoldiketone system is essentially planar, and it is the AB ring system that can undergo the most significant conformational changes. All the tetracyclines have identical conformations at physiological pH (Mitscher *et al.*, 1972) with hydrogen bonding between the 12*a*-hydroxyl group and the 4-dimethyla-

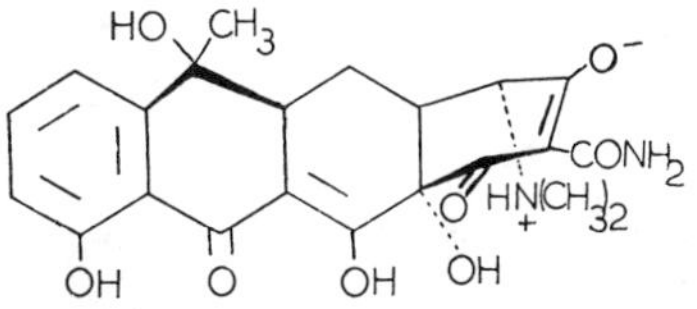

FIG. 6. Conformation of tetracyclines at physiological pH. The dimethyl amino group is below the plane of the BCD system (which is essentially flat) with the possibility of H-bonding between this dimethylamino group and the 12*a*-OH. (From Mitscher *et al.*, 1972.)

mino group giving a flattening of ring A (Fig. 6). Although this is the conformation at physiological pH, it may not be the active conformation. All tetracyclines should, therefore, be designed to contain ring A such that all possible conformations of the AB system can be attained. This implies that ring A must be retained in the form present in the tetracyclines. The most important consideration is the nature of the chelate with magnesium ions since this interaction is vital to tetracycline action. The magnesium ion may lock the tetracycline in a specific conformation, and so tetracycline analogs must be able to adopt this specific conformation. The site of chelation of magnesium on the tetracycline molecule has only recently been resolved. Proton magnetic resonance and ^{13}C-NMR studies in dimethylsulfoxide suggested that tetracyclines can chelate rare earths at the ring A oxygen functions (Williamson and Everett, 1975; Gulbis and Everett, 1975, 1976). However, it is found that these chelated ions can be easily displaced by monovalent ions such as Na^+ (Gulbis *et al.*, 1976) and the studies assumed a zwitterionic form whereas in fact the nonionic form occurs in the media used (Stezowski, 1976; Prewo and Stezowski, 1977). Recent X-ray crystallographic studies suggest it is the C1, C11, and C12 oxygen functions which are involved in chelation (Jogun and Stezowski, 1976). Subsequently, optical rotatory dispersion (ORD) studies have shown that it is the C11, C12, diketone moiety which is the site of magnesium chelation, a 1:1 complex being formed (Newman and Frank, 1977). At pH values greater than 9.0, when the *N*-dimethyl group is unionized, an additional magnesium ion chelates with the ring A oxygen functions. The ORD studies in buffer appear the most relevant to the *in vivo* situation, and so it is probable that at physiological pH the 1:1 complex involving the phenoldiketone group predominates with a small contribution from the 1:2 complex (Mitscher *et al.*, 1968, 1969). The nature of the chelate depends on the ion; with Ca, one molecule chelates at the C10, C11 oxygens and another at the C12, C1 oxygens (Newman and Frank,

1977). The conclusions to be drawn are that the potential for chelation must be retained, namely, the C10, C11, and C12 oxygen functions; also that ring A must be retained in the form present in the natural antibiotics.

In the design of new tetracycline analogs, the semisynthetic approach has been widely used since the total synthesis of tetracyclines is an immense problem. Most synthetic studies have concentrated on synthesis of the natural antibiotics themselves. The earliest approaches to tetracycline synthesis (Muxfeldt *et al.*, 1960; Fields *et al.*, 1961; Korst *et al.*, 1968) paralleled the biosynthetic route and involved successive Claisen condensations to assemble the ring system using an aromatic precursor of ring D as the starting point. These were naturally multistage reactions, for example the synthesis of 6-demethyl-6-deoxytetracycline by Korst *et al.* (1968) involved twenty-two stages. A major improvement in this type of route was pioneered by Muxfeldt (Muxfeldt and Rogalski, 1965). The first complete synthesis of a natural tetracycline, oxytetracycline, was achieved by this improved route in 1968 (Muxfeldt *et al.*, 1968), and, by variation of the precursors, different totally synthetic tetracyclines are being prepared (Dürckheimer, 1975). Mention should also be made of the work of Shemyakin who, for example, used a Diels–Alder reaction to add the B ring in a seventeen-stage reaction yielding a tetracycline precursor (Gurevich *et al.*, 1967). An entirely novel approach has been pioneered by Barton (reviewed by Barton, 1971) in which a tetracycline analog aromatic in both rings A and D is prepared, the final sequence being to convert the A ring to the required level of oxygenation. It is not feasible in this review to give a full account of these elegant studies on the synthesis of tetracyclines, but they have been recently reviewed by Hlavka and Boothe (1973) and Dürckheimer (1975). Although they have led to the development of routes to the tetracyclines, these synthetic studies have not as yet provided new information on the structural requirements for tetracycline activity. The advantage of semisynthesis has been that it readily yields new derivatives.

However, the range of reactions that can be carried out in semisynthesis is limited. One drawback of basing an analysis of structural requirements for tetracycline action on semisynthetic compounds is that it will only give an indication of which ensemble of groups present in these analogs is the minimum requirement for activity. Total synthesis would extend the scope of possible analogs. Indeed, on consideration of the requirements for molecular action, it is possible to envisage structures that do not directly contain the *full* tetracycline structure and yet that still fulfill the criteria for tetracycline activity outlined in this and the previous section. One example is the hypothetical compound

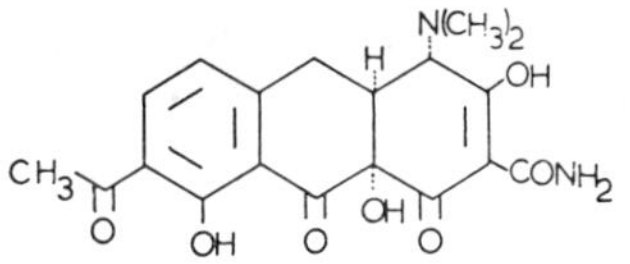

(XIV)

which retains all the essential elements for activity (Ireland and Brown, 1977). Evidence that this type of compound could have tetracycline-like activity is provided by the finding that the pillaromycins (for example, pillaromycin A, XV) (Asai *et al.*, 1970; Pezzaniti *et al.*, 1975) and chelocardin (XVI) (Mitscher *et al.*, 1970)

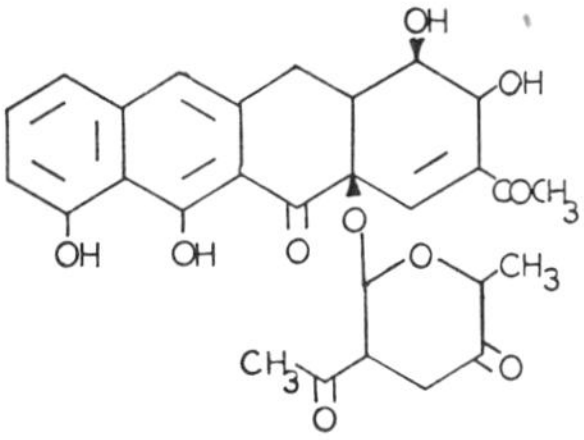

(XV) 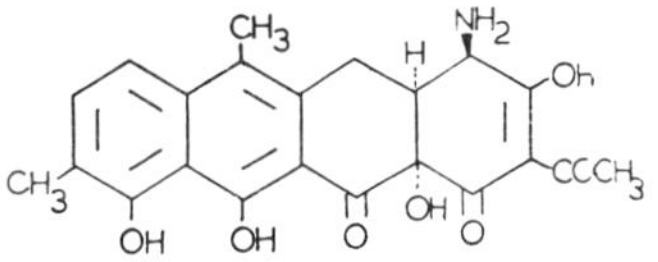 (XVI)

have antibacterial activity. A similar mode of action is indicated since chelocardin competes with chlortetracycline for binding sites on the bacterial ribosomes (Mao and Robishaw, 1971). Synthesis of this type of compound would allow further correlations of structure with activity. A study of the molecular action of the pillaromycins would also be informative since they are stated to have the unnatural configurations at the 4, 4*a*, and 12*a* positions (Kamiya *et al.*, 1971).

B. Selectivity of Action

Tetracyclines are active against *in vitro* protein synthesis by mammalian ribosomes as well as against protein synthesis by bacterial ribosomes (Weisberger *et al.*, 1964), although much higher concentrations of drug are required. Specificity of action does not, therefore, reside totally in a difference in ribosome structure between mammalian and bacterial systems. The selective antimicrobial activity of tetracyclines is mainly due to the suicidal ability of bacteria to accumulate the antibiotics by an active (energy-dependent) transport system that is absent in mammalian cells (Franklin and Higginson, 1969; Reynard and Nellis, 1972). The tetracyclines cross the nonpolar region of the membrane in this energy-linked process as a complex with magnesium ions (Dockter and Magnuson, 1973). A membrane-bound protein has been implicated (O'Hara and Kono, 1975), and the mobility of the carrier is markedly affected by changes in the membrane phospholipids (Dockter and Magnuson, 1975). Chelation is essential, therefore, not only for action at the site but also for transport into the bacterial cell. The existence of this active uptake process explains the lack of correlation between hydrophobic nature and *in vitro* antibacterial activity (Collett *et al.*, 1970) which was mentioned earlier. A correlation would only be expected if the tetracyclines were distributed into bacterial cells by passive diffusion.

The incidence of tetracycline-resistant organisms gives some insight into the uptake process, since ribosomes from tetracycline-resistant cells are just as sensitive to tetracycline as those from tetracycline-sensitive cells (Laskin and Chan, 1964). This suggests that resistance is due to the deletion of the process that actively transports the tetracyclines into the cells, and this has been shown to be the case (Izaki and Arima, 1963; Franklin and Godfrey, 1965). There may be an increased binding of the drugs at the cell surface as well (Sompolinsky and Krausz, 1973). However, the 7-dimethylamino compound, minocycline, is still active against organisms resistant to other tetracyclines, (Redin, 1966; Steigbigel *et al.*, 1968), suggesting that, due to the increased lipophilicity of this compound, there is a modified uptake system. This would explain the apparently anomalous increase in activity resulting from substitution at the 7-position with an electron-donating group [a decrease in activity being anticipated (see earlier)].

To summarize, the magnesium chelation reaction discussed in the foregoing is as important to the transport of tetracyclines (possibly excluding minocycline) into bacterial cells as it is to the action on protein synthesis once the drug is within the cells. The necessity for the "ideal" tetracycline to contain the structural requirements for chelation, stressed in the previous section, therefore applies equally to insure uptake into bacterial cells.

IV. Effect of Structural Variation on Pharmacokinetic Properties

In the previous sections, the structural features of the tetracyclines that are essential for their antibacterial activity have been delineated. Attention will now be focused on the requirements for optimal absorption of the tetracyclines and optimal disposition to the area within the body where they are required. This is a most important facet of structural variation within this group of antibiotics. Although molecular manipulation has not *markedly* improved the spectrum or intensity of the antibacterial effect, it has resulted in the development of drugs with significantly improved therapeutic properties due to improved pharmacokinetics. The structural requirements for antibacterial activity and for favorable disposition may not always coincide and so a balance must be maintained between these two sets of requirements.

One major point of incompatibility is the chelation properties of the tetracyclines. It was seen earlier that chelation of magnesium ions is fundamental to the uptake of tetracyclines into bacterial cells and to their molecular action, and yet chelation of divalent ions in the gastrointestinal tract leads to a dramatic reduction in the oral absorption of tetracyclines (Dearborn *et al.*, 1957). Furthermore, once the drug has been absorbed, these chelation properties lead to undesirable location of the tetracyclines in bone and teeth. This conflict in requirements emphasizes the need, when considering the action of a particular drug or group of drugs, to consider conjointly their mode of action and their disposition rather than each in isolation. For clarity in this discussion of the pharmacokinetics of the tetracyclines, only four compounds will be considered. Tetracycline [Fig. 1(III)] and oxytetracycline [Fig. 1(II)] are the naturally occurring compounds that have been used the most extensively and so probably have the best clinical properties of the older tetracyclines. These two biosynthetic tetracyclines will be compared with the semisynthetic compounds doxycycline [Fig. 2(IX)] and minocycline [Fig. 2(X)]. The former is claimed to have improved properties *in vivo* and the latter has altered distribution properties. Comparison of these four compounds will serve to demonstrate all the major effects that structural variation can have on pharmacokinetic properties. There is a considerable amount of data on the disposition of these four drugs in man and a relatively large degree of variation in the values quoted. This variation is not altogether unexpected and could be due to problems of bioavailability, to normal variation in response, to variation in the assay methods or their reliability, or to problems of sampling, for example, the selection of the most appropriate sampling times. Nevertheless, consideration of the data reveals significant differences in the *in vivo* properties of these four drugs.

These pharmacokinetic data will be considered here under the headings: absorption, plasma protein binding, excretion and metabolism, tissue distribution, and half-life. It should be noted at the outset that the data should only be extrapolated to the therapeutic situation with caution as most of the studies relate to healthy volunteers. There may, in fact, be differences between this artificial experimental situation and the clinical situation. It is known, for example, that tetracyclines will only penetrate the meninges when they are inflamed. Also the state of the patient may alter the pharmacokinetic properties; for example, blood levels of minocycline in volunteers resting in bed were recorded 60% higher than levels found in ambulatory volunteers when equivalent doses of the antibiotic had been taken (Bernard *et al.*, 1971). Also, the plasma half-life of tetracycline was found to be significantly reduced in under-nourished subjects (Shastri and Krishnaswamy, 1976).

A. Absorption

Early literature on the oral absorption of tetracycline is contradictory: during the late 1950's it was suggested that absorption could be enhanced by coadministration of glutamine or citric acid or phosphates. It was subsequently shown that the recorded variability in absorption was really due to the usual procedure of adding supposedly inert tablet lubricants or fillers. These contain divalent metal ions, particularly magnesium and calcium, that hinder the absorption of tetracycline due to the formation of poorly soluble chelates (Weinberg, 1957; Finland 1958). Concurrent administration of any preparation containing polyvalent metal ions, such as antacids, milk, or iron preparations, will consequently reduce oral absorption of tetracycline (Dearborn *et al.*, 1957; Neuvonen *et al.*, 1970).

The presence of food will also hinder absorption, this is particularly so for the older tetracyclines, although for doxycycline and minocycline it is claimed that absorption is not affected by food or dairy products *to the same degree* as with the older antibiotics tetracycline and oxytetracycline (Rosenblatt *et al.*, 1966; Schach von Wittenau, 1968; Brogden *et al.*, 1975; Welling *et al.*, 1977). Indeed, it is often recommended that doxycycline should be taken with food to reduce the incidence of nausea associated with its administration; ingestion with milk is not, however, advised. The greater deleterious effect of food on the absorption of tetracycline and oxytetracycline is probably partially a consequence of the slower rate of absorption of these drugs. Doxycycline and minocycline have a more rapid rate of absorption (peak blood levels attained within 2 hours) (MacDonald *et al.*, 1973) than tetracycline and oxytetracycline (peak blood levels achieved after 3–4 hours) (Dolusio and Dittert, 1969). Doxycycline and minocycline will, therefore, be less affected by any reduction in transit time down the intestine.

The tetracyclines are administered as their hydrochloride salts as these are more water-soluble than the bases themselves over most of the pH range (Miyazaki *et al.*, 1975) and problems of absorption are not likely to be due to problems of dissolution. Nevertheless, it should be noted here that there are variations in the bioavailability of different preparations for both tetracycline and oxytetracycline (Brice and Hammer, 1969; Blair *et al.*, 1971; Barr *et al.*, 1972). It was seen earlier that the tetracyclines are ionized over the whole of the pH range, and it has been suggested that it is only the neutral species, present as only a very minute fraction of the total drug, that partitions across membranes (Terada and Inagi, 1975). This is consistent with the suggestion that only the nonionized form, and not the zwitterionic, occurs in hydrophobic regions (Stezowski, 1976; Prewo and Stezowski, 1977). This fact coupled with the finding that absorption mainly occurs in the duodenum with much less absorption further down the intestine (Pindell *et al.*, 1959; Fabre *et al.*, 1971) explains the problems associated with the absorption of tetracyclines. There is a slow rate of partition and only a limited region of the gut involved in absorption of these drugs. The duodenum is presumably the major site of absorption since at the pH of the duodenal contents the tetracyclines are in their most lipophilic form (Colaizzi and Klink, 1969).

Even under optimum conditions, tetracycline and oxytetracycline are not fully absorbed, whereas, by contrast, doxycycline and minocycline are almost totally absorbed (Table II). There are two reasons for this difference. First, the semisynthetic compounds, doxycycline and minocycline, are more lipophilic than the natural antibiotics, tetracycline and oxytetracycline (Table II) and this increased lipophilicity enhances transfer across the gut wall. Second, they do not contain the 6-hydroxy group which is responsible for the acid and alkali lability of the natural compounds (Fig. 4). Because tetracycline and oxytetracycline do con-

TABLE II

ORAL ABSORPTION OF THE FOUR TETRACYCLINES

Drug	% absorbed	Lipophilicity[a]	6-Hydroxy group
Tetracycline	58[b]	0.025	Present
Oxytetracycline	77–80[b]	0.036	Present
Doxycycline	93[b]	0.600	Absent
Minocycline	Completely[c]	1.100	Absent

[a] Apparent partition between octanol and pH 7.5 buffer (Colaizzi and Klink, 1969).

[b] Fabre *et al.* (1971).

[c] MacDonald *et al.* (1973).

tain this group, they are degraded to a certain extent in the gastrointestinal tract, yielding inactive and unabsorbed degradation products. The natural compounds have the added disadvantage that these degradation products and the unabsorbed fraction of the dose administered may irritate the mucosa of the intestine and the unabsorbed antibiotic will suppress the normal gut flora. This, of course, does not occur with doxycycline and minocycline.

Important improvements have, therefore, been achieved within this group of antibiotics by deletion of the 6-hydroxy function and by increasing the lipophilic nature. The notable results of these modifications are that it is possible to get almost total absorption, with a lessened deleterious effect by the presence of food, and that the side effects due to incomplete absorption are avoided. As a result, lower doses are needed to achieve equivalent blood levels.

B. Plasma Protein Binding

The tetracyclines have been found to bind *reversibly* to plasma proteins (Fabre *et al.*, 1971) and the degree of binding is significant for three main reasons. First, on passage through the kidney, only nonprotein-bound drug will be filtered in the glomeruli, and, as active secretion is not a major means of excretion for these drugs (see later), this protein binding will delay excretion. Second, tetracycline that is protein-bound is temporarily inactivated since only unbound drug posssesses antibacterial activity (Sirota and Saltzman, 1950; Abraham, 1951; Remington and Finland, 1962). Third, assuming a steady-state situation, the concentration of unbound drug in extravascular fluids will be the same as the concentration of unbound drug in the plasma since only unbound drug can equilibrate across membranes. By analogy, drug bound in tissues will not possess antibacterial activity, and so it is the concentration of unbound tetracycline in the fluid surrounding the bacteria, and from which the bacteria absorb tetracycline, that is important in determining the effectiveness of tetracycline. The bacteria can be envisaged as competing with tissue-binding sites for tetracycline unbound in the environment of the bacteria. This oversimplification illustrates that it is not the total amount of tetracycline in a tissue that is important but the concentration of unbound tetracycline available. This is likely to be closer to the concentration of unbound antibiotic in plasma than to the averaged concentration over a tissue, assuming that near equilibrium conditions are achieved and that there is no active uptake mechanism for the concentration of tetracyclines in extravascular fluids. These appear to be valid assumptions on current evidence.

Although the binding of tetracyclines in plasma has been studied extensively, there is a wide variation in the results. This could be due to variation in the pH of the plasma samples as binding varies with pH (Williamson, 1969). Only those studies carried out at pH 7.4 are thus valid for the normal situation. Errors may be introduced due to the techniques used; for example, ultrafiltration may overestimate the degree of binding since the drug will bind to the ultrafiltration membrane. Bioassay methods are variable and spectroscopic or radiochemical assay methods may assay degradation products as well as active antibiotic. For all these reasons care must be taken in interpreting the results. Representative values are given in Table III. It is apparent that oxytetracycline is about 20–35% bound, tetracycline about 25–55%

TABLE III

PLASMA BINDING OF THE FOUR TETRACYCLINES[a]

Drug	% bound	Reference
Tetracycline, ultrafiltration	54	Remington and Finland (1962)
	55	Schach von Wittenau and Yeary (1963)
	58	Kirby *et al.* , (1961)
	65	Bennett *et al.* (1966)
equilibrium dialysis	24	Kunin *et al.* (1959b)
	36	Wozniak (1960)
	35	Green *et al.* (1976a)
	36	Kunin (1962)
	53	Powis (1974)
	56	Schach von Wittenau and Yeary (1963)
Oxytetracycline, ultrafiltration	34	Schach von Wittenau and Yeary (1963)
	35	Bennett *et al.* (1966)
equilibrium dialysis	20	Kunin *et al.* (1959b)
	24	Green *et al.* (1976a)
	27	Kaplan *et al.* (1960)
	35	Schach von Wittenau and Yeary (1963)
Doxycycline, ultrafiltration	82	Schach von Wittenau and Yeary (1963)
	91	Williamson (1969)
	93	Rosenblatt *et al.* (1966)
equilibrium dialysis	60	Green *et al.* (1976a)
	82	Schach von Wittenau and Yeary (1963)
Minocycline, ultrafiltration	35–66	Raff *et al.* (1977)
equilibrium dialysis	76	MacDonald *et al.* (1973)
not specified	55	Green *et al.* (1976a)
	59	Miura *et al.* (1969)

[a] Adapted from Green *et al.* (1976a).

bound, doxycycline about 60–90% bound, and minocycline about 55–75% bound; it is assumed that these values can be extrapolated to the therapeutic condition. Excluding minocycline, binding increases with increasing lipophilicity and, from comparison with other series of drugs, this would be expected. The lower than anticipated value for minocycline (the most lipophilic of the group) suggests there is an optimum lipophilicity for binding or more probably that a steric effect of the *N*-dimethyl group leads to a lower affinity than doxycycline for some plasma constituent.

The nature of the binding of tetracycline in plasma has been investigated by Powis (1974) who showed that just over half (54%) of the bound tetracycline is associated with albumin, 38% is bound to lipoproteins, and the remaining 8% to other proteins such as globulins. The binding to lipoproteins is probably a nonspecific attraction to lipid material, whereas the binding to albumin appears to be to specific sites on the protein. Powis (1974) found that there are two sites on albumin for tetracycline: a low-capacity high-affinity site and a high-capacity low-affinity site. Until substantiated it can be assumed that the reduced plasma binding of minocycline with respect to doxycycline is most likely due to a reduction in the specific binding to albumin rather than in the nonspecific sequestration into lipoprotein. The binding to albumin is hydrophobic in nature and chelation is not involved (Popov *et al.*, 1972; Ma *et al.*, 1973). The binding forces are not solely hydrophobic, however; a charge-transfer mechanism may also be involved (Zia and Price, 1976). The overall trend emerging is that the lipophilic nature of the tetracycline is the major factor in determining the degree of binding in the plasma. Comparing tetracycline (assuming it is 40% bound) and doxycycline (assuming it is 70% bound) then, if dosage gives *equal blood levels*, twice as much tetracycline than doxycycline would be "available." Balanced against this is the fact that the rate of excretion would be expected to be higher for tetracycline than for doxycycline. These two factors must therefore be equated in deciding the optimum value for lipophilicity within the tetracycline groups of antibiotics.

C. Excretion and Metabolism

The major route of excretion for the more polar tetracyclines is via the kidney: 70% of a given dose of tetracycline and 60% of a given dose of oxytetracycline is excreted in the urine (Fabre *et al.*, 1971). By contrast, only 33% of a given dose of doxycycline is eliminated by this route (Fabre *et al.*, 1971). This reduced urinary excretion is due to the increase in lipophilicity. In accord with this it is found that only 11% of a given dose of the even more lipophilic minocycline is excreted in the urine (Brogden *et al.*, 1975). These differences in excretion will be partially due to differences in the degree of plasma protein binding of these drugs since protein and, therefore, protein-bound drug cannot be filtered in the glomeruli. Only the unbound drug can be excreted.

A second major determinant is the net extent of tubular reabsorption. This is the amount of reabsorption occurring in the kidney tubules minus the active secretion of drug into the urine. To understand the effect of changes in lipophilicity on these processes, it is necessary to consider the renal plasma clearance value for each drug. This is calculated by dividing the amount of drug excreted in the urine in unit time by the plasma concentration of drug. Hence it corresponds to a hypothetical volume of plasma completely denuded of drug in unit time. Literature values for renal plasma clearance of the four tetracyclines are given in Table IV. Since only unbound drug is available for excretion, values calculated using the total plasma concentration may be misleading. The most meaningful values, therefore, are those which are calculated using the concentration of unbound drug, and which are, therefore, corrected for plasma protein binding. Assuming that a value of 125–130 ml/min is a typical rate for glomerular filtration, then a renal plasma clearance value of this order would indicate that the plasma was totally cleared of unbound drug by the kidney and that no net tubular reabsorption was occurring. It can be seen from Table IV that the values for tetracycline and especially oxytetracycline approach the rate of glomerular filtration. This means the kidney efficiently extracts unbound drug from the plasma and that little net reabsorption occurs.

On increasing the lipophilicity, as in the case of doxycycline and minocycline, there is a dramatic reduction in clearance showing that extensive reabsorption occurs. Thus, the lipophilic nature of the tetracycline controls the overall degree and rate of urinary excretion. Because tetracyclines are most lipophilic between pH 5.0 to 6.5 (Colaizzi and Klink, 1969), alkalinization of the urine will increase urinary excretion, the effect being greater for doxycycline than for tetracycline, as expected (Jaffe *et al.*, 1973). Urinary excretion is the major route of elimination for tetracycline and oxytetracycline and they will, therefore, accumulate in cases of renal impairment. Indeed, the half-life of tetracycline has been reported to increase from the normal value of about 10 hours to 4–5 days in cases of anuria (Kunin *et al.*, 1959a). For doxycycline and minocycline, however, this route is not the major route of elimination. A major advantage of doxycycline is that although there is normally some urinary excretion, there is no accumulation of drug if there is renal impairment (Ao *et al.*, 1974; Whelton *et al.*, 1974) and

TABLE IV

RENAL CLEARANCE VALUES FOR THE FOUR TETRACYCLINES

Drug	Renal clearance (ml/min)	Reference
Tetracycline	50	Kunin (1962)
	68	Chulski *et al.* (1963)
	74	Kunin *et al.* (1959b)
	73	Fabre *et al.* (1971)
	80	Barr *et al.* (1972)
	72 109[a]	Green *et al.* (1976b)
Oxytetracycline	99	Kunin *et al.* (1959b)
	102	Kunin and Finland (1961)
	98	Fabre *et al.* (1971)
	83 111[a]	Green *et al.* (1976b)
Doxycycline	20	MacDonald *et al.* (1973)
	24	Fabre *et al.* (1971)
	28	Laurencet and Fabre (1968)
	18 45[a]	Green *et al.* (1976b)
Minocycline	5	Bernard *et al.* (1971)
	9	Macdonald *et al.* (1973)
	15 33[a]	Green *et al.* (1976b)

[a] Values corrected for protein binding.

there is no difference in the level of drug in normal and diseased kidneys (Whelton *et al.*, 1975). It can, therefore, be used in cases of renal insufficiency but is not indicated for urinary tract infections. There is some confusion over the effect of minocycline in cases of renal impairment; there may or may not be accumulation of drug (Bernard *et al.* 1971; Carney *et al.*, 1974) and, until the situation is clarified, it is advisable not to use this drug in renal insufficiency (Brogden *et al.*, 1975). Consequently, doxycycline is the only tetracycline that can be used without concern over renal function.

The major route of excretion for doxycycline is thought to be direct diffusion from the blood to the lumen of the intestine where it complexes with the feces (Schach von Wittenau and Twomey, 1971; Schach von Wittenau *et al.*, 1972). Because it is sequestered it will not markedly affect the gut flora. It is also metabolized to a limited extent, in contrast to tetracycline and oxytetracycline which are apparently not metabolized significantly (Fabre *et al.*, 1971), and there is some excretion (a few percent) of doxycycline in the bile (Alestig, 1974). With minocycline there is an even greater degree of metabolism (MacDonald *et al.*, 1973), and biliary excretion is a more important route of elimination than for the other tetracyclines. All the tetracyclines are, in fact, found in the bile and there is an enterohepatic circulation (Kunin and Finland, 1961). Studies in the rat suggest that for tetracycline all the drug excreted in the bile is reabsorbed (Adir, 1975). This recycling is particularly evident in the case of minocycline (Green *et al.*, 1976b).

In conclusion, the most important factor governing excretion is lipophilicity. As the lipophilic nature increases, renal clearance decreases and the extent of metabolism increases. The ideal tetracycline should be sufficiently lipophilic to ensure that extensive tubular reabsorption occurs thus producing a prolonged half-life and preferably there should be no accumulation in renal impairment. Doxycycline is the only known tetracycline that fulfils these criteria and, on this basis, most closely approaches the requirements for the ideal tetracycline. In cases where urinary excretion is desired, then, a more polar tetracycline, such as tetracycline itself, could be substituted.

D. Tissue Distribution

It is well documented that the tetracyclines are widely distributed into most body tissues (André, 1956; Fabre *et al.*, 1971; MacDonald *et al.*, 1973). Some measure of the relative overall distribution of the four tetracyclines under consideration here can be obtained by comparison of their volumes of distribution (Table V). This is the hypothetical volume that would be occupied by the drug present in tissue if it were at the same concentration as drug in the plasma. This value is then expressed as a percentage of body weight. Despite the variation in the values quoted, it can be seen that once again lipophilicity is of cardinal importance. Values over 100% of body weight are recorded for the more polar compounds, tetracycline and oxytetracycline, showing that extensive binding to tissues occurs. For doxycycline and minocycline, a larger fraction of total drug in the body is present in the plasma than is the case for tetracycline or oxytetracycline. As only free drug can equilibrate across membranes, it is instructive to calculate volumes of distribution using free drug concentration in plasma rather than concentration of total drug. These values corrected for protein binding are also given in Table V and the result is qualitatively the same. The volume of

TABLE V

VOLUMES OF DISTRIBUTION OF THE FOUR TETRACYCLINES

Drug	Volume of distribution (% of body weight)	Reference
Tetracycline	95	Spitzy and Hitzenberger (1957)
	101	Chulski *et al.* (1963)
	159	Kunin *et al.* (1959b)
	306 473[a]	Green *et al.* (1976b)
Oxytetracycline	90	Spitzy and Hitzenberger (1957)
	189	Kunin *et al.* (1959b)
	305 407[a]	Green *et al.* (1976b)
Doxycycline	63 158[a]	Green *et al.* (1976b)
Minocycline	74 164[a]	Green *et al.* (1976b)

[a] Values corrected for protein binding.

distribution does not show, however, where the drug is distributed in the body and so data on the tissue levels of tetracyclines are important.

In general, tetracyclines penetrate well into extravascular and intracellular fluids with penetration increasing with increasing lipophilicity (Schach von Wittenau and Delahunt, 1966). This apparently contradicts the fact that tetracycline and oxytetracycline have higher volumes of distribution and must mean that the latter two antibiotics are much more highly bound than doxycycline and minocycline to some tissue component not shown in the tissue distribution studies. In all cases, except fatty tissue and the CNS, drug levels higher than blood levels are attained, but only minocycline achieves satisfactory levels in the CNS. Even so the levels are not as high as those found in other tissues (only 25% of the blood level after 12 hours) (MacDonald *et al.*, 1973). It was stressed earlier that the tissue level of an antibiotic is an averaged value for the tissue and so does not accurately reflect the concentration of antibiotic available to the bacteria. Nevertheless, the tissue binding can serve as a temporary store of antibiotic and ensure that the level of unbound drug is maintained in the tissue.

Probably the most important aspect of distribution is the rate of penetration of the drug into poorly vascularized tissue. The rate and degree of penetration will increase with an increase in lipophilic nature; for example, doxycycline will penetrate into the mucous membranes of the maxillary sinus and into the bronchial wall (Eneroth *et al.*, 1975; Gartmann, 1975). One important feature of tissue penetration of tetracyclines is their accumulation in teeth and bone (reviewed by Storey, 1973; Skinner and Nalbandian, 1975). They are deposited into newly formed areas of bone (Bevelander *et al.*, 1961; Saxén, 1965) persisting for at least 10 weeks (Milch *et al.*, 1957). They will permanently discolor the first permanent molars and even the incisors, particularly if given in the first 3 years of life and may lead to an increased incidence of dental caries (Baker, 1975). They will affect the growth of the fetus as they can cross the placenta (Kline *et al.*, 1964; Moya, 1965). It is suggested that doxycycline has a lower degree of complexation with calcified tissue than tetracycline and oxytetracycline (Schach von Wittenau, 1968). This may be the reason for the diminished volume of distribution. The most lipophilic member of the series, minocycline, has recently been reported to have no cumulative effect on bone and teeth growth in rhesus monkeys (Yen and Shaw, 1975). It appears, therefore, that this detrimental effect on bone and teeth is reduced as lipophilicity increases.

There is some confusion over the relevance of tissue levels, tissue binding, plasma levels, and plasma binding of tetracyclines. Certainly the total blood level is not the sole criterion for comparing a group of antibiotics, as differing degrees of plasma binding occur. Similarly, averaged tissue levels are not the only criterion of activity. The major concern is that adequate levels of drug are achieved in the vicinity of the bacteria. The tetracyclines are so well distributed into most tissues that enhanced penetration due to more favorable partition properties as lipophilicity increases is only of benefit in poorly vascularized areas of the body. Moreover, as lipophilicity increases the volume of distribution decreases. Since the plasma accounts only for a low proportion of the total body weight, this finding is not merely a consequence of the localization of a bigger fraction of drug in the plasma due to increased binding to plasma proteins. It appears that the ideal tetracycline would have a lipophilicity between that of tetracycline and doxycycline. A slightly more lipophilic compound than tetracycline would not have the disadvantage of the high protein binding found with doxycycline, would have a higher volume of distribution than doxycycline, would penetrate into inaccessible tissues better than tetracycline, and have a greater degree of tubular reabsorption than tetracycline.

E. Half-Life

In common with the other pharmacokinetic parameters, there is a wealth of information on the half-lives of the individual tetracyclines. Representative values are quoted in Table VI for both single-dose and repeat-dose studies. The latter are more relevant to the clinical situation as the tetracyclines are taken as a course of treatment. On repeat dosing, a steady-state situation can be achieved and the half-life apparently increases during repeat dosing (Dolusio and Dittert, 1959; Fabre *et al.*, 1971). Notari (1973) has indicated that, if anything, a shorter half-life would be expected in the steady state compared to the single-dose studies and suggests that the discrepancy is due to inclusion of part of the distribution phase with the elimination phase in calculating the half-life in a single-dose study.

Tetracyclines with prolonged half-lives are desirable as they would have a reduced frequency of administration compared to tetracycline itself. More stable blood levels would be produced with less risk of the level falling below the minimum acceptable level of 0.8 μg/ml (Fabre *et al.*, 1971). A decrease in rate of excretion or an increase in plasma binding or an increase in volume of distribution will serve to prolong half-life. Therefore an increase in lipophilic nature would be expected to give an overall increase in half-life as the resulting decreased excretion and increased plasma binding should outweight the decrease in volume of distribution. This is what is found to occur in practice: the more lipophilic tetracyclines have longer half-lives. Notari (1973) has stressed, however, that the half-lives are not too dissimilar (about 11 hours for tetracycline compared to about 17 hours for doxycycline) and that, with correctly designed dosage schedules, adequate and comparable blood levels could be achieved for all the tetracyclines on twice daily dosage. Or sustained-release preparations could be used (Lucas *et al.*, 1977).The shorter half-life found for tetracycline with respect to doxycycline is not, therefore, so great a disadvantage as the incomplete oral absorption of the former drug.

V. Conclusions

Study of the structure–activity relationships of the semisynthetic tetracyclines shows that both the tricarbonylmethane and phenoldiketone systems (see Fig. 3) must be retained intact otherwise antibacterial activity is lost. This is confirmed by studies on the mode of action of the tetracyclines. The conformation of ring A and the *N*-dimethylamino group must also be retained. By contrast, the region of the molecule from C5 to C9 can be modified so long as there is no interference with

TABLE VI

HALF-LIVES OF THE FOUR TETRACYCLINES (ORAL ADMINISTRATION)

Drug	Half-life (hours)	Reference
	A. Single Dose	
Tetracycline	6	Dolusio and Dittert (1969)
	14	Waddington *et al.* (1954)
	8	Chulski *et al.* (1963)
	9	Kunin *et al.* (1959b)
Oxytetracycline	7	Green *et al.* (1976b)
	9	Kunin *et al.* (1959b)
Doxycycline	8	Dolusio and Dittert (1969)
	9	Green *et al.* (1976b)
	15	Rosenblatt *et al.* (1966)
	18	Fabre *et al.* (1971)
	22	Schach von Wittenau (1968)
Minocycline[a]	10–16	Bernard *et al.* (1971)
	16	MacDonald *et al.* (1973)
	16	Simon *et al.* (1976)
	7–8 during first 12–18 hr 13–15 during subsequent period	Heine (1969) quoted in Brogden *et al.* (1975)
	4–5 during first phase 17 during second phase	La Verge *et al.*, (1976)
	B. Repeat Dosage	
Tetracycline	10	Dolusio and Dittert (1969)
	11	Olon and Holvey (1968)
	12	Green *et al.* (1976b)
Oxytetracycline	9	Barker and Prescott (1973)
	9	Green *et al* . (1976b)
Doxycycline	15	Dolusio and Dittert (1969)
	17	Green *et al.* (1976b)
	20	Fabre *et al.* (1971)
Minocycline[a]	11	Green *et al.* (1976b)
	25	Heine (1969), quoted in Brogden *et al.* (1975)

[a] Determination of the half-life of minocycline is complicated by biliary recycling of the drug.

the above-stated essential features. Once the minimum structural requirements essential for antibacterial activity are defined, the next consideration is to see how modification of physicochemical properties can maximize clinical effectiveness. Notari (1973) and Dürckheimer (1975) have outlined several goals for optimization within a group of orally active antibiotics.

These goals can be summarized as follows:

1. Reduced side effects.
2. Improved antibacterial effectiveness due to a decrease in the minimum inhibitory concentration (MIC) or by an improvement in the spectrum of activity.
3. Increased stability.
4. Improved pharmacokinetic properties due to (*a*) an increase in the degree or rate of oral absorption and a decrease in the effect of food on absorption; (*b*) an increase in the distribution into tissue; (*c*) an increase in the half-life to maintain higher post-distribution levels; and (*d*) a decrease in the binding to plasma proteins.

A. Side Effects

It has been possible by increasing the lipophilic nature of the drug to prevent the undesirable inhibition of the normal gut flora. However, it has not been possible to abolish completely the binding of tetracyclines in bone and teeth, although this effect appears to be considerably lessened as lipophilicity increases.

B. Antibacterial Effectiveness

The aim in antibacterial therapy is to maintain levels of drug above the MIC and so, in this respect, any change in activity is not really significant unless there can be substantial reduction in dosage and, therefore, an increase in the therapeutic index. Extensive studies have been carried out demonstrating what are on the whole only small differences in activity against pathogenic organisms between the individual tetracyclines. On balance, doxycycline is a little more active than tetracycline and oxytetracycline (Williamson, 1969; Redin, 1966; Steigbigel *et al.*, 1968), and minocycline is even more active (Redin, 1966; Brogden *et al.*, 1975; Chow *et al.*, 1975). Because variability in blood levels of drugs is found in practice, dosages are selected so that levels well above the MIC are achieved. These differences in activity, therefore, are not nearly so important as the differences in disposition properties. The most important change in antibacterial activity that has been effected by structural modification is undoubtedly the broadened spectrum of activity of minocycline with respect to the other tetracyclines. Minocycline is active against organisms resistant to the other tetracyclines; for example, Kuck *et al.* (1971) showed that of 101 clinically isolated strains of *Staphylococcus aureus,* 48 were resistant to tetracycline at a concentration of 4 μg/ml but all were sensitive to minocycline at this concentration.

C. Stability

One of the major successes in the development of new tetracyclines has been the production of more stable compounds due to deletion of the 6-hydroxy group. The goal of improved stability has, therefore, been achieved, although epimerization at the 4-position at low pH (Hoener *et al.*, 1974), yielding the inactive epimer, is still a property of newer tetracyclines.

D. Pharmacokinetic Properties

Once the basic requirements for tetracycline activity had been determined, major improvements within this series of antibiotics came about by optimization of the pharmacokinetic properties. The two major structural modifications that led to these improvements are, first, the aforementioned increase in stability and, second, the increase in lipophilic nature up to an optimum value. Compounds with a higher degree of lipophilicity than the natural antibiotics, tetracycline and oxytetracycline, are completely absorbed orally with less interference by the presence of food and are able to penetrate better into poorly perfused regions of the body. They also have an increased half-life. The overall result is that lower and less frequent dosage is necessary. Typical doses for adults, recommended by manufacturers for oxytetracycline and tetracycline are 250 or 500 mg, 4× daily, whereas for doxycycline and minocycline the manufacturers recommend a loading dose of 200 mg followed by 100 mg daily. One advantage of the reduced frequency of dosing is that there is less likelihood of a dose being missed and there is also less possibility of the blood level falling below the accepted level. The only drawbacks of increasing the lipophilicity are that protein binding increases and very lipophilic compounds have a much reduced antibacterial activity (Blackwood and English, 1970). There is, therefore, an optimum value for lipophilicity, and this must be defined.

E. The Ideal Tetracycline

Of the *currently available* drugs, doxycycline and minocycline most closely fulfil the criteria for the ideal tetracycline, and doxycycline would be preferred except when treating tetracycline-resistant bacteria or when there is a requirement for the unique penetrative powers of minocycline. [Minocycline is the only tetracycline that reaches satisfactory levels in the CNS or in "inaccessible" regions of the body (MacDonald *et al.*, 1973; Hoeprich and Warshauer, 1974).] Doxycycline would normally be preferred to minocycline since it has a greater half-life and because minocycline causes vestibular effects such as dizziness and vertigo in a relatively high number of patients (Gould and Brookler, 1972; Williams *et al.*, 1974; Jacobson and Daniel, 1975), although these effects are reversible. Furthermore, doxycycline is the only tetracycline that can be safely used in cases of renal insufficiency.

In comparing tetracycline and doxycycline, the major differences chemically are that only tetracycline possesses the labile 6-hydroxy group, and doxycycline is more lipophilic. As a result, doxycycline has on balance the more favorable properties of the two drugs. Tetracycline is not completely absorbed, whereas doxycycline is almost totally absorbed; and tetracycline is mainly excreted by the kidney, whereas this is not the major route of excretion for doxycycline. The result is that the half-life of doxycycline is half as much again as that for tetracycline. Doxycycline, however, is much more highly bound to plasma proteins than is tetracycline and, therefore, for equal blood levels, more tetracycline would be available than doxycycline in the vicinity of the bacteria where it is required. For this reason the optimum level of lipophilicity of a tetracycline is intermediate between the values for tetracycline and doxycycline. On this basis methacycline should be an improved drug as it is intermediate in lipophilicity (Blackwood and English, 1970), but only 50% of a given dose of methacycline is absorbed (Fabre *et al.*, 1971), the reason being obscure. It may be that a lipophilic pro-drug that is completely absorbed and then hydrolyzed *in vivo* to a tetracycline possessing the essential features for antibacterial activity, with no 6-hydroxy group, and with lipophilicity intermediate between doxycycline and tetracycline would be the ultimate refinement in this group of antibiotics.

This discussion of the tetracycline group of antibiotics shows that, in drug design based on a lead compound, the priorities are to identify the minimum structural requirements for pharmacological activity and then to optimize the disposition characteristics by structural variation, while retaining these basic features. In retrospect, it can be seen that consideration of data on *all* the aspects of a group of drugs is meaningful in the development of improved analogs; this is an important lesson for future studies in drug design.

References

Abraham, E. P. (1951). *J. Pharm. Pharmacol.* **3,** 257–270.

Adir, J. (1975). *J. Pharm. Sci.* **64,** 1847–1850.

Alestig, K. (1974). *Scand. J. Infect. Dis.* **6,** 265–271.

André, T. (1956). *Acta Radiol.* **142,** 1–89.

Ao, N. K., Taneja, O. P., Bhatia, V. N., and Aggarwal, D. S. (1974). *Chemotherapy (Basel)* **20,** 129–140.

Asai, M., Mizuta, E., Mizuno, K., Miyake, A., and Tatsuoka, S. (1970). *Chem. Pharm. Bull.* **18,** 1720–1723.

Baker, K. L. (1975). *Med. J. Aust.* **2,** 301–304.

Barker, B. M., and Prescott, F. (1973). "Antimicrobial Agents in Medicine," p. 156. Blackwell, Oxford.

Barr, W. H., Gerbracht, L. M., Letcher, K., Plaut, M., and Strahl, N. (1972). *Clin. Pharmacol. Ther.* **13,** 97–108.

Barrett, G. C. (1963). *J. Pharm. Sci.* **52,** 309–330.

Barton, D. H. R. (1971). *Pure Appl. Chem.* **25,** 5–23.

Bennett, J. V., Mickelwait, J. S., Barrett, J. E., Brodie, J. L., and Kirby, W. M. M. (1966). *Antimicrob. Agents Chemother.* pp. 180–182.

Bernard, B., Yin, J. E., and Simon, H. J. (1971). *J. Clin. Pharmacol. New Drugs* **11,** 332–348.

Bernardi, L., De Castiglione, R., Colonna, V., Masi, P., and Mazzoleni, R. (1974). *Farmaco, Ed. Sci.* **29,** 902–909.

Bernardi, L., De Castiglione, R., Masi, P., Mazzoleni, R., and Scarponi, U. (1975). *Farmaco, Ed. Sci.* **30,** 1025–1030.

Bevelander, G., Rolle, G. K., and Cohlan, S. Q. (1961). *J. Dent. Res.* **40,** 1020–1024.

Blackwood, R. K., and English, A. R. (1970). *Adv. Appl. Microbiol.* **13,** 237–266.

Blackwood, R. K., and English, A. R. (1977). In "Structure–Activity Relationships among the Semisynthetic Antibiotics" (D. Perlman, ed.), pp. 397–426. Academic Press, New York.

Blackwood, R. K., and Stephens, C. R. (1964). *J. Am. Chem. Soc.* **86,** 2736–2737.

Blackwood, R. K., Beerebohm, J. J., Rennhard, H. H., Schach von Wittenau, M., and Stephens, C. R. (1963). *J. Am. Chem. Soc.* **85,** 3943–3953.

Blair, D. C., Barnes, R. W., Wildner, E. L., and Murray, W. J. (1971). *J. Am. Med. Assoc.* **215,** 251–254.

Bodley, J. W., and Zieve, P. J. (1969). *Biochem. Biophys. Res. Commun.* **36,** 463–468.

Boothe, J. H. (1962). *Antimicrob. Agents Chemother.* pp. 213–225.

Boothe, J. H., Morton, J., Petisi, J. P., Wilkinson, R. G., and Williams, J. H. (1953). *J. Am. Chem. Soc.* **75,** 4621.

Boothe, J. H., Bonvicino, G. E., Waller, C. W., Petisi, J. P., Wilkinson, R. W., and Broschard, R. B. (1958). *J. Am. Chem. Soc.* **80,** 1654–1657.

Brice, G. W., and Hammer, H. F. (1969). *J. Am. Med. Soc.* **208,** 1189–1190.

Brogden, R. N., Speight, T. M., and Avery, G. S. (1975). *Drugs* **9,** 251–291.

Cammarata, A., Yau, S. J., Collett, J. H., and Martin, A. N. (1970). *Mol. Pharmacol.* **6,** 61–66.

Carney, S., Butcher, R. A., Dawborn, J. K., and Pattison, G. (1974). *Clin. Exp. Pharmacol. Physiol.* **1,** 299–308.

Chow, A. W., Patten, V., and Guze, L. B. (1975). *Antimicrob. Agents & Chemother.* **7,** 46–49.

Chulski, T., Johnson, R. H., Schlagel, C. A., and Wagner, J. G. (1963). *Nature (London)* **198,** 450–453.

Cid-Dresdner, H. (1965). *Z. Kristallogr., Kristallgeom., Kristallphys., Kristallchem.* **121,** 170–189.

Clive, D. L. J. (1968). *Q. Rev., Chem. Soc.* **22,** 435–456.

Colaizzi, J. L., and Klink, P. R. (1969). *J. Pharm. Sci.* **58,** 1184–1189.

Collett, J. H., Collett, C., Martin, A. N., and Cammarata, A. (1970). *J. Pharm. Pharmacol.* **22,** 672–678.

Connamacher, R. H., and Mandel, H. G. (1964). *Fed. Proc., Fed. Am. Soc. Exp. Biol.* **23,** 388.

Connamacher, R. H., and Mandel, H. G. (1965). *Biochem. Biophys. Res. Commun.* **20,** 98–103.

Conover, L. H., Moreland, W. T., English, A. R., Stephens, C. R., and Pilgrim, F. J. (1953). *J. Am. Chem. Soc.* **75,** 4622–4623.

Conover, L. H., Butler, K., Johnston, J. D., Korst, J. J., and Woodward, R. B. (1962). *J. Am. Chem. Soc.* **84,** 3222–3224.

Day, L. E. (1966). *J. Bacteriol.* **92,** 197–203 and 1263.

Dearborn, E. H., Litchfield, T. J., Eisner, H. J., Corbett, J. J., and Bunnett, C. W. (1957). *Antibiot. Med.* **4,** 627–641.

Dockter, M. E., and Magnuson, J. A. (1973). *Biochem. Biophys. Res. Commun.* **54,** 790–795.

Dockter, M. E., and Magnuson, J. A. (1975). *Arch. Biochem. Biophys.* **168,** 81–88.

Doerschuk, A. P., McCormick, J. R. D., Goodman, J. J., Szumski, S. A., Growich, J. A., Miller, P. A., Bitler, B. A., Jensen, E. R., Petty, M. A., and Phelps, A. S. (1956). *J. Am. Chem. Soc.* **78,** 1508–1509.

Dolusio, J. T., and Dittert, L. W. (1969). *Clin. Pharmacol. Ther.* **10,** 690–701.

Donohue, J., Dunitz, J. D., Trueblood, K. N., and Webster, M. S. (1963). *J. Am. Chem. Soc.* **85,** 851–856.

Duggar, B. M. (1948). *Ann. N.Y. Acad. Sci.* **51,** 177–181.

Dürckheimer, W. (1975). *Angew. Chem.* **87,** 751–764.

Eneroth, C. M., Lundberg, C., and Wretlind, B. (1975). *Chemotherapy (Basel)* **21,** Suppl. 1, 1–7.

Esse, R. C., Lowery, J. A., Tamorna, C. R., and Steger, G. M. (1964). *J. Am. Chem. Soc.* **86,** 3875–3877.

Fabre, J., Milek, E., and Kaliopoulos, P. (1971). *Schweiz. Med. Wochenschr.* **101,** 539–598 and 625–633.

Fey, G., Reiss, M., and Kersten, H. (1973). *Biochemistry* **12,** 1160–1164.

Fields, T. L., Kende, A. S., and Boothe, J. H. (1961). *J. Am. Chem. Soc.* **83,** 4612–4618.

Finland, M. (1958). *Antibiot. Med.* **5,** 359–363.

Finland, M. (1974). *Clin. Pharmacol. Ther.* **15,** 3–8.

Finlay, A. C., Hobby, G. L., P'an, S. Y., Regna, P. P., Routien, J. B., Seeley, D. B., Shull, G. M., Sobin, B. A., Solomons, I. A., Vinson, J. W., and Kane, J. H. (1950). *Science* **111,** 85.

Franklin, T. J. (1964). *Biochem. J.* **90,** 624–628.

Franklin, T. J. and Godfrey, A. (1965). *Biochem. J.* **94,** 54–60.

Franklin, T. J. and Higginson, B. (1969). *Biochem. J.* **112,** 12P.

Free, S. M., and Wilson, J. W. (1964). *J. Med. Chem.* **7,** 395–399.

Gale, E. F., and Folkes, J. P. (1953). *Biochem. J.* **53,** 493–498.

Gartmann, J. (1975). *Chemotherapy (Basel)* **21,** Suppl. 1, 19–26.

Gatenbeck, S., (1961). *Biochem. Biophys. Res. Commun.* **6,** 422–426.

Gottstein, W. J., Minor, W. F., and Cheney, L. C. (1959). *J. Am. Chem. Soc.* **81,** 1198–1201.

Gould, W. J., and Brookler, K. H. (1972). *Arch. Otolaryngol.* **96,** 291.

Green, A., and Boothe, J. H. (1960). *J. Am. Chem. Soc.* **82,** 3950–3953.

Green, R., Brown, J. R., and Calvert, R. T. (1976a). *J. Pharm. Pharmacol.* **28,** 514–515.

Green, R., Brown, J. R., and Calvert, R. T. (1976b). *Eur. J. Clin. Pharmacol.* **10,** 245–250.

Gulbis, J., and Everett, G. W. (1975). *J. Am. Chem. Soc.* **97,** 6248–6249.

Gulbis, J., and Everett, G. W. (1976). *Tetrahedron* **32,** 913–917.

Gulbis, J., Everett, G. W., and Frank, C. W. (1976). *J. Am. Chem. Soc.* **98,** 1280–1281.

Gurevich, A. I., Karapetyan, M. G., Kolosov, M. N., Korobko, V. G., Onoprienko, V. V., Popravko, S. A., and Shemyakin, M. M. (1967). *Tetrahedron Lett.* pp. 131–134.

Hash, J. H., Wishnik, M., and Miller, P. A. (1964). *J. Biol. Chem.* **239,** 2070–2078.

Hirowaka, S., Okaya, Y., Lovell, F. M., and Pepinsky, R. (1959). *Acta Crystallogr.* **12,** 811–812.

Hlavka, J. J., and Boothe, J. H. (1973). *Fortschr. Arzneimittelforsch.* **17,** 210–240.

Hlavka, J. J., Schneller, A., Krazinski, H., and Boothe, J. H. (1962). *J. Am. Chem. Soc.* **84,** 1426–1430.

Hoener, B.-A., Sokoloski, T. D., Mitscher, L. A., and Malpeis, L. (1974). *J. Pharm. Sci.* **63,** 1901–1904.

Hoeprich, P. D., and Warshauer, D. M. (1974). *Antimicrob. Agents & Chemother.* **5,** 330–336.

Hughes, D. W., Wilson, W. L., Butterfield, A. G., and Pound, N. J. (1974). *J. Pharm. Pharmacol.* **26,** 79–80.

Ireland, D. S., and Brown, J. R. (1977). *J. Chem. Soc., Perkin Trans.* **1,** 467–470.

Izaki, K., and Arima, K. (1963). *Nature (London)* **200,** 384–385.

Jacobson, J. A., and Daniel, B. (1975). *Antimicrob. Agents & Chemother.* **8,** 453–456.

Jaffe, J. M., Colaizzi, J. L., Poust, R. I., and MacDonald, R. H. (1973). *J. Pharmacokinet. Biopharm.* **1,** 267–282.

Jogun, K. H., and Stezowski, J. J. (1976). *J. Am. Chem. Soc.* **98,** 6018–6026.

Kaji, A. (1973). *Prog. Mol. Subcell. Biol.* **3,** 85–158.

Kamiya, K., Asai, M., Wada, Y., and Nishikawa, M. (1971). *Experientia* **27,** 363–365.

Kaplan, S. A., Yuceoglu, A. M., and Strauss, J. (1960). *J. Appl. Physiol.* **15,** 106–108.

Kellaway, I. W., and Mariott, C. (1977). *J. Pharm. Pharmacol.* **28,** 8P.

Kende, A. S., Fields, T. L., Boothe, J. H., and Kushner, S. (1961). *J. Am. Chem. Soc.* **83,** 439–449.

Kirby, W. M. M., Roberts, C. E., and Burdick, R. E. (1961). *Antimicrob. Agents Chemother.* pp. 286–292.

Kline, A. H., Blattner, R. J., and Lunin, M. (1964). *J. Am. Med. Assoc.* **188,** 178–180.

Korst, J. J., Johnston, J. D., Butler, K., Bianco, E. J., Conover, L. H., and Woodward, R. B. (1968). *J. Am. Chem. Soc.* **90,** 439–457.

Koschel, K., Hartmann, G., Kersten, W., and Kersten, H. (1966). *Biochem. Z.* **344,** 76–86.

Kuck, N. A., Redin, G. S., and Forbes, M. (1971). *Proc. Soc. Exp. Biol. Med.* **136,** 479–481.

Kunin, C. M. (1962). *Proc. Soc. Exp. Biol. Med.* **110,** 311–315.

Kunin, C. M. and Finland, M. (1961). *Clin. Pharmacol. Ther.* **2,** 51–69.

Kunin, C. M. Rees, S. B., Merrill, J. P., and Finland, M. (1959a). *J. Clin. Invest.* **38,** 1487–1497.

Kunin, C. M., Dornbush, A. C., and Finland, M. (1959b). *J. Clin. Invest.* **38,** 1950–1963.

Laskin, A. I. (1967). *In* "Antibiotics" (D. Gottlieb and P. D. Shaw, eds.), Vol. 1, pp. 331–359. Springer-Verlag, Berlin and New York.

Laskin, A. I., and Chan, W. M. (1964). *Biochem. Biophys. Res. Commun.* **14,** 137–142.
Last, J. A. (1969). *Biochim. Biophys. Acta* **195,** 506–514.
Laurencet, F. R., and Fabre, J. P. (1968). *J. Urol. Nephrol.* **74,** 1038–1047.
La Verge, R., Javaudin, L., Quesnier, L. R., Trebaul, L., Scarabin, M., and Devissagnet, J. P. (1976). *Therapie* **31,** 105–119.
Leeson, L. J., Krueger, J. E., and Nash, R. A. (1963). *Tetrahedron Lett.* pp. 1155–1160.
Lucas, C. R., Mugglestone, C. J., and Thomas, D. R. (1977). *J. Int. Med. Res.* **5,** 124–127.
Ma, J. K. H., Jun, H. W., and Luzzi, L. A. (1973). *J. Pharm. Sci.* **62,** 1261–1264.
McCormick, J. R. D. (1965). *In* "Biogenesis of Antibiotic Substances" (Z. Vanek and Z. Hostalek, eds.), pp. 73–91. Academic Press, New York.
McCormick, J. R. D. (1967). *In* "Antibiotics" (D. Gottlieb and P. Shaw, eds.), Vol. 2, pp. 113–122. Springer-Verlag, Berlin and New York.
McCormick, J. R. D., Fox, S. M., Smith, L. L., Bitler, B. A., Reichenthal, J., Origoni, V. E., Muller, W. H., Winterbottom, R., and Doerschuk, A. P. (1957a). *J. Am. Chem. Soc.* **79,** 2849–2858.
McCormick, J. R. D., Sjölander, N. O., Hirsch, U., Jensen, E. R., and Doerschuk, A. P. (1957b). *J. Am. Chem. Soc.* **79,** 4561–4563.
McCormick, J. R. D., Miller, P. A., Growich, J. A., Sjölander, N. O., and Doerschuk, A. P. (1958). *J. Am. Chem. Soc.* **80,** 5572–5573.
McCormick, J. R. D., Jensen, E. R., Miller, P. A., and Doerschuk, A. P. (1960). *J. Am. Chem. Soc.* **82,** 3381–3386.
McCormick, J. R. D., Reichenthal, J., Johnson, S., and Sjölander, N. O. (1963). *J. Am. Chem. Soc.* **85,** 1694–1695.
MacDonald, H., Kelly, R. G., Allen, E. S., Noble, J. F., and Kanegis, L. A. (1973). *Clin. Pharmacol. Ther.* **14,** 852–861.
Mao, J. C.-H., and Robishaw, E. E. (1971). *Biochim. Biophys. Acta* **238,** 157–160.
Martell, M. J., and Boothe, J. H. (1967). *J. Med. Chem.* **10,** 44–46.
Martell, M. J., Ross, A. S., and Boothe, J. H. (1967). *J. Am. Chem. Soc.* **89,** 6780–6781.
Maxwell, I. H., (1968). *Mol. Pharmacol.* **4,** 25–37.
Milch, R. A., Rall, D. P., and Tobie, J. E. (1957). *J. Natl. Cancer Inst.* **19,** 87–93.
Miller, G. H., Smith, H. L., Rock, W. L., and Hedberg, S. (1977). *J. Pharm. Sci.* **66,** 88–92.
Miller, M. W., and Hochstein, F. A. (1962). *J. Org. Chem.* **27,** 2525–2528.
Miller, P. A., McCormick, J. R. D., and Doerschuk, A. P. (1956). *Science* **123,** 1030–1031.
Minieri, P. P., Firman, M. C., Mistretta, A. G., Abbey, A., Bricker, C. E., Rigler, N. E., and Sokol, H. (1953). *Antibiot. Annu.,* pp. 81–87.
Mitscher, L. A. (1968). *J. Pharm. Sci.* **57,** 1633–1649.
Mitscher, L. A., Bonacci, A. C., and Sokoloski, T. D. (1968). *Antimicrob. Agents Chemother.* pp. 78–86.
Mitscher, L. A., Bonacci, A. C., Slater-Eng, B., Hacker, A. K., and Sokoloski, T. D. (1969). *Antimicrob. Agents Chemother.,* pp. 111–115.
Mitscher, L. A., Juvarkar, J. V., Rosenbrook, W., Andres, W. W., Schenk, J., and Egan, R. S. (1970). *J. Am. Chem. Soc.* **92,** 6070–6071.
Mitscher, L. A., Slater-Eng, B., and Sokoloski, T. D. (1972). *Antimicrob. Agents & Chemother.* **2,** 66–72.
Miura, Y., Mizumoto, T., and Shibaki, H. (1969). *Jpn. J. Antibiot.* **22,** 483–487.
Miyazaki, S., Nakano, M., and Arita, T. (1975). *Chem. Pharm. Bull.* **23,** 1197–1204.
Money, T., and Scott, A. I. (1968). *Prog. Org. Chem.* **7,** 1–34.
Moya, F. (1965). *Antimicrob. Agents & Chemother.* **5,** 1051–1057.
Muxfeldt, H., and Rogalski, W. (1965). *J. Am. Chem. Soc.* **87,** 933–934.
Muxfeldt, H., Rogalski, W., and Striegler, K. (1960). *Angew. Chem.* **72,** 170–171.
Muxfeldt, H., Hardtmann, G., Kathwala, F., Vedejs, E., and Moeberry, J. B. (1968). *J. Am. Chem. Soc.* **90,** 6534–6536.

Neuvonen, P. J., Gothoni, G., Hackmann, R., and Björksten, K. (1970). *Br. Med. J.* **4,** 532–534.

Newman, E. C., and Frank, C. W. (1977). *J. Pharm. Sci.* **65,** 1728–1732.

Notari, R. E. (1973). *J. Pharm. Sci.* **62,** 865–880.

O'Hara, K., and Kono, M. (1975). *J. Antibiot.* **28,** 607–608.

Olon, L. P., and Holvey, D. N. (1968). *Clin. Med.* **75,** 33–44.

Peradejordi, F., Martin, A. N., and Cammarata, A. (1971). *J. Pharm. Sci.* **60,** 576–582.

Pestka, S. (1971). *Annu. Rev. Microbiol.* **25,** 487–562.

Petisi, J., Spencer, J. L., Hlavka, J. J., and Boothe, J. H. (1962). *J. Med. Chem.* **5,** 538–546.

Pezzaniti, J. O., Clardy, J., Lau, P.-Y., Wood, G., Walker, D. L., and Fraser-Reid, B. (1975). *J. Am. Chem. Soc.* **97,** 6250–6251.

Pindell, M. H., Cull, K. M., Doran, K. M., and Dickinson, H. L. (1959). *J. Pharmacol. Exp. Ther.* **125,** 287–294.

Popov, P. G., Vaptzarova, K. I., Kossekova, G. P., and Nikolov, T. K. (1972). *Biochem. Pharmacol.* **21,** 2363–2372.

Powis, G. (1974). *J. Pharm. Pharmacol.* **26,** 113–118.

Prewo, R., and Stezowski, J. J. (1977). *J. Am. Chem. Soc.* **99,** 1117–1121.

Purcell, W. P., Bass, G. E., and Clayton, J. M. (1973). "Strategy of Drug Design. A Molecular Guide to Biological Activity." Wiley, New York.

Purich, S. D., Colaizzi, J. L., and Poust, R. I. (1973). *J. Pharm. Sci.* **62,** 545–549.

Raff, M. J., Summersgill, J. T., Fontana, F. J., Barnwell, P. A., Wateman, N. G., and Scharfenberger, L. (1977). *J. Antibiot.* **30,** 593–596.

Redin, G. S. (1966). *Antimicrob. Agents Chemother.* pp. 371–376.

Remington, J. S., and Finland, M. (1962). *Clin. Pharmacol. Ther.* **3,** 284–304.

Reynard, A. M., and Nellis, L. F. (1972). *Biochem. Biophys. Res. Commun.* **48,** 1129–1132.

Rigler, N. E., Bag, S. P., Leyden, D. E., Sudmeier, J. L., and Reilley, C. N. (1965). *Anal. Chem.* **37,** 872–875.

Rogalski, W., Kirchlechner, R., Seubert, J., Gottschlich, R., Hameister, W., Bergmann, R., and Wahlig, H. (1976). Ger. Offen. 2, 437, 487.

Rosenblatt, J. E., Berrett, J. E., Brodie, J. L., and Kirby, W. M. M. (1966). *Antimicrob. Agents Chemother.* pp. 134–141.

Sarkar, S., and Thach, R. E. (1968). *Proc. Natl. Acad. Sci. U.S.A.* **60,** 1479–1486.

Saxén, L. (1965). *Science* **149,** 870–872.

Schach von Wittenau, M. (1968). *Chemotherapy (Basel)* **13,** Suppl., 41–50.

Schach von Wittenau, M., and Blackwood, R. K. (1966). *J. Org. Chem.* **31,** 613–615.

Schach von Wittenau, M., and Delahunt, C. S. (1966). *J. Pharmacol. Exp. Ther.* **152,** 164–169.

Schach von Wittenau, M., and Twomey, T. M. (1971). *Chemotherapy (Basel)* **16,** 217–228.

Schach von Wittenau, M., and Yeary, R. (1963). *J. Pharmacol. Exp. Ther.* **140,** 258–266.

Schach von Wittenau, M., Beereboom, J. J., Blackwood, R. K., and Stephens, C. R. (1962). *J. Am. Chem. Soc.* **84,** 2645–2647.

Schach von Wittenau, M., Hochstein, F. A., and Stephens, C. R. (1963). *J. Org. Chem.* **28,** 2454–2456.

Schach von Wittenau, M., Blackwood, R. K., Conover, L. H., Glavert, R. H., and Woodward, R. B. (1965). *J. Am. Chem. Soc.* **87,** 134–135.

Schach von Wittenau, M., Twomey, T. M., and Swindell, A. C. (1972). *Chemotherapy (Basel)* **17,** 26–39.

Schlecht, K. D., and Frank, C. W. (1975). *J. Pharm. Sci.* **64,** 352–354.

Sensi, P., DeFerrari, G. A., Gallo, G. G., and Roland, G. (1955). *Farmaco, Ed. Sci.* **10,** 337–345.

Shastri, R. A., and Krishnaswamy, K. (1976). *Clin. Chim. Acta* **66,** 157–164.

Simon, C., Malerczyk, V., Preuss, I., Schmidt, K., and Grahmann, H. (1976). *Arzneim-Forsch.* **26,** 556–560.
Sirota, J. H., and Saltzman, A. (1950). *J. Pharmacol. Exp. Ther.* **100,** 210–218.
Skinner, H. C. W., and Nalbandian, J. (1975). *Yale J. Biol. Med.* **48,** 377–397.
Snell, J. F., Wagner, R. L., and Hochstein, F. A. (1956). *Proc. Int. Conf. Peaceful Uses At. Energy, 1st, 1955* Vol. 12, pp. 431–434.
Sompolinsky, D., and Krausz, J. (1973). *Antimicrob. Agents & Chemother.* **4,** 237–247.
Spitzy, K. H., and Hitzenberger, G. (1957). *Antibiot. Annu.* pp. 996–1003.
Steigbigel, N. H., Reed, C. W., and Finland, M. (1968). *Am. J. Med. Sci.* **255,** 179–195.
Stephens, C. R., Conover, L. H., Pasternack, R., Hochstein, F. A., Moreland, W. T., Regna, P. P., Pilgrim, F. J., Brunings, K. J., and Woodward, R. B. (1954). *J. Am. Chem. Soc.* **76,** 3568–3575.
Stephens, C. R., Murai, K., Brunings, K. J., and Woodward, R. B. (1956). *J. Am. Chem. Soc.* **78,** 4155–4158.
Stephens, C. R., Beereboom, J. J., Rennhard, H. H., Gordon, P. N., Murai, K., Blackwood, R. K., and Schach von Wittenau, M. (1963). *J. Am. Chem. Soc.* **85,** 2643–2652.
Stezowski, J. J. (1976). *J. Am. Chem. Soc.* **98,** 6012–6018.
Stezowski, J. J. (1977). *J. Am. Chem. Soc.* **99,** 1122–1129.
Storey, E. (1973). *Drugs* **6,** 321–323.
Suarez, G., and Nathans, D. (1965). *Biochem. Biophys. Res. Commun.* **18,** 743–750.
Takeuchi, Y., and Buerger, M. J. (1960). *Proc. Natl. Acad. Sci. U.S.A.* **46,** 1366–1370.
Terada, H., and Inagi, T. (1975). *Chem. Pharm. Bull.* **23,** 1960–1968.
Tritton, T. R. (1977). *Biochemistry* **16,** 4133–4138.
Turley, R. H., and Snell, J. F. (1966). *In* "Biosynthesis of Antibiotics" (J. F. Snell, ed.), Vol. 1, pp. 95–120. Academic Press, New York.
Tute, M. S. (1975). *Chem. Ind. (London)* pp. 100–105.
Vasquez, D. (1965). *Biochim. Biophys. Acta* **114,** 277–288.
Waddington, W. S., Bergy, G. G., Nielsen, R. L., and Kirby, W. M. M. (1954). *Am. J. Med. Sci.* **228,** 164–173.
Waller, C. W., Hutchings, B. L., Wolf, C. F., Goldman, A. A., Proschard, R. W., and Williams, J. H. (1952). *J. Am. Chem. Soc.* **74,** 4981.
Weinberg, E. D. (1957). *Bacteriol. Rev.* **21,** 46–68.
Weisberger, A. S., Wolfe, S., and Armentrout, S. (1964). *J. Exp. Med.* **120,** 161–181.
Weisblum, B., and Davies, J. (1968). *Bacteriol. Rev.* **32,** 493–528.
Welling, P. G., Koch, P. A., Lau, C. C., and Craig, W. A. (1977). *Antimicrob. Agents Chemother.* **11,** 462–469.
Whelton, A., Schach von Wittenau, M., Twomey, T. M., Walker, W. G., and Blanchine, J. R. (1974). *Kidney Int.* **5,** 365–371.
Whelton, A., Nightingale, S. D., Carter, G. C., Gordon, L. S., Bryant, H. H., and Walker, W. G. (1975). *J. Infect. Dis.* **132,** 467–471.
White, J. P., and Cantor, C. R. (1971). *J. Mol. Biol.* **58,** 397–400.
Williams, D. N., Laughlin, L. W., and Lee, Y.-H. (1974). *Lancet* **2,** 744–746.
Williamson, D. E. , and Everett, G. W. (1975). *J. Am. Chem. Soc.* **97,** 2397–2405.
Williamson, G. M. (1969). *Bull. Chim. Ther.* **1,** 53–60.
Wozniak, L. A. (1960). *Proc. Soc. Exp. Biol. Med.* **105,** 430–433.
Yen, P. K.-J., and Shaw, J. H. (1975). *J. Dent. Res.* **54,** 423.
Zia, H., and Price, J. C. (1976). *J. Pharm. Sci.* **65,** 226–230.

Neurotransmitter Mechanisms during Mental Illness Induced by Alterations in Thyroid Function

RADHEY L. SINGHAL AND RAM B. RASTOGI*

Department of Pharmacology
Faculty of Medicine
University of Ottawa
Ottawa, Ontario, Canada

* Present address; Nordic Research Laboratories, Connlab Holdings Limited, Montreal, Quebec, Canada.

I. Introduction

There is ample evidence to support the view that there is an association between mental disturbances and altered levels of hormones such as adrenal corticoids, thyroid hormones, androgens, and estrogens (Rubin and Mandell, 1966; Mandell and Mandell, 1967; Glass *et al.*, 1971; Wheatley, 1972; Dewhurst *et al.*, 1969). Although it is only recently that neuroendocrinologists have become interested in studying the effects of hormones on the functioning of the brain, psychiatrists for many years have felt that the solution of several etiological problems in psychiatry would come only from a better understanding of the neuroendocrinological mechanisms. During the twenties, an endocrine psychology was evolved that attempted to explain the variations of normal personality on a hormonal basis (Freud, 1905). Within the last decade, however, advances in methodology and diagnosis resulted in a flush of enthusiasm, which led to the realization that the psychiatric illnesses, such as depression, mania, anxiety, and schizophrenia, could not be treated overnight. This has enabled researchers to focus attention on the specific aspect of the relationship that may exist between endocrine function and mental disorders.

Over the past few years, investigators in the fields of neurochemistry and psychopharmacology have begun a more systematic inquiry into the potential relationship between brain biogenic amines and various types of altered behavior in experimental animals. More recently, workers using specific pharmacological tools have even made it possible to implicate a single neurotransmitter substance in the control of a specific type of behavior (Reis *et al.*, 1970; Bartholini *et al.*, 1969; Ernst, 1967; Butcher and Engel, 1969; Kane, 1970; Hole, 1972). However, since the "single amine single disease" hypothesis for psychiatric illness now seems less tenable (Davis, 1975), indications are that we must employ an integrative approach in order to elucidate the role of various putative neurohumors in the control of mental functioning and behavior.

Clinical studies have revealed that there are significant alterations in the levels of circulating hormones during affective disorders (Dewhurst *et al.*, 1969; Board *et al.*, 1957; McClure, 1966; Gibbons, 1964). Since evidence also suggests that hormones affect the metabolism of putative neurotransmitters (Azmitia *et al.*, 1970; Shen and Ganong, 1976; Singhal *et al.*, 1977; Luine *et al.*, 1977), particularly during vulnerable periods of development, it is likely that changes in the mental state during certain endocrine disorders might be the sequelae of alterations in central monoamine metabolism produced by altered levels of hormones. Additionally, it has been shown that neurotransmitters, such as catecholamine and indoleamine (which are associated with depressive disorders and mania) play a major role in the regulation of neuroendocrine function (Anton-Tay and Wurtman, 1971). Hence, it is difficult to conceive as to which one of the two abnormalities (i.e., changes in hormonal secretion induced by altered levels of central amines or aberrant metabolism of putative neurotransmitters induced by altered hormonal levels) has the prime role in the pathophysiology of affective illness. The major aim of this contribution is to focus attention on studies concerning the relationship between varying levels of hormones and brain biogenic amine metabolism and behavior. Specifically, our own interest has centered on investigating the influence of variations in thyroid hormone levels on the metabolism of brain norepinephrine (NE), dopamine (DA), 5-hydroxytryptamine (5-HT), and acetylcholine (ACh). Because there is some similarity between hyperthyroidism and mania (Maletzky and Blachley, 1971), hyperthyroid animals have been employed in an experimental model to examine the intraneuronal basis of the mechanism of action of drugs clinically used for this affective disorder.

II. Evidence for Neuroendocrine Abnormalities in Mental Dysfunction

A. Adrenocortical Hormones

The study of possible interaction between emotion and the adrenocortical system was revived in the 1950s. Bliss *et al.* (1956) concluded that a psychiatric disorder accompanied by emotional turmoil is likely to be associated with increased 17-hydroxycorticoid levels. Board *et al.* (1957) found 60% higher mean plasma 17-hydroxycorticosteroid level in depressed patients as compared to the normal values. The change seemed specific because clinical recovery produced by either electroconvulsive therapy or imipramine was accompanied by a drop in plasma corticosteroid levels (Gibbons and McHugh, 1962). Even though the activity of adrenal cortex during pure manic state (which is distinct from emotional excitement seen during other psychiatric conditions) has not yet been extensively studied, available data indicate decreased urinary 17-hydroxycorticosteroid output in manic patients (Rizzo *et al.*, 1954).

In order to ascertain whether alterations in behavior during affective disorders are, at least in part, associated with altered biogenic amine metabolism induced by changes in corticosteroid level, the effects of bilateral adrenalectomy and subsequent corticosterone treatment on brain NE and DA were investigated in our laboratory. Data presented in

Table I demonstrate that surgical removal of adrenals resulted in increased synthesis and, possibly, release of NE and DA as evidenced by increased activity of the rate-limiting enzyme tyrosine hydroxylase (TH), and decreased levels of endogenous NE and DA in discrete brain regions. The changes in various parameters appeared specific to adrenocortical hormone, since replacement therapy with corticosterone decreased synthesis and release and restored amine levels and TH activity to normal limits. Our results are consistent with the findings of Javoy *et al.* (1968) who reported increased turnover of brain NE at 6 days after adrenalectomy. Furthermore, Caesar *et al.* (1970) reported that following adrenalectomy, there was an increase in the urinary excretion of 4-hydroxy-3-methoxyphenylglycol (MOPEG) and homovanillic acid (HVA), the chief metabolites of NE and DA, respectively. The histochemical studies that demonstrated enhanced monoamine disappearance in most parts of the brain, particularly in hypothalamus and cerebral cortex of adrenalectomized animals (Fuxe *et al.*, 1970; Olson and Fuxe, 1971), also support the hypothesis that low corticosteroid levels result in a general rise of brain catecholamine turnover.

B. Sex Hormones

There is also evidence to show that female sex hormones play an important role in the development of the central nervous system, particularly during vulnerable periods of growth (Timiras, 1971). This action is, in part, reflected biochemically by alterations in electrolyte distribution (Valcana *et al.*, 1967) and precocious laying down of the myelin sheath around the nerve fibers in brain tissue (Curry and Heim, 1966; Casper *et al.*, 1967). Estradiol treatment in developing rats significantly elevated the brain protein content and the activity of choline acetyltransferase and acetylcholinesterase. Conversely, a significantly lower activity of choline acetyltransferase and acetylcholinesterase was observed in brains of ovariectomized rats (Cavallotti and Luigi, 1972). Furthermore, ovariectomy in neonatal rats retarded the electrophysiological, behavioral, and biochemical maturation of the brain (Bisanti and Cavallotti, 1972). Evidence indicates that ovariectomy at 2 weeks of age reduced brain protein, lipid, cerebroside, and sulfatide levels with the difference becoming statistically significant at 21 days. It is generally assumed that the incidence of mental disorders in women is increased at times when the delicate balance between estrogen and progesterone levels is disturbed (Smith, 1975). Earlier workers had indicated that the premenstrual woman is more likely to be hyperactive, aggressive, violent, and possibly criminal (Morton *et al.*, 1953). To many

TABLE I

EFFECT OF ADRENALECTOMY (ADX) AND REPLACEMENT THERAPY WITH CORTICOSTERONE ON STRIATAL TH AND NE AND DA LEVELS IN CERTAIN BRAIN REGIONS[a]

Treatment	Striatal TH (nmol dopa/gm/hr)	NE (μg/gm)			DA (μg/gm)		
		Brain stem	Hypothalamus	Striatum	Brain stem	Hypothalamus	Striatum
Sham-operated	63.3 ± 4.2 (100)	0.61 ± 0.02 (100)	1.92 ± 0.10 (100)	0.26 ± 0.01 (100)	1.23 ± 0.08 (100)	0.55 ± 0.02 (100)	7.87 ± 0.51 (100)
ADX (7 days)	76.6 ± 5.1 (121)[b]	0.65 ± 0.02 (107)	2.00 ± 0.07 (104)	0.26 ± 0.01 (100)	1.15 ± 0.07 (94)	0.53 ± 0.02 (97)	7.24 ± 0.62 (92)
ADX (15 days)	82.9 ± 3.8 (131[b]; 100)	0.54 ± 0.04 (89; 100)	1.40 ± 0.08 (73[b]; 100)	0.20 ± 0.01 (76[b]; 100)	1.02 ± 0.05 (83[b]; 100)	0.51 ± 0.03 (93; 100)	6.06 ± 0.28 (77[b]; 100)
ADX + corticosterone (3 days)	84.6 ± 4.8 (131[b]; 102)	0.55 ± 0.03 (90; 102)	1.54 ± 0.07 (80[b]; 110)	0.22 ± 0.01 (85; 111)	1.09 ± 0.05 (89; 107)	0.60 ± 0.02 (109; 117[c])	7.03 ± 0.31 (99; 116[c])
ADX + corticosterone (7 days)	65.5 ± 3.6 (103; 79[c])	0.62 ± 0.04 (102; 114)	1.74 ± 0.06 (91; 124[c])	0.23 ± 0.02 (88; 115)	1.19 ± 0.04 (97; 117[c])	0.61 ± 0.02 (110; 119[c])	7.33 ± 0.39 (104; 121[c])

[a] Each value represents the mean ± S.E.M. of 6 rats in the group. Rats were killed at 7 or 15 days after adrenalectomy. Groups of adrenalectomized rats were injected with corticosterone (10 mg/kg/day, i.p.) for either 3 or 7 days, beginning from 12 or 8 days, respectively, after adrenalectomy and killed 15 days after surgical removal of adrenals. The controls (adrenalectomized) received an equal volume of the vehicle (5:1 mixture of 95% ethanol and saline). The activity of TH was determined in particulate fraction in the absence of pteridine cofactor according to the methods of McGeer *et al.* (1967). Data in parentheses express results in percentages taking the values of sham-operated and 15 days ADX rats as 100%. The DA levels in this study were determined according to the procedure of Hrdina *et al.* (1975) modified from Spano and Neff (1971). It is possible that the relatively higher DA levels reported in Table IV may have been due to an artifact of the assay method (Laverty and Taylor, 1968) that we were then employing.

[b] Statistically significant difference when compared with the values of sham-operated rats ($p < 0.05$).

[c] Statistically significant difference when compared with the values of ADX (15 days) animals ($p < 0.05$).

investigators, the striking fact that depression occurs premenstrually, during postpartum menopause, and while using oral contraceptive agents has been suggestive of a relationship between female sex hormones and depression (Hegarty, 1955; Rees, 1953; Dalton, 1971; Yalmon *et al.*, 1968; Kane, 1968). The chain of events whereby estrogens and/or progestogens in oral contraceptive medications trigger depression in predisposed individuals is not certain. There is conflicting evidence with regard to the question as to whether it is the predominantly progestogenic or the predominantly estrogenic medication that is more likely to produce dysphoric effect. So far as the neurochemical basis of the oral contraceptive-induced depression is concerned, it has been speculated that this may result from interference with brain tryptophan metabolism so as to decrease the amount of 5-HT produced (Rose, 1969). This is probably accomplished by diminishing the availability of pyridoxine, a necessary cofactor in the synthesis of 5-HT from tryptophan. There have been reports on the use of oral pyridoxine to combat the depressive side effect of the contraceptive pill (Blumblatt and Winston, 1970), but, as yet, no conclusive results have been presented.

Greengrass and Tongue (1971, 1972, 1973, 1974a,c) demonstrated that the central monoamine metabolism was significantly altered in mice during estrous cycle, pregnancy, postpartum period, administration of sex hormones to intact females as well as following gonadectomy. Recently, these investigators demonstrated that administration of ethinyloestradiol to ovariectomized rats inhibited the reuptake of NE, whereas progesterone interfered with that of 5-HT (Greengrass and Tongue, 1974b). It has been speculated that beneficial effects on mood and motivation induced by estrogens in estrogen-deficient subjects (Greenblatt, 1965) may be associated with enhanced levels of NE in the vicinity of pre- and postsynaptic receptors. By contrast, the tranquilizing action of progesterone seen in females (Merryman *et al.*, 1954) might, in part, be related to its diminishing effect on NE levels within the synaptic clefts (Greengrass and Tongue, 1974c).

C. Thyroid Hormones

An abundance of information now exists emphasizing the importance of thyroid hormones in the structural and biochemical ontogeny of the central nervous system, and they are considered to be determinants of the adult neurophysiological and behavioral processes. Using developing rat cerebellum as a model, hyperthyroidism was shown to result in a premature termination of cell division (Balazs *et al.*, 1971; Gourdon *et al.*, 1973; Nicholson and Altman, 1972; Weichsel, 1974) as well as a shift to an earlier age in the developmental time course of DNA biosynthesis and the activity of thymidine kinase (Weichsel, 1974). Conversely, hypothyroidism resulted in a delay in cerebellar cell acquisition (Balazs, 1971; Gourdon *et al.*, 1973; Hamburgh *et al.*, 1971; Nicholson and Altman, 1972) as well as in the maximum activity of thymidine kinase (Weichsel and Dawson, 1976). Gelber *et al.* (1964) observed that, whereas administration of L-thyroxine significantly enhanced the leucine-^{14}C incorporation into protein of developing brain, it elicited no such effect in brains of adult rats. Functional dissimilarities in mitochondrial fractions have been presumed to be responsible for the varying effects on adult and immature rats as the mitochondria of mature brain have been shown to be rather insensitive to the action of thyroxine (Klee and Sokoloff, 1964). Thyroid hormone has also been shown to stimulate RNA polymerase activity and the synthesis of ribosomal and, perhaps, messenger RNA. This chain of reactions ultimately enhances the cellular contents of functional ribosomes subsequently leading to increased synthesis of brain proteins (Tata *et al.*, 1963).

By contrast, neonatal thyroidectomy has been shown to decrease the metabolism of protein and nucleic acids (Geel and Timiras, 1967a). A decreased incorporation of isotopic leucine into protein has been shown in the cerebral cortex of rats made hypothyroid at 1 day of age (Geel *et al.*, 1967). Because the incorporation of labeled amino acid into microsomal or ribosomal protein *in vitro* is markedly dependent on Mg^{2+}, K^+, and Na^+ concentrations, it has been suggested that the reduced incorporation of amino acids into proteins in neonatally thyroidectomized rats may be associated with altered Na^+–K^+ pump (Geel *et al.*, 1967).

Several investigators have also demonstrated marked alterations in enzyme activity of the nervous system in thyroid-deficient animals. Geel and Timiras (1967b) found a decrease in the activity of choline acetyltransferase in the cerebral cortex and acetylcholinesterase activity in the hypothalamus. Garcia Argiz *et al.* (1967) reported that thyroid deprivation at birth leads to an altered developmental pattern of glutamate decarboxylase, Mg^{2+} and Na^+–K^+ ATPase and γ-aminobutyric acid transaminase, and Na^+–K^+ ATPase in the cerebellum. The decreased levels of several of these brain enzymes in neonatally thyroidectomized rats were restored following administration of thyroid hormone (Krawiec *et al.*, 1969). Siegel and Sisler (1964) demonstrated that cycloheximide, an inhibitor of protein synthesis, prevented the L-triiodothyronine-induced rise in the activities of several brain enzymes in neonatally hypothyroid rats, supporting the view that thyroid hormone enhances protein biosynthesis in the brain. Since cycloheximide inhibits protein synthesis by preventing the transfer of aminoacetyl transfer RNA to ribosomes, it seems possible that thyroid hormone affects brain protein synthesis at the translational level.

The process of myelination is an important aspect of brain development. Deposition of myelin accounts for considerable increase in brain dry weights postnatally. The timing of myelination seems to be specified in the genetic code, because it always occurs at a particular time in a given species. In rats, it usually starts somewhere between 12 to 20 days of life (Curry and Heim, 1966; Jacobson, 1963). As early as 1948, Barnett had reported that hypothyroidism in developing rats markedly retarded the process of myelination. Thyroid hormone deprivation in early life also reduced the cerebroside, sulfatide and cholesterol content of the brain as well as delayed the onset of sulfatide biosynthesis (Walravens and Chase, 1969). Balazs *et al.* (1969) have assessed myelin deposition by determining cholesterol content and showed that the amount of myelin was significantly reduced in thyroid-deprived rats. By contrast, administration of thyroxine to normal animals during early life resulted in an accelerated rate of myelination (Schapiro, 1966).

III. Hyperthyroidism and Related Mental Illness

A number of recent studies in human and subhuman primate subjects have supported the view that the pituitary–thyroidal system can be stimulated under psychologically stressful conditions. Johansson *et al.* (1970) found significantly elevated plasma protein-bound-iodine (PBI) levels in a group of army officers subjected to a simulated military stress situation. Mason *et al.* (1973) reported increases in both plasma thyrotropin (TSH) and thyroxine levels in all of the 8 normal young men during the 20-minute anticipatory period immediately before their first experimental session involving exercise to the point of exhaustion on a bicycle ergometer. More recently, elevation of plasma TSH levels also has been found in relation to both the chair-restraint and conditioned-avoidance situations in the monkey (Mason, 1975).

In addition, studies have demonstrated that excessive thyroid secretion produces psychological symptoms including emotional lability, restlessness, irritability, over-reactiveness with predominant anxiety and tension (Eayrs, 1960; Whybrow and Ferrell, 1974). More severe mental disorders may also be seen in hyperthyroid patients if left untreated with antithyroid drugs. Psychoses of the acute organic type have frequently been encountered in severe cases and also during thyroid crisis. The incidence of other psychoses in hyperthyroid individuals has been under some dispute (Bursten, 1961). At one extreme, Lidz and Whitehorn

(1949) detected evidence of psychosis in 20% of thyrotoxic patients attending an out-patient clinic, whereas Kleinschmidt *et al.* (1956) considered that 20% of their 84 thyrotoxics were schizophrenic or borderline psychotics. Evidence also exists suggesting some behavioral similarities (such as hypermobility and sleeplessness, exaggerated responses to environmental stimuli, etc.) between hyperthyroidism and mania (Maletzky and Blachley, 1971). Even though considerable research has been carried out to delineate the neuronal basis of mania, the exact nature of underlying disturbances in the metabolism of various putative neurotransmitters is not clearly understood. In humans, moral and ethical reasons preclude the direct biochemical assay of brain tissue in patients suffering from affective disorder. Therefore, the development of an appropriate animal model does not only provide insight of the neuronal mechanisms underlying the pathophysiology of mania, but may also be useful in eliminating the mode of action of antimanic agents clinically used to combat this psychiatric illness. Recent work carried out in our laboratory has been concerned with examining the complete profile of NE, DA, 5-HT, and ACh metabolism in brains of developing rats treated with L-triiodothyronine (T_3). Neonatal animals were chosen for these studies since earlier workers had demonstrated that thyroid hormone influences the maturation of central aminergic neurons as well as protein and lipid metabolism only during the early periods of growth (Klee and Sokoloff, 1964; Gelber *et al.*, 1964; Walravens and Chase, 1969; Rastogi and Singhal, 1974a,b).

A. Relevance of Animal Experimentation

1. *Experimental Hyperthyroidism—Physical and Behavioral Manifestations in Developing Rats*

In neonates, hyperthyroidism was induced by daily administration of 10 μg/100 gm of T_3. This dose regimen seemed to accelerate a rush toward adulthood in the neonates. There was an advancement in the appearance of incisors and opening of the eyes by 2 to 3 days. The elevation of pinnae and snout elongation were advanced in comparison to littermate controls. After 15 days of treatment, the animals had the appearance of "miniature adults." This rapid approach toward adulthood tended to decrease the body weight (82%) and brain weights (86%). Grave *et al.* (1973) reported similar decreases in body weights of hyperthyroid rats. The neurophysiological precocity was evidenced by earlier appearance of startle, righting, and placing reflexes and a more coordinated feeding behavior. The animals were hyperactive as reflected in their spontaneous locomotor activity. Treatment with T_3 tended to slow down the rats during the first 10 days of life. However, at 15 days of age, hyperthyroid animals showed 192% increase in their sponaneous locomotor activity, which remained elevated throughout the entire period of thyroid hormone administration (45 days). Neonatally induced hyperthyroidism seemed to leave a fairly permanent effect on the locomotor activity since it remained significantly higher than control even 60 days after the discontinuation of T_3 treatment (Rastogi and Singhal, 1976a).

2. *Effects on Certain Amino Acid Levels in Brain*

Available evidence supports the role of amino acid precursors in the modulation of their respective amine synthesis in the brain. For example, the Michaelis constant of tryptophan hydroxylase (TPH) for tryptophan (TP) in presence of pteridine cofactor is 300 μM, which is higher than the endogenous concentration of TP present in the brain (30 μM) (Jequier *et al.*, 1969). Thus, TP seems to play a modulatory role in the synthesis of 5-HT. In fact, it has been demonstrated that pharmacological agents that elevate the concentration of free TP in plasma and its synaptosomal uptake in brain also enhance the synthesis of 5-HT (Hamon and Glowinski, 1974). Moreover, TP is the only essential amino acid that is partially bound to albumin in plasma (McMenamy and Oncley, 1958), and it is only the free TP that is available to brain for 5-HT synthesis. Under normal conditions, plasma–brain TP ratio is 5:1. Pharmacological agents that enhance brain TP levels do so by displacing this amino acid from binding site in the albumin. It is suggested that T_3, which also binds to albumin, displaces TP from the binding site, making more of it available in free form to cross the blood–brain barrier and reach neuronal tissue. Our data that neonatal T_3 treatment enhanced the level of this important amino acid in midbrain suggest that this hormone accelerated the uptake of TP across the synaptic membrane (Rastogi and Singhal, 1976b). It has previously been shown that neonatal thyroid deficiency has a severe effect on the maturation of nerve cells and dendritic ramification (Eayrs, 1968; Legrand, 1967). The number of nerve terminals per nerve cell is markedly reduced in neonatal hypothyroid rats. Perhaps it can be hypothesized that if the converse is also true, the enhanced levels of brain TP may, in part, be due to increased amounts of TP being taken up presumably by more ramified nerve endings.

In addition to TP, repeated T_3 treatment in neonatal rats increased tyrosine (TR) level in striatum. Recently, Wurtman *et al.* (1974) presented evidence that agents increasing or decreasing brain TR concentration also produce parallel changes in the rate at which the brain synthesizes catecholamines. It has been shown that Michaelis constant (K_m) of TH for TR [0.14 mM for whole rat brain (Coyle, 1972) and 0.1 mM for sheep caudate nuclei (Poillon, 1971)] is higher relative to brain TR concentrations (0.08 mM) (Wurtman *et al.*, 1974). It is reasonable to suppose that T_3 treatment in neonatal rats enhanced catecholamine synthesis by increasing TR levels in brain tissue in addition to exerting effects on the rate-limiting enzyme, TH.

3. *Increased Catecholaminergic Activity*

Administration of L-triiodothyronine in early life increased the activity of the rate-limiting enzyme TH, in both particulate and soluble fractions (Table II). In order to gain additional evidence for the influence of neonatal hyperthyroidism on catecholamine metabolism, another method involving the recapture of $^{14}CO_2$ (Gershon *et al.*, 1974) evolved during the synthesis of catecholamine from L-tyrosine-(1-^{14}C) was employed. Data presented in Table III demonstrate that repeated administration of T_3 during neonatal life augmented the rate of catecholamine synthesis in P_2 pellet (synaptosomes) by 44%. Furthermore, the level of MOPEG, an important metabolite of NE was markedly enhanced (Table III). This is consistent with the data of Keller *et al.* (1974) who also reported a rise in MOPEG levels in T_3-treated rats. Because the level of

TABLE II

EFFECT OF NEONATAL HYPERTHYROIDISM ON STRIATAL TH, HVA, AND DOPAC LEVELS[a]

Treatment	Soluble TH (nmol dopa/mg/hr)	Particulate TH (nmol dopa/gm/hr)	HVA (μg/gm)	DOPAC (μg/gm)
Control	13.48 ± 0.60 (100)	82.43 ± 7.3 (100)	1.73 ± 0.14 (100)	2.29 ± 0.18 (100)
Hyperthyroidism	17.12 ± 0.91 (127)[b]	112.10 ± 8.5 (136)[b]	4.34 ± 0.33 (251)[b]	5.50 ± 0.39 (240)[b]

[a] Each value represents the mean ± S.E.M. of 6 animals in the group. Neonatal rats were injected subcutaneously with T_3 (10 μg/100 gm/day) for 30 days and killed 24 hr after the last injection. Data in parentheses indicate results in percentages taking the values of control rats as 100%. The activity of particulate TH was determined in the absence of pteridine cofactor according to the method of McGeer *et al.* (1967), whereas that of soluble fraction in the presence of BH_4, according to the method of Rastogi *et al.* (1977e) modified from Black (1975).

[b] Statistically significant difference when compared with the values of control rats ($p <$ 0.05).

TABLE III

EFFECT OF NEONATAL HYPERTHYROIDISM ON WHOLE-BRAIN MOPEG LEVELS AS WELL AS CATECHOLAMINE SYNTHESIS AND NE-^{3}H UPTAKE IN SYNAPTOSOMES[a]

Treatment	MOPEG (μg/gm)	Catecholamine synthesis	NE-^{3}H uptake
Control	0.56 ± 0.02 (100)	4.05 ± 0.26 (100)	3.22 ± 0.29 (100)
Hyperthyroidism	1.00 ± 0.07 (179)[b]	5.81 ± 0.43 (144)[b]	3.06 ± 0.18 (95)

[a] Each value represents the mean ± S.E.M. of 6 rats in the group. For experimental details, see footnote *a* of Table II. Catecholamine synthesis is expressed in picomoles $^{14}CO_2$ formed per milligram protein per 25 min, whereas the uptake of NE is expressed in nanocuries NE-^{3}H per milligram protein per 5 min.

[b] Statistically significant difference when compared with the values of control rats ($p < 0.05$).

MOPEG seems to reflect the amount of NE present at the receptor site, it seems that the neuronal release of NE was increased in neonatally hyperthyroid rats, even though no conspicuous change was seen in the steady-state levels of this catecholamine in the discrete brain regions examined (Table IV). By contrast, the endogenous levels of brain DA were increased. Since hyperthyroidism failed to alter the synaptosomal uptake of NE-^{3}H (Table III) and as NE and DA are presumed to be taken up into the presynaptic neurons by a similar uptake mechanism, it is possible that the high levels of DA in brain might not be due to enhanced uptake of DA. It is likely that the rate of DA synthesis exceeded the rate of its neuronal release from dopaminergic neurons resulting in partial accumulation of this monoamine. The rise in HVA, the extraneuronal metabolite of DA, is due to increased turnover of DA in T_3-treated rats. Beley *et al.* (1975) and Engström *et al.* (1974) also reported a similar rise in DA turnover in brains of rats treated with thyroxine.

Several interpretations can be offered with regard to the importance of elevated levels of DA (Table IV) and its metabolites, HVA and dihydroxyphenylacetic acid (DOPAC) (Table II), in aroused behavior seen in T_3-exposed neonatal rats. Dopaminergic neurons are critical components of the locomotor system, and studies suggest that increased dopaminergic activity produces hypermobility (Bartholini *et al.*, 1969). It is possible that increased spontaneous locomotor activity in hyperthyroid rats may be the result of increased synthesis and turnover of DA induced by thyroid hormone. For reasons cited by previous workers (Bliss and Ailion, 1971), one would expect that the rise in striatal HVA and DOPAC levels in neonatal hyperthyroid rats may also be related to disturbed emotion.

Previous workers have shown that a lowering of NE in the hypothalamus results in a marked decrease in spontaneous locomotor activity. Alternatively, the injection of minute amounts of NE has been found to induce hyperactivity (Broitman and Donoso, 1971). Reis and Fuxe (1969) demonstrated that sham-rage behavior induced by brain-stem transection is dependent on the activation of central NE receptors. Evidence also indicates that overstimulation of pre- and/or postsynaptic receptors for NE with concurrent administration of nialamide and DOPA is associated with aggressive behavior (Randrup and Munkvad, 1968). The finding that thyroxine augmented the rate of disappearance of NE-^{3}H administered intracisternally (Schildkraut *et al.*, 1971) supports the contention that accelerated behavioral activity in T_3-treated rats might, at least in part, be associated with increased turnover of brain NE. Catechol-*O*-methyltransferase (COMT) is known to be a presynaptic enzyme that *O*-methylates both NE and DA. The possibility, therefore, remains that, owing to low activity of COMT in midbrain and cerebral cortex of hyperthyroid rats, the released NE and DA may remain within the synaptic cleft for a relatively longer period of time and thus prolong the bombardment of amines at their corresponding receptors and, in turn, facilitate neural transmission in noradrenergic and dopaminergic

TABLE IV

EFFECT OF NEONATAL HYPERTHYROIDISM ON NE AND DA LEVELS IN CERTAIN BRAIN REGIONS[a]

Region examined	NE (μg/gm)		DA (μg/gm)	
	Control	Hyperthyroid	Control	Hyperthyroid
Hypothalamus	2.27 ± 0.21 (100)	2.47 ± 0.26 (109)	—	—
Pons-medulla	0.59 ± 0.03 (100)	0.63 ± 0.02 (107)	0.89 ± 0.06 (100)	1.28 ± 0.06 (144)[b]
Midbrain	0.62 ± 0.04 (100)	0.53 ± 0.05 (85)	1.20 ± 0.09 (100)	1.62 ± 0.07 (135)[b]
Striatum	0.30 ± 0.01 (100)	0.28 ± 0.01 (96)	12.41 ± 1.03 (100)	16.88 ± 1.07 (136)[b]
Hippocampus	0.41 ± 0.02 (100)	0.46 ± 0.03 (113)	0.74 ± 0.06 (100)	0.90 ± 0.06 (121)[b]

[a] Each value is the mean ± S.E.M. of 6 animals in the group. For experimental details, see footnote *a* of Table II. The DA was assayed according to the procedure of Laverty and Taylor (1968).

[b] Statistically significant difference when compared with control rats ($p < 0.05$).

neurons. It is interesting to note that clinical studies conducted by previous workers have shown increased turnover of NE in brains of manic patients (Goodwin and Sack, 1973). Furthermore, Messiha *et al.* (1970) have reported enhanced urinary excretion of DA during manic illness.

4. *Increased 5-Hydroxytryptaminergic Activity*

Hyperthyroidism induced in neonatal life enhanced the functioning of 5-hydroxytryptaminergic neurons, as evidenced by increased activity of the rate-limiting enzyme TPH in midbrain (Table V) and 5-hydroxyindoleacetic acid (5-HIAA) levels, the major metabolite of 5-HT, in several discrete areas of the brain examined (Table VI). The effect of hyperthyroidism on the rate of 5-HT synthesis in synaptosomes also was studied employing the method of Gershon *et al.* (1974) in which $^{14}CO_2$ evolved during the synthesis of 5-HT from L-tryptophan-(1-^{14}C) was recaptured. Data presented in Table V demonstrate that neonatal T_3 treatment increased the synthesis of 5-HT in nerve endings as well. Although this endocrine disorder tended to decrease 5-HT-^{3}H uptake (by 14%) in synaptosomes, the change was statistically nonsignificant (Table V).

In view of the conflicting data presented over the past few years (Grahame-Smith, 1971; Foldes and Costa, 1975), it is difficult to interpret the existing evidence for the involvement of 5-HT in behavioral activity. Administration of TP in conjunction with MAO inhibitor enhanced locomotor activity and produced enhanced synthesis of 5-HT (Grahame-Smith, 1971). By contrast, treatment with *p*-chlorophenylalan-

TABLE V

EFFECT OF NEONATAL HYPERTHYROIDISM ON MIDBRAIN TPH AND SYNAPTOSOMAL 5-HT SYNTHESIS AND 5-HT-^{3}H UPTAKE[a]

Treatment	TPH (nmol/gm/hr)	5-HT .synthesis	5-HT-^{3}H uptake
Control	10.78 ± 0.96 (100)	15.32 ± 1.10 (100)	17.38 ± 1.34 (100)
Hyperthyroid	13.79 ± 1.10 (128)[b]	18.38 ± 1.31 (120)[b]	14.94 ± 1.29 (86)

[a] Each value is the mean ± S.E.M. of 6 animals in the group. For experimental details, see footnote *a* of Table II. The 5-HT synthesis rate is expressed in picomoles $^{14}CO_2$ formed per milligram protein per 25 min, whereas the uptake of 5-HT-^{3}H is expressed in nanocuries 5-HT-^{3}H per milligram protein per 5 min.

[b] Statistically significant difference when compared with the values of control rats ($p < 0.05$).

TABLE VI

EFFECT OF NEONATAL HYPERTHYROIDISM ON 5-HT AND 5-HIAA LEVELS IN CERTAIN BRAIN REGIONS[a]

Region examined	5-HT (μg/gm)		5-HIAA (μg/gm)	
	Control	Hyperthyroid	Control	Hyperthyroid
Cerebellum	0.55 ± 0.03 (100)	0.47 ± 0.03 (86)[b]	0.41 ± 0.08 (100)	0.48 ± 0.07 (116)
Hypothalamus	2.49 ± 0.17 (100)	1.97 ± 0.18 (79)[b]	1.95 ± 0.19 (100)	2.96 ± 0.24 (152)[b]
Pons-medulla	1.48 ± 0.07 (100)	1.45 ± 0.08 (98)	1.36 ± 0.12 (100)	1.81 ± 0.13 (133)[b]
Midbrain	1.76 ± 0.09 (100)	1.71 ± 0.11 (97)	1.64 ± 0.07 (100)	1.98 ± 0.09 (121)[b]
Striatum	1.52 ± 0.18 (100)	1.16 ± 0.17 (76)	1.37 ± 0.08 (100)	2.32 ± 0.11 (169)[b]
Hippocampus	1.32 ± 0.12 (100)	1.19 ± 0.15 (90)	1.26 ± 0.10 (100)	1.49 ± 0.09 (118)[b]

[a] Each value is the mean ± S.E.M. of 6 animals in the group. For experimental details, see footnote *a* of Table II.

[b] Statistically significant difference when compared with the values of control rats ($p < 0.05$).

ine, an inhibitor of 5-HT synthesis, was found to result in suppressed behavioral arousal (Hole, 1972). Our previous data also demonstrated that radio- or chemical thyroidectomy in neonatal rats decreased brain 5-HT metabolism as well as spontaneous locomotor activity (Rastogi and Singhal, 1974c; Singhal *et al.*, 1976). Recently, it was also shown that neonatal exposure to cadmium significantly augmented not only NE, DA, and 5-HT metabolism in certain brain areas, but also the behavioral activity of rats (Rastogi *et al.*, 1977a). Green and Kelly (1976) have presented direct correlation between serotonergic activity and locomotor performance in experimental rats. Clinical studies by Post *et al.* (1973) demonstrated enhanced levels of 5-HIAA in cerebrospinal fluid of man subjected to increased psychomotor activity. The finding that TP administration enhanced not only 5-HT and 5-HIAA concentrations but also caused a rise in HVA levels of cerebrospinal fluid (Moir, 1971) suggests that there may be some relationship between the metabolism of cerebral DA and TP. It remains to be shown whether enhanced uptake of TP in nerve endings of hyperthyroid animals produces increased metabolism of 5-HT and, in turn, locomotor performance or whether it is altered by interfering with brain DA metabolism.

5. *Increased Cholinergic Activity*

The traditional "single-transmitter catecholamine theory" of affective disorder has postulated that whereas mania is associated with high levels of NE, depression is accompanied by decreased concentrations of this brain amine. However, the contemporary investigational evidence, suggesting that virtually every behavioral process is controlled by a homeostatic system involving intricate balances of mutual regulations among various neurotransmitter-metabolizing systems, makes this hypothesis less tenable. The finding that Parkinson's disease is associated with a deficit of DA and excess of ACh led us to reason for "two-factor hypothesis" of behavioral abnormalities seen during altered thyroidal status. It was postulated that hyperthyroidism, which shares certain features common with mania (Maletzky and Blachley, 1971) is associated with a high catecholamine–low acetylcholine level (or function), whereas hypothyroidism, which shares certain features common with depression (Whybrow *et al.*, 1969; Libow and Durrell, 1965; Whybrow and Ferrell, 1974), is accompanied by low catecholamine-high acetylcholine concentration.

Following this reasoning, the effects of neonatal hypothyroidism and hyperthyroidism were investigated on catecholamine and ACh metabolism of rat brain. Data demonstrate that thyroid deficiency at birth decreased the steady-state levels as well as the metabolism of NE and DA, but enhanced the accumulation of brain ACh (Hrdina *et al.*, 1975; Singhal *et al.*, 1975). In fact, the ratio of ACh:DA was increased in hypothyroid state (Rastogi *et al.*, 1975) which may be associated with suppressed behavior in thyroid-deficient animals. However, neonatal hyperthyroidism increased not only the synthesis and turnover of NE and DA, but also that of ACh (Rastogi *et al.*, 1977b), as evidenced by increased endogenous level of this neurohormone as well as enhanced activity of its synthesizing enzyme, cholineacetyltransferase (ChAT), in the brain stem (Table VII). Similar changes, although statistically nonsignificant, also were noted in cerebral cortices of hyperthyroid rats. These data would seem to contradict the hypothesis that high catecholamine and low acetylcholine levels may be the underlying cause of hypermobility in neonatally T_3-treated rats. However, it is possible that simultaneous increase in cholinergic and dopaminergic function, without marked alterations in the ratio of these putative neurohumors, would only produce quantitative changes in spontaneous locomotion as seen during hyperthyroidism without producing abnormal movements characteristic of Parkinson's disease or Huntington's chorea (Aquiltonius and Sjoström, 1971; Klawans and Rubowitz, 1972).

TABLE VII

EFFECT OF NEONATAL HYPERTHYROIDISM ON ACH, ACHE, AND CHAT LEVELS IN BRAIN STEM AND CORTEX[a]

Treatment	ChAT		ACh (nmole/gm)		AChE	
	Cortex	Brain stem	Cortex	Brain stem	Cortex	Brain stem
Control	2.05 ± 0.12 (100)	2.84 ± 0.21 (100)	4.00 ± 0.34 (100)	13.00 ± 0.70 (100)	2.68 ± 0.14 (100)	7.46 ± 0.26 (100)
Hyperthyroid	2.32 ± 0.09 (113)	3.98 ± 0.18 (140)[b]	4.50 ± 0.50 (112)	20.80 ± 1.10 (160)[b]	2.92 ± 0.05 (109)	10.33 ± 0.42 (138)[b]

[a] Values represent the means ± S.E.M. of 6 animals in the group. One-day-old rats were injected daily with T_3 (10 μg/100 gm/day, s.c.) for 15 days and sacrificed 24 hr after the last injection. Data in parentheses express results in percentages taking the values of control rats as 100%. The activity of ChAT is expressed as micromoles of ACh formed per hour per gram tissue, whereas that of AChE as micromoles of substrate (acetylthiocholine) hydrolyzed per minute per gram tissue.

[b] Statistically significant difference when compared with the control values ($p < 0.05$).

Our data on the effect of neonatal hyperthyroidism on brainstem ACh are in line with the finding of Khanna and Pandhi (1972) who reported a marked increase of heart ACh in rats treated with thyroxine. It has been shown that neonatal administration of T_3 not only accelerates maturation of body form and innate behavioral patterns (Eayrs, 1964), but also influences the brain metabolism of specific proteins and nucleic acids that are important constituents of the entire catalytic apparatus of neuronal cells (Sokoloff, 1970). The increase in the biosynthetic capacity for ACh may be additional evidence for the more rapid biochemical maturation of the brain in hyperthyroid animals. Because choline is known to play a rate-limiting role in the biosynthesis of ACh (Cohen and Wurtman, 1976) and neonatal T_3-treatment enhances the endogenous level of TP in midbrain as well as in synaptosomes (nerve endings), it would be desirable to know the influence of hyperthyroidism on high-affinity choline uptake in the brain.

IV. Lithium: Influence on Behavior and Brain Monoamines in Neonatally Hyperthyroid Rats

The promise offered by lithium in combating mania or hypomania has added considerable impetus to investigations of the mechanisms by which this alkali metal elicits its beneficial effect. However, there have been only a handful of attempts to lay out a unified neurochemical mechanism of action for this antimanic drug. Unfortunately, most of the animal studies have so far been carried out only in normal subjects. It may be recognized that the metabolism of a drug may not necessarily be the same in normal individuals as in manic patients who are under psychological stress and display abnormal metabolism of certain neurotransmitters. In order to elucidate the precise mode of antimanic action of lithium, it would, therefore, be desirable to employ an appropriate animal model that is analogous to the affective disorder.

The finding that hyperthyroidism produced certain neurochemical and behavioral changes that were comparable to those seen in manic subjects (Beley *et al.*, 1975; Engström *et al.*, 1974; Rastogi and Singhal, 1976a; Goodwin and Sack, 1973; Messiha *et al.*, 1970; Maletzky and Blachley, 1971) led us to investigate neuronal mechanisms underlying the behavioral suppressant effect of lithium in neonatally hyperthyroid animals. Data presented in Fig. 1 demonstrate that, whereas administration of lithium carbonate (60 mg/kg/day) for 10 days beginning from 20 days of age failed to alter significantly behavioral activity in normal animals, it reduced the rise in locomotor performance seen in T_3-treated

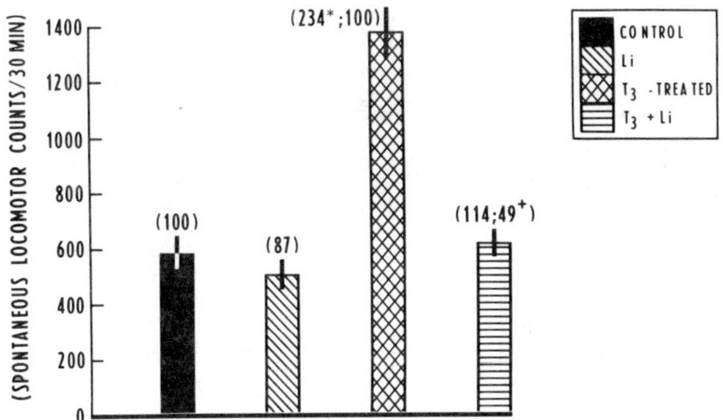

FIG. 1. Effect of lithium treatment on spontaneous locomotor activity in young hyperthyroid rats. Each bar represents the mean ± S.E.M. of 8 rats in the group. One-day-old rats were injected subcutaneously with T_3 (10 μg/100 gm/day) for 30 days (hyperthyroid rats). Groups of rats pretreated with the vehicle or T_3 for 20 days since birth were injected with lithium (60 mg/kg, i.p.) alone or in conjunction with T_3, respectively, for the remaining 10 days. The spontaneous locomotor activity was determined 24 hours after the last injection of T_3 or lithium for a 30-minute session as described in the text. Data in parentheses express results in percentages taking the values for controls or T_3-treated rats as 100%. (*) Statistically significant difference when compared with the values of control rats ($p < 0.05$); (†) statistically significant difference when compared with the values of T_3-treated rats ($p < 0.05$).

rats. It is of interest that other workers have demonstrated that lithium antagonized the amphetamine- (Segal *et al.*, 1975) and L-dopa-stimulated increases in locomotor activity in rats (Smith, 1976).

A. EFFECT ON THE BIOSYNTHETIC CAPACITY OF NE AND DA

Results illustrated in Fig. 2 demonstrate that chronic injection of lithium for 10 days in normal rats increased the activity of striatal TH by 29%. Segal *et al.* (1975) reported an elevated TH activity in substantia nigra and caudate putamen of rats receiving lithium chronically. Additionally, increased turnover and possibly deamination of brain NE have been observed in animals treated acutely or chronically with this antimanic drug (Schildkraut *et al.*, 1969a; Poitou and Bohuon, 1975). In contrast to these effects in normal rats, administration of lithium in hyperthyroid animals decreased the activity of TH in striatum as well as pons-medulla and restored values to the control range (Fig. 2).

Data in Fig. 3 show that despite increased activity of TH, the steady-state levels of NE in several brain areas except pons-medulla of normal rats failed to change in response to chronic lithium treatment. Schildkraut *et al.* (1966) and Schanberg *et al.* (1967) suggested that administra-

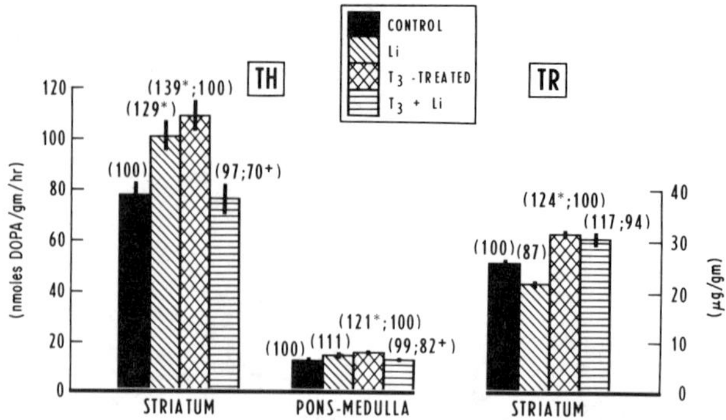

FIG. 2. Effect of lithium treatment on TH and TR levels in young hyperthyroid animals. Each bar is the mean ± S.E.M. of 7 animals in the group. One-day-old rats were injected subcutaneously with T_3 (10 μg/100 gm/day) for 30 days. Groups of rats pretreated with the vehicle or T_3 for 20 days since birth were injected with lithium (60 mg/kg, i.p.) alone or in conjunction with T_3, respectively, for the remaining 10 days. Animals were killed 24 hours after the last injection. Data in parentheses express results in percentages taking the values for control or T_3-treated animals as 100%. The TH activity was assayed in particulate fraction in the absence of pteridine cofactor according to the method of McGeer *et al.* (1967). (*) Statistically significant difference when compared with the values of control rats ($p < 0.05$); (†) statistically significant difference when compared with the values of T_3-treated rats ($p < 0.05$).

tion of lithium increased intraneuronal deamination of NE. These investigators found that administration of lithium in normal rats pretreated with NE-^{3}H by intracisternal route decreased normetanephrine, but elevated (51%) the levels of deaminated catechols in the brain. It is, therefore, possible that unaltered levels of NE in lithium-treated normal rats, in face of increased TH activity and presumably decreased evoked liberation of this amine (Katz *et al.*, 1968; Katz and Kopin, 1969; Bindler *et al.*, 1971) could be due to enhanced deamination of intraneuronally accumulated NE by MAO whose activity was significantly increased in cerebral cortex (17%) and midbrain (23%) (Fig. 4).

Data in Fig. 4 also demonstrate that lithium decreased the activity of COMT in these brain areas. It may be noted that in neonatally hyperthyroid rats, lithium administration in conjunction with T_3 for 10 days beginning from 20 days of age, elevated NE concentration in hypothalamus, pons-medulla, midbrain, and striatum. Furthermore, MAO activity failed to change in lithium-treated hyperthyroid animals. The finding that lithium treatment in T_3-treated rats significantly decreased brain MOPEG levels supports the view that this antimanic drug diminished the neuronal release of NE in hyperthyroid animals (Rastogi and Singhal, 1977a). The levels of DA also failed to alter in lithium-

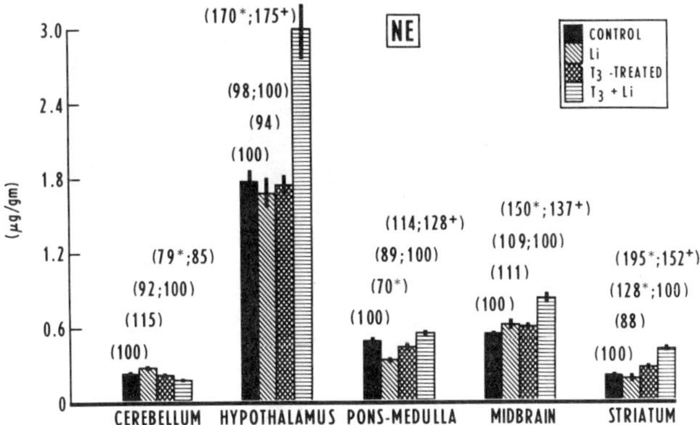

FIG. 3. Effect of lithium treatment on NE levels in certain brain regions of neonatally hyperthyroid rats. (For experimental details, see Fig. 2. caption.) (*) Statistically significant difference when compared with the values of control rats ($p < 0.05$); (†) statistically significant difference when compared with the values of T_3-treated rats ($p < 0.05$).

treated normal rats except in striatum where these were decreased to 77% of control values (Fig. 5). However, the concentration of striatal DOPAC, the intraneuronal metabolite of DA, was increased (34%) (Fig. 4), suggesting that lithium enhanced the deamination of DA as well. In hyperthyroid rats, lithium decreased the T_3-stimulated rise in DA as well as DOPAC to values that were not significantly different from normal controls (Rastogi and Singhal, 1977b). In 1974, Messiha *et al.* found that

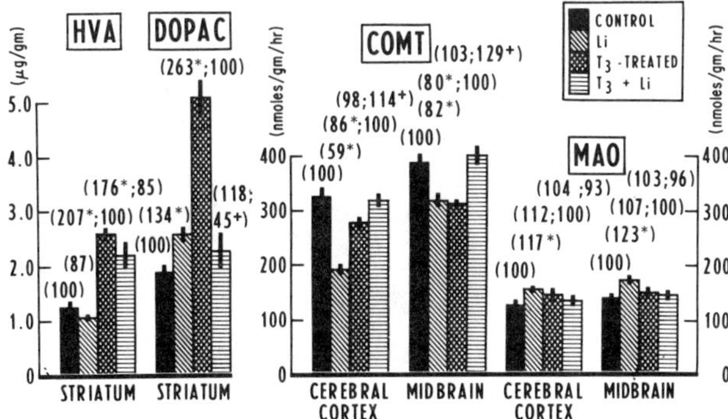

FIG. 4. Effect of lithium treatment on HVA, DOPAC, MAO, and COMT activity in neonatally hyperthyroid rats. (For experimental details, see Fig. 2 caption.) (*) Statistically significant difference when compared with the values of control rats ($p < 0.05$); (†) statistically significant difference when compared with the values of T_3-treated rats ($p < 0.05$).

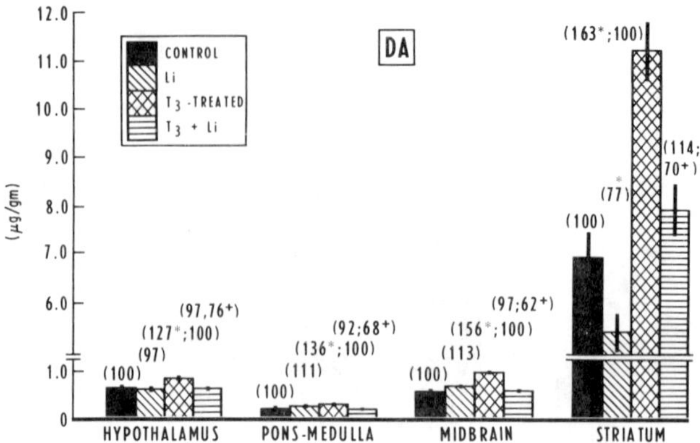

FIG. 5. Effect of lithium on DA levels in certain brain regions of neonatally hyperthyroid rats. (For experimental details, see Fig. 2 caption.) The DA levels were assayed according to the procedure of Hrdina *et al.* (1975), modified from Spano and Neff (1971). It is possible that the relatively higher DA levels reported in Table IV may have been due to an artifact of the assay method (Laverty and Taylor, 1968) that we were then employing. (*) Statistically significant difference when compared with the values of control rats ($p < 0.05$)· (†) statistically significant difference when compared with the values of T_3-treated rats ($p < 0.05$).

increased DA excretion in the manic state diminished toward normal subsequent to stabilization on lithium therapy.

Our finding that lithium produced effects on various neuronal components of the catecholaminergic system in hyperthyroid animals that were different from those seen in normal rats is quite interesting. It would seem that in normal individuals lithium produces changes in noradrenergic and dopaminergic systems that may not be the same as those seen in patients suffering from affective illnesses since they are under psychological stress and display abnormal catecholamine metabolism (Goodwin and Sack, 1973) as well as hormonal imbalance (Dewhurst *et al.*, 1969).

B. Effect on 5-HT Metabolism

Data in Fig. 6 demonstrate that administration of lithium not only enhanced midbrain TPH and TP levels in normal rats, but also in T_3-treated animals. Results in Fig. 7 show that lithium treatment elevated the levels of 5-HT in certain regions of the brain of normal as well as T_3-treated rats. Furthermore, chronic treatment with lithium for 10 days increased 5-HIAA levels of pons-medulla, midbrain, and striatum (Fig. 8). By contrast, this alkali metal decreased the T_3-induced increases in 5-

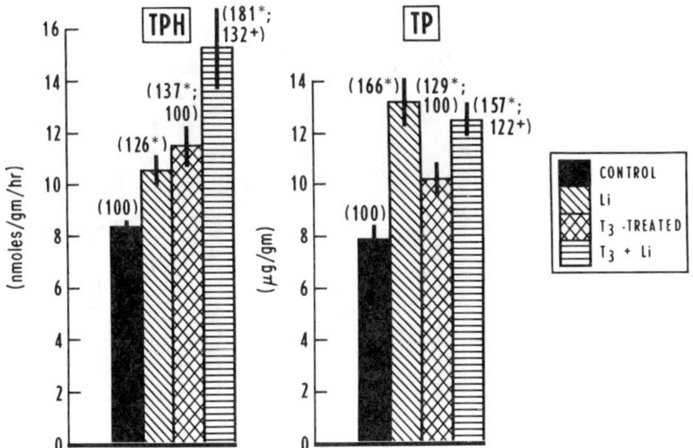

FIG. 6. Effect of lithium treatment on TPH and TP levels in midbrain of neonatally hyperthyroid rats. (For experimental details, see Fig. 2 caption.) (*) Statistically significant difference when compared with the values of control rats ($p < 0.05$); (†) statistically significant difference when compared with the values of T_3-treated rats ($p < 0.05$).

HIAA concentrations of hypothalamus, pons-medulla, midbrain, and striatum. The maximal change was seen in hypothalamus where the concentration of this indoleamine metabolite attained subnormal limits. It may be emphasized that, unlike the effects of lithium on catecholaminergic system, this psychotropic drug manifested effects on serotonergic system of neonatally T_3-treated rats that were generally comparable to

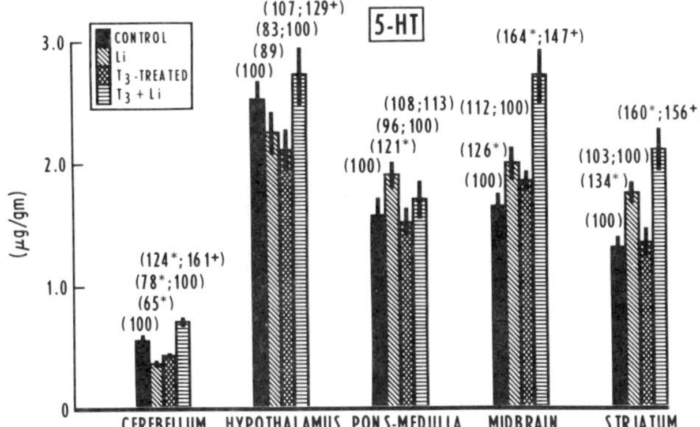

FIG. 7. Effect of lithium treatment on 5-HT levels in certain brain regions of neonatally hyperthyroid rats. (For experimental details, see Fig. 2 caption.) (*) Statistically significant difference when compared with the values of control rats ($p < 0.05$); (†) statistically significant difference when compared with the values of T_3-treated rats ($p < 0.05$).

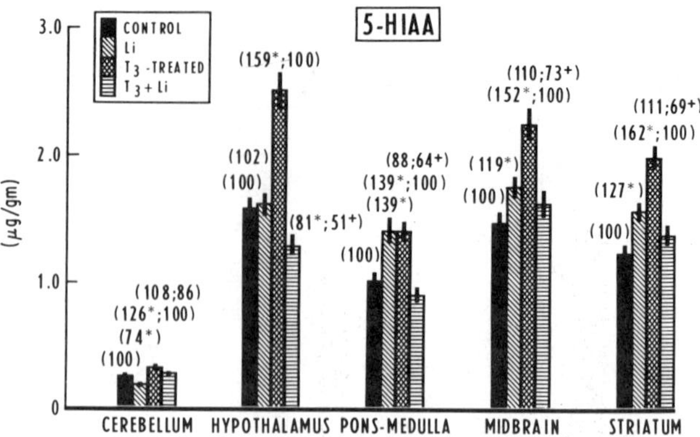

FIG. 8. Effect of lithium treatment on 5-HIAA levels in certain brain regions of neonatally hyperthyroid rats. (For experimental details, see Fig. 2 caption.) (*) Statistically significant difference when compared with the values of control rats ($p < 0.05$); (†) statistically significant difference when compared with the values of T_3-treated rats ($p < 0.05$).

those seen in normal animals of the corresponding age group, except that the 5-HIAA levels were consistently lowered in lithium-treated hyperthyroid animals.

Several investigators (Perez-Cruet *et al.*, 1971; Poitou *et al.*, 1974; Schubert, 1973) have reported that chronic administration of lithium enhances the synthesis as well as deamination of brain 5-HT. It is also known that lithium suppresses the impulse-induced release of 5-HT from serotonergic neurons (Schubert, 1973). Indeed, Schildkraut *et al.* (1969b) demonstrated that lithium slowed the rate of disappearance of intracisternally administered radioactive 5-HT. Under these circumstances, it is possible that lithium elevated 5-HT by impairing its neuronal release in brains of normal as well as hyperthyroid rats. The accumulated 5-HT is presumably not protected against degradation by MAO, particularly in normal rat brain in which the activity of this deaminating enzyme was significantly increased. However, in lithium-treated hyperthyroid rats, 5-HIAA levels were consistently decreased, which is difficult to explain, particularly in view of no change in the activity of MAO. The decrease in 5-HIAA in lithium-treated hyperthyroid rats is in line with the data of Goodwin *et al.* (1973) who found lowered indoleamine metabolite in cerebrospinal fluid of manic patients chronically treated with lithium. The possibility also exists that lithium might have accelerated the active transport of 5-HIAA in T_3-treated rats which show a variety of biochemical and histological changes in brain. Although the issue of feedback regulation of brain 5-HT synthesis is still controversial, it is not unlikely that the increased TPH activity may not be in direct response to lithium treatment in both normal and hyperthyroid rats but may reflect an adaptive change as a consequence of decreased levels of 5-HT reaching to the receptor sites (Rastogi and Singhal, 1977a).

The elevated tryptophan levels in midbrain of lithium-treated normal as well as hyperthyroid rats are in agreement with the data of Perez-Cruet *et al.* (1971) and Poitou *et al.* (1974). Because tryptophan is not synthesized by mammalian tissue, an increase in its concentration could be due to altered protein binding in serum, blockade of its catabolism, or an enhancement in the uptake and transport to the brain. Administration of lithium in normal rats failed to alter the ratio between the free and total tryptophan in the serum (Schubert, 1973). Furthermore, lithium, when given to normal rats, produced no significant change in the activity of liver tryptophan pyrrolase, the rate-limiting enzyme involved in the conversion of tryptophan to kynurenine (Schubert, 1973; Yamaguchi *et al.*, 1967). If such were also the case in neonatally T_3-treated rats, then the altered uptake and/or transport of this essential amino acid may be one of the mechanisms responsible for increased levels of midbrain tryptophan (Knapp and Mandell, 1973) which is known to modulate 5-HT synthesis.

Available data indicate that inhibition of brain DA synthesis (Friedman and Gershon, 1973; Messiha *et al.*, 1974) may be involved in the psychomotor action of lithium during mania in addition to a more fundamental effect on brain electrolyte levels (Baer *et al.*, 1970a,b). Further, since lithium facilitates the neuronal uptake of NE (Colburn *et al.*, 1967; Katz *et al.*, 1968), the suppressed locomotor activity may, in part, be due to postulated decrease of effective NE levels in the synaptic clefts. In view of recent evidence implicating 5-HT in hypermobility (Green and Kelly, 1976; Hole, 1972), the role of 5-HT-ergic neurons in mediating some of the antimanic effects of lithium also cannot be overlooked.

How does lithium exert behavioral suppressant effect in hyperthyroid rats? Studies indicate that lithium alters thyroid function probably by causing a decrease in the amount of thyroxine secreted by the gland (Fieve and Platman, 1968; Shopsin *et al.*, 1969). Cooper and Simpson (1969) demonstrated that lithium produced a significant drop in protein-bound iodine (PBI), elevation of radioactive iodine uptake (RAIU), and a lowering of circulating free thyroxine. However, it is still difficult to say whether lithium alters the central amine metabolism and behavioral activity directly by acting at neuronal levels or indirectly by lowering the concentration of thyroid hormone in the circulation.

V. Diazepam: Influence on Locomotor Performance and Brain Biogenic Amines in Hyperthyroid Rats

It is generally accepted now that hormonal secretory patterns and responses might be influenced during affective disorder (Sachar, 1975). The occurrence of psychiatric symptoms in patients suffering from hyperthyroidism has been reported (Eayrs, 1961; Maletzky and Blachley, 1971). Furthermore, Wheatley (1972) noted the presence of anxiety in hyperthyroid subjects. Despite extensive studies directed toward elucidating the mechanism of action of diazepam, only a very few investigators have examined the effect of this tranquilizing drug in animals that were previously subjected to stress or are hyperactive. The influence of chronic diazepam on behavioral activity as well as amine metabolism and uptake in the synaptosomal fraction were recently examined in our laboratory in hyperthyroid rats by Dr. Rastogi.

A. Effect on Behavioral Activity

A group of normal and hyperthyroid rats were injected with diazepam in conjunction with saline or T_3, respectively, for 15 days beginning from 15 days of age. Locomotor activity was quantitated 18 hours after the last injection of benzodiazepine. Administration of diazepam decreased the mobility in both normal as well as T_3-treated rats. In point of fact, the locomotor activity in T_3-treated rats was restored to normal values (Table VIII). These data are in contrast to the effects of lithium that suppressed only the T_3-stimulated rise in spontaneous locomotor activity and exerted no appreciable influence in normal rats.

B. Effect on NE, DA, and 5-HT Metabolism

In normal rats, diazepam treatment for 15 days produced no effect on soluble TH in striatum as well as on catecholamine synthesis in synaptosomes (Table IX). However, diazepam elevated the endogenous levels of both NE and DA in several discrete brain regions examined (Table X). Because diazepam treatment failed to alter synaptosomal uptake of NE-^{3}H (Table IX), the elevated endogenous levels of NE and DA cannot be attributed to this neuronal phenomenon. Administration of barbiturates was found to decrease the number of protuberances that the presynaptic membrane makes into boutons, an action that may contribute to a reduction of transmitter release (Pfenninger *et al.*, 1971). Furthermore, ultrastructural studies have demonstrated that phenobarbital increases the absolute number of NE vesicles found in adrenergic nerve terminals of the vas deferens (Cote *et al.*, 1970). If this is also true for brain exposed to a tranquilizing agent, it is conceivable that elevated

TABLE VIII

EFFECT OF DIAZEPAM TREATMENT ON SPONTANEOUS LOCOMOTOR ACTIVITY IN YOUNG HYPERTHYROID RATS[a]

Treatment	Spontaneous locomotor counts/25 min	% Change
Control	228 ± 20	(100)
Diazepam	112 ± 12	(49)[b]
T_3-treated	484 ± 58	(212[b]; 100)
T_3 + diazepam	218 ± 19	(95; 45[c])

[a] Each value represents the mean ± S.E.M. of 6 rats in the group. One-day-old rats were injected daily with T_3 (10 μg/100 gm, s.c.) for 30 days to induce hyperthyroidism. A group of T_3-treated rats were injected daily with diazepam (10 mg/kg, s.c.) in conjunction with T_3 for 15 days beginning from 15 days of age. Spontaneous locomotor activity of each rat was quantitated 18 hr after the last injection. Data in parentheses express results in percentages taking the values of control and T_3-treated rats as 100%.

[b] Statistically significant difference when compared with the values of control rats ($p < 0.05$).

[c] Statistically significant difference when compared with the values of T_3-treated animals ($p < 0.05$).

TABLE IX

EFFECT OF DIAZEPAM TREATMENT ON BRAIN MOPEG, STRIATAL TH, AND SYNAPTOSOMAL UPTAKE AND SYNTHESIS OF CATECHOLAMINE IN HYPERTHYROID RATS[a]

Treatment	Soluble TH (nmol dopa/mg/hr)	Catecholamine synthesis	NE-^{3}H uptake	MOPEG (μg/gm)
Control	13.48 ± 0.6 (100)	4.05 ± 0.26 (100)	3.22 ± 0.29 (100)	0.47 ± 0.05 (100)
Diazepam	12.40 ± 0.91 (92)	4.13 ± 0.34 (102)	3.09 ± 0.31 (96)	0.34 ± 0.02 (72)[b]
T_3-treated	17.12 ± 0.90 (127[b]; 100)	5.81 ± 0.43 (144[b]; 100)	3.06 ± 0.18 (95; 100)	0.91 ± 0.07 (193[b]; 100)
T_3 + diazepam	12.66 ± 0.70 (94; 74[c])	3.24 ± 0.42 (80; 56[c])	2.54 ± 0.29 (79; 83)	0.55 ± 0.04 (117; 61[c])

[a] Each value represents the mean ± S.E.M. of 6 rats in the group. One-day-old rats were injected daily with T_3 (10 μg/100 gm, s.c.) for 30 days to induce hyperthyroidism. A group of T_3-treated rats was injected daily with diazepam (10 mg/kg, s.c.) in conjunction with T_3 for 15 days beginning from 15 days of age. The animals were sacrificed 18 hr after the last injection. Data in parentheses express results in percentages taking the values of control and T_3-treated rats as 100%. The TH activity was determined in soluble fraction in presence of BH_4, according to the method of Rastogi *et al.* (1977e) modified from Black (1975). Catecholamine synthesis is expressed in picomoles $^{14}CO_2$ per milligram protein per 25 min, whereas NE uptake is expressed in nanocuries per milligram protein per 5 min.

[b] Statistically significant difference when compared with control rats ($p < 0.05$).

[c] Statistically significant difference when compared with T_3-treated rats ($p < 0.05$).

TABLE X

EFFECT OF DIAZEPAM ON NE AND DA LEVELS IN CERTAIN BRAIN REGIONS OF HYPERTHYROID RATS[a]

Treatment	NE (μg/gm)				DA (μg/gm)			
	Hypo-thalamus	Striatum	Pons-medulla	Midbrain	Hypo-thalamus	Striatum	Pons-medulla	Midbrain
Control	1.86 ± 0.17 (100)	0.24 ± 0.02 (100)	0.48 ± 0.03 (100)	0.54 ± 0.03 (100)	0.59 ± 0.04 (100)	6.62 ± 0.41 (100)	0.32 ± 0.01 (100)	0.54 ± 0.03 (100)
Diazepam	3.08 ± 0.23 (166)[b]	0.31 ± 0.02 (131)[b]	0.61 ± 0.03 (127)[b]	0.64 ± 0.02 (118)[b]	0.78 ± 0.04 (132)[b]	8.53 ± 0.63 (129)[b]	0.42 ± 0.03 (130)[b]	0.62 ± 0.07 (114)
T_3-treated	1.41 ± 0.19 (76; 100)	0.27 ± 0.02 (114; 100)	0.40 ± 0.02 (83; 100)	0.69 ± 0.12 (127; 100)	1.10 ±0.09 (187[b]; 100)	9.32 ± 0.72 (139[b]; 100)	0.41 ± 0.02 (128[b]; 100)	0.67 ± 0.03 (124[b]; 100)
T_3 + diazepam	2.91 ± 0.22 (156[b]; 206[c])	0.41 ± 0.04 (170[b]; 152[c])	0.63 ± 0.08 (131; 158[c])	0.49 ± 0.06 (91; 71)	0.59 ± 0.03 (100; 54[c])	5.86 ± 0.34 (89; 63[c])	0.44 ± 0.03 (138[b]; 107)	0.50 ± 0.03 (92; 74[c])

[a] Values represent the means ± S.E.M. of 6 rats in each group. For experimental details, see footnote *a* of Table IX. The DA levels in this study were determined according to the procedure of Hrdina *et al.* (1975) modified from Spano and Neff (1971). It is possible that the relatively higher DA levels reported in Table IV may have been due to an artifact of the assay method (Laverty and Taylor, 1968) that we were then employing.

[b] Statistically significant difference when compared with the values of control rats ($p < 0.05$).

[c] Statistically significant difference when compared with the value of T_3-treated rats ($p < 0.05$).

levels of NE and DA in various brain regions may, in part, be associated with increased binding capacity of storage vesicles and/or suppressed release of NE and DA from the corresponding presynaptic nerve fibers (Rastogi *et al.*, 1976a, 1977c). This view gains support from the significantly decreased levels of brain MOPEG in diazepam-treated rats (Table IX). Chronic administration of diazepam or bromazepam, a relatively new benzodiazepine, for 22 days also was found to decrease significantly HVA levels in rat striatum (Rastogi *et al.*, 1977c). These changes in metabolite levels did not seem to be due to increased activity of *O*-methylating enzyme that remained completely unaffected following benzodiazepine treatment.

In constrast to the effect on catecholamine uptake, chronic diazepam treatment enhanced the synaptosomal uptake of 5-HT-^{3}H (Fig. 9). This may account for elevated levels of 5-HT in different brain regions (Rastogi *et al.*, 1977d), in addition to impaired release of this indoleamine by benzodiazepine, as has been suggested by previous workers (Stein *et al.*, 1975).

The amount of TP present in the brain is directly proportional to the amount of free TP present in the circulation. Since both TP and benzodiazepines bind avidly to albumin in plasma (McMenamy and Oncley, 1958; Goodman and Gilman, 1975), the elevated levels of midbrain TP (Fig. 9) might be the result of displacement of TP from the binding site in albumin molecule by diazepam (Agarwal *et al.*, 1977a). In a study of Grahame-Smith and Parfitt (1970), it was shown that TP is

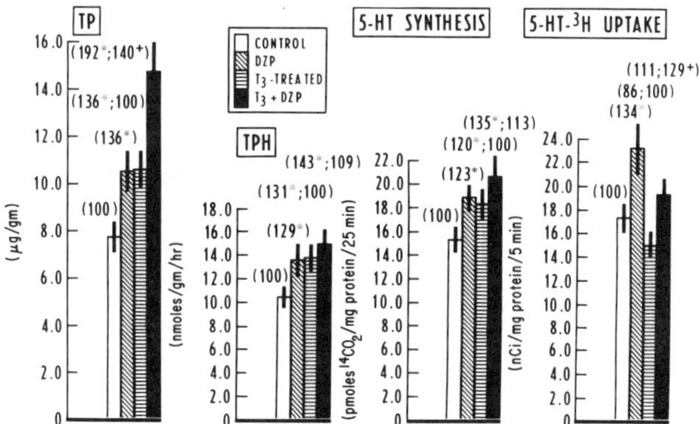

FIG. 9. Effect of diazepam (DZP) treatment on midbrain TP, TPH, and uptake and synthesis of 5-HT in brain synaptosomes of neonatally T_3-treated rats. (For experimental details, see footnote *a* of Table IX.) (*) Statistically significant difference when compared with control rats ($p < 0.05$); (†) statistically significant difference when compared with T_3-treated rats ($p < 0.05$).

actively transported into synaptosomes. It can, therefore, be assumed that diazepam treatment might accelerate the transport of TP across the nerve membrane, as observed in the synaptosomal preparation (R. B. Rastogi, unpublished data). The enhanced TPH activity seen in the midbrain region of diazepam-treated rats seems to reflect an adaptive change. When neuronal uptake of 5-HT is accentuated by diazepam, the synaptic gap concentration of this amine for bombardment of corresponding receptor sites is diminished. This, by a negative feedback mechanism, increases TPH activity in cell bodies of 5-HT-ergic neurons, which are known to be localized in the raphe nucleus. Since intraneuronal TPH is not saturated with regard to the substrate TP (Jequier *et al.*, 1969), the augmented uptake of TP results in increased synthesis of 5-HT as seen in the synaptosomal fraction (Fig. 9). A similar compensatory change in 5-HT synthesis in brains of animals treated with other psychoactive drugs including lithium has been reported by Knapp (1975). Despite the secondary rise in 5-HT synthesis with diazepam, there seems to be a deficiency of 5-HT in the synaptic cleft probably because of decreased neuronal liberation of this indoleamine as shown by previous workers (Wise *et al.*, 1972). Stein *et al.* (1975) found increased concentration of 5-HT-^{14}C after its intraventricular injection to rats that had been treated with oxazepam for 6 days. The reported increase in 5-HIAA levels (Chase *et al.*, 1970; Wise *et al.*, 1972) may be due to "spilling over" of excess 5-HT on to the deaminating enzyme MAO whose activity remained unchanged following diazepam administration (Agarwal *et al.*, 1977a) in addition to its impeded efflux from the brain (Chase *et al.*, 1970).

In contrast to the effects noted in normal rats, administration of diazepam to neonatally hyperthyroid animals decreased soluble TH activity in striatum as well as the rate of catecholamine synthesis in synaptosomes to values that were statistically not different from controls (Table IX). Additionally, DA levels were decreased in diazepam-treated hyperthyroid rats attaining values within normal range, except in pons-medulla (Table X). Despite decreased synthesis, the steady-state levels of NE in hypothalamus, striatum and pons-medulla were significantly enhanced (Table X), which is probably due to decreased release of this monoamine by diazepam in brains of hyperthyroid rats. The finding that diazepam decreased the T_3-stimulated increase in the concentration of MOPEG (Table IX) also provides evidence that diazepam manifests its tranquilizing effect by reducing the turnover of brain NE.

Unlike the effects of diazepam on catecholaminergic system of young hyperthyroid rats, in the serotonergic system of T_3-treated rats, this minor tranquilizer produced changes that were generally comparable to those in normal animals of the corresponding age group. The synaptosomal uptake of 5-HT was significantly increased in diazepam-treated hyperthyroid rats as was the case with normal animals. The net effect of diazepam in hyperthyroid rats was to reduce the turnover and, thus, the availability of 5-HT in the synaptic cleft resulting in marked intraneuronal accumulation of 5-HT and 5-HIAA (Figs. 10 and 11).

Several lines of evidence have emerged implicating 5-hydroxytryptaminergic neurons in anxiety (Stein *et al.*, 1975). Wise *et al.* (1972), employing the "conflict test" (in which drug-induced increases in the rate of punished responses are taken as an index of anxiety-reducing activity, whereas decreases in the rate of nonpunished responses are taken as an index of depressed activity), have shown that benzodiazepines exerted their anxiety-reducing effects by decreasing the turnover of brain 5-HT. These investigators observed punishment-lessening effects with methisergide in the rat "conflict test" (Stein *et al.*, 1973). Studies also indicate that *p*-chlorophenylalanine, a 5-HT synthesis inhibitor, suppressed punishment behavior (Robichaud and Sledge, 1969; Geller and Blum, 1970; Stein *et al.*, 1973). Because evidence points to some similarity between hyperthyroidism and anxiety (Wheatley, 1972), it is probable that increased synthesis and presumably release of 5-HT in hyperthyroid subjects may be associated with anxiety, whereas enhanced catecholaminergic activity may be equated with the hyperactivity response. Further, it has been shown that intraventricular injection of NE increased, rather than decreased, the punishment-lessening activity of systemically administered benzodiazepines (Wise *et al.*, 1972). In the same study, it was also found that intraventricular injection of NE

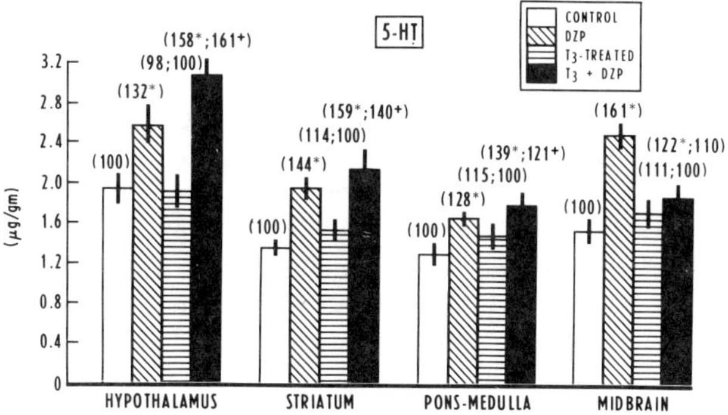

FIG. 10. Effect of diazepam treatment on 5-HT levels in certain brain regions of neonatally T_3-treated rats. (For experimental details, see footnote *a* of Table IX.) (*) Statistically significant difference when compared with control rats ($p < 0.05$); (†) statistically significant difference when compared with T_3-treated rats ($p < 0.05$).

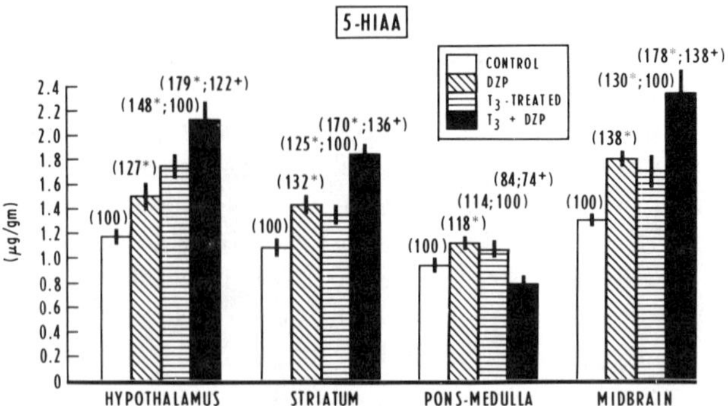

FIG. 11. Influence of diazepam treatment on 5-HIAA levels in certain brain regions of neonatally T_3-treated rats. (For experimental details, see footnote *a* of Table IX.) (*) Statistically significant difference when compared with control rats ($p < 0.05$); (†) statistically significant difference when compared with T_3-treated rats ($p < 0.05$).

antagonized the depressant effect of oxazepam on nonpunished behavior (Wise *et al.*, 1972). All these data suggest that behavioral tranquilization observed in diazepam-treated hyperthyroid rats might, at least in part, be related to decreased turnover of NE and possibly DA (Lapierre *et al.*, 1977).

VI. Depression vs Hypothyroidism

Evidence from clinical as well as animal studies indicate that a number of metabolic and psychic disturbances may be common to thyroid deficiency and affective illness. Biochemical studies have demonstrated that hypothyroidism and depression, both show a diminished response to infused norepinephrine (Prange *et al.*, 1967; Schneckloth *et al.*, 1953) and both probably show a high urinary output of catecholamines and their metabolites (Bunney *et al.*, 1967; Wiswell *et al.*, 1963). Disturbances in sodium, potassium, and calcium metabolism also have been found in affective illness (Coppen, 1965) as well as thyroid dysfunction (Rawson, 1953; Frizel *et al.*, 1967). Furthermore, psychological studies have suggested that the symptoms of myxedema, a severe form of hypothyroidism, make an insidious appearance and are generally characterized by listlessness, lack of energy, slowness of speech, reduced sensory capacity, impairment of memory, somnolence, social withdrawal, and an altered sleep pattern (Eayrs, 1960; Kales *et al.*, 1967). Several of these psychological symptoms are commonly seen in depressed patients as well, for example, somnolence, slowness of speech, reduced sensory capacity, lack of energy, social withdrawal, and altered sleep pattern (Whybrow *et al.*, 1969; Libow and Durrell, 1965; Whybrow and Ferrell, 1974).

Although hypothyroidism in man was found to produce no significant differences in rapid eye movement sleep or total sleep time, the duration of time spent in stages 3 and 4 were consistently decreased (Taber, 1963). The observed changes in sleep pattern seemed to be thyroid hormone specific since treatment with desiccated thyroid increased these sleep phases in hypothyroid patients. In addition, there is indirect evidence suggesting that depressed patients may have actually lower thyroid hormone levels than are normally present (Prange *et al.*, 1969b, 1970; Wilson *et al.*, 1970). Indeed, Dewhurst *et al.* (1969) have observed abnormally high levels of thyrotropic hormone in the blood of depressed patients, although it was suggested that the emotional stress associated with psychiatric illness might have been the cause of this hormonal increase. Thus, even though there is evidence to implicate thyroid dysfunction with depression, it is impossible at present to pinpoint whether abnormal thyroid function is the result or the cause of affective disorder. In order to gain evidence whether abnormalities in putative neurotransmitter function might be the underlying cause of suppressed behavior and learning deficit (Davenport and Dorcey, 1972; Davenport *et al.*, 1976) seen during hypothyroidism, alterations in brain NE, DA, and 5-HT metabolism were studied during this endocrine disorder.

VII. Neurochemical Correlates of Suppressed Behavior during Hypothyroidism

A. Effect of Neonatal Radiothyroidectomy on Brain NE, DA, 5-HT, and ACh

Radio and chemical thyroidectomy at birth resulted in marked interference with ontogenic increases of spontaneous locomotor activity (Rastogi and Singhal, 1975a; Rastogi *et al.*, 1976b), as well as the production of several monoamines in rat brain (Fig. 12). Whereas 50 μCi of ^{131}I exerted only little effect on thyroid gland, a 200-μCi dose of radioisotope produced almost total thyroidectomy without producing any significant effect on parathyroid. This dose of ^{131}I also inhibited the developmental increases in TH and TPH activity as well as NE, DA, and 5-HT levels. However, the levels of 5-HIAA were consistently increased in brains of neonatally hypothyroid rats. Toth and Csaba (1966) also reported a significant reduction in 5-HT levels in brain stem and blood of thyroidectomized rabbits.

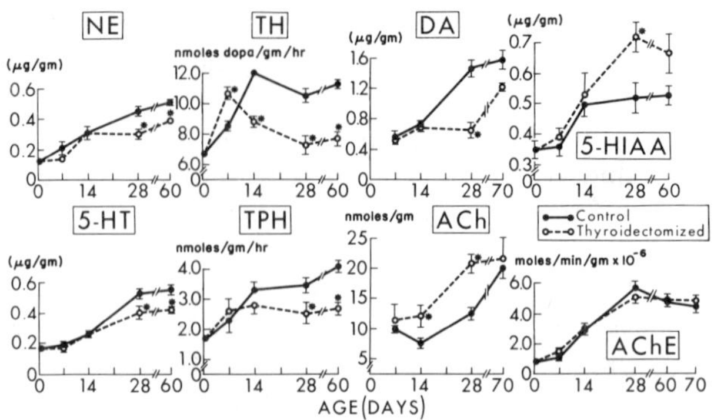

FIG. 12. Influence of neonatal thyroidectomy on the ontogenesis of brain biogenic amines. Each point represents the mean ± S.E.M. of 6 rats in the group. One-day-old rats were injected intraperitoneally with 200 μCi of ^{131}I and killed after 0, 7, 14, 28, 60, and 70 days. (*) Statistically significant alterations when compared to the values of littermate controls of the corresponding age group ($p < 0.05$).

In contrast to the observed changes in steady-state levels of brain NE, DA, and 5-HT, the endogenous level of ACh was consistently increased in hypothyroid rats. The rise in the concentration of this neurohormone does not seem to be due to decreased metabolism since the ontogenic pattern of acetylcholinesterase (AChE) remained unaltered during hypothyroidism (Fig. 12). However, Hamburgh and Flexner (1957) reported a slight decrease in AChE activity (5–14%) in the cerebral cortex of hypothyroid rats between the tenth and thirtieth day of age. Also, a significant reduction in this ACh-hydrolyzing enzyme in the cerebral cortex (25%) and hypothalamus (10%) of 22-day-old hypothyroid rats was reported by Geel and Timiras (1967b). Valcana (1971) found a suppression (17%) of AChE activity in the cerebral cortex, but an increase (27%) in the activity of this enzyme in the cerebellum of 29-day-old neonatally thyroidectomized rats. However, in none of these reports were the levels of brain ACh measured simultaneously. In our studies, the activity of AChE at early developmental stages was found to be unaltered by thyroidectomy and was only moderately (about 10%) depressed on the thirtieth day (Hrdina *et al.*, 1974, 1975). The possibility exists that when the activity of AChE is measured in the whole brain, as was the case in our experiments, slight but significant changes in discrete brain areas may become masked. This may explain the apparent differences that seem to exist between our findings and those reported by earlier workers (Hamburgh and Flexner, 1957; Valcana, 1971; Geel and Timiras, 1967b).

It is probable that high levels of ACh observed in our study did not result directly from an effect of thyroidectomy on the metabolism of this neurohormone but may have been due to some other mechanism, such as a decrease in the utilization of ACh. It is known that ACh levels vary inversely with the degree of functional activity of the brain and are higher than normal during sleep, under anesthesia, and in certain states of behavioral depression (Richter and Crossland, 1949; Crossland and Slater, 1968). As described by previous workers, hypothyroid animals show marked impairment in various functional and behavioral tests (Eayrs, 1960; Bradley *et al.*, 1960; Davenport *et al.*, 1976; Sobrian *et al.*, 1976). The findings that chemical thyroidectomy induced by daily administration of methimazole to neonatal rats produced a marked rise in the ratio of brain ACh:DA (Rastogi *et al.*, 1975) is of interest. It is, therefore, conceivable that the functional hypoactivity may have resulted in the observed accumulation of brain ACh. Further studies to examine simultaneously the changes in the activity of choline acetyltransferase and AChE as well as the levels of ACh in discrete brain areas are needed to clarify whether (*a*) thyroid hormone deficiency exerts a direct effect on the metabolism of brain ACh or whether (*b*) the observed changes in individual components of the ACh system are secondary to some functional changes in the CNS and/or to alterations in other neurotransmitter systems.

Richardson *et al.* (1970) suggested that excess of brain ACh is associated with certain depressive states in experimental animals. Similarly, Janowsky *et al.* (1972) observed a reversal of manic symptoms into depression in humans following intravenous injection of physostigmine, an AChE inhibitor, and suggested that, whereas a low ACh level is associated with mania, higher levels of this neurohumor may be present in depressive illness. Because catecholamine-containing neurons also play an important role in locomotor performance, it is possible that decreased metabolism and functioning of NE- and DA-containing neurons in conjunction with increased levels of ACh may underlie the suppressed behavior seen in hypothyroid animals.

It has been suggested that studies using the whole brain generally reflect changes of larger brain regions, such as the cortex, which may mask even the most pronounced alterations seen in specific brain regions. The effects of neonatal radiothyroidectomy were, therefore, investigated on NE and 5-HT metabolism in various discrete brain areas. Data demonstrate that neonatal radiothyroidectomy markedly reduced the endogenous levels of NE in hypothalamus (31%), pons-medulla (33%), and striatum (46%) (Fig. 13). Although most of the cerebellum

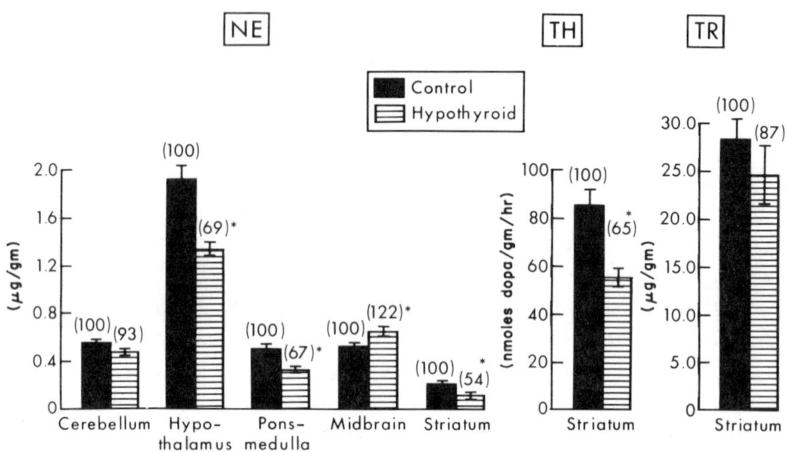

FIG. 13. Effect of neonatal hypothyroidism on NE levels in certain brain regions and on striatal TH and TR. Each bar represents the mean ± S.E.M. of 6 animals in each group. One-day-old rats were injected intraperitoneally with 200 μCi of ^{131}I and killed at 30 days of age. Control rats received an equal volume of physiological saline. Data in parentheses express results in percentages taking the values of control rats as 100%. The activity of TH enzyme was determined in particulate fraction in absence of pteridine cofactor, according to the procedure of McGeer *et al.* (1967). (*) Statistically significant difference when compared with the values of control animals ($p < 0.05$).

develops after birth, neonatal thyroidectomy failed to produce any change in NE levels of this region. A 22% rise in the level of this neurohumor was noted in midbrain. Furthermore, hypothyroidism led to a 35% decrease in the activity of particulate TH in the striatal region. Although the concentration of striatal TR, the precursor of catecholamines, seemed to be lowered, the change was statistically nonsignificant.

Neonatal radio-iodine treatment reduced DA levels in striatum. A slight rise of DA was seen in midbrain; however, the change was statistically nonsignificant. Hypothyroidism also resulted in significant decreases in midbrain TPH enzyme as well as 5-HT levels in cerebellum, midbrain, and striatum. Whereas the concentration of this indoleamine remained unchanged in hypothalamus, a significantly higher level of 5-HT was noted in pons-medulla of thyroid-deficient rats. The activity of TPH was decreased by 24% in midbrain of hypothyroid rats. Of interest are the changes in 5-HIAA levels: they were enhanced in all brain areas examined except the hypothalamus and pons-medulla (Fig. 14).

Since the level and the turnover of brain 5-HT are profoundly dependent on the uptake of tryptophan in the brain (Fernström and

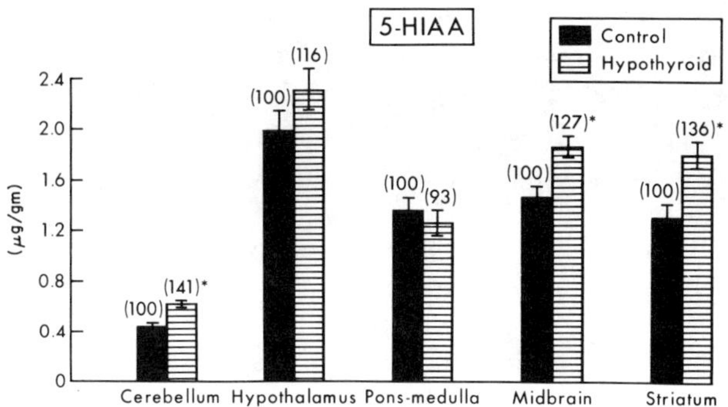

FIG. 14. Effect of neonatal hypothyroidism on 5-HIAA levels in certain brain regions. Bars represent the means ± S.E.M. of 6 animals in each group. One-day-old rats were injected intraperitoneally with 200 μCi of ^{131}I and killed at 30 days of age. Control rats received an equal volume of physiological saline. Data in parentheses express results in percentages taking the values of control rats as 100%. (*) Statistically significant difference when compared with the values of control rats ($p < 0.05$).

Wurtman, 1971), it is possible that the synthetic rate of 5-HT might change in response to altered levels of its precursor. In order to examine whether the observed decrease in the rate of synthesis of the indoleamine might be related to the lack of available precursor, the effect of neonatal thyroidectomy was studied on TP levels of midbrain. It was found that neonatal thyroidectomy produced no significant change in the concentration of this important amino acid in midbrain area (Rastogi, 1975).

One aspect of 5-HT metabolism after neonatal thyroidectomy that warrants consideration is the fact that, in contrast to the observed reduction in 5-HT levels, the concentration of 5-HIAA was significantly increased in whole brain as well as in discrete areas of the brain. In order to gain deeper insight into the mechanism(s) responsible for the elevated levels of 5-HIAA in the face of low levels of 5-HT in thyroid-deficient rats, changes in the activity of the catabolizing enzyme, MAO, were studied in various brain regions. Whereas radiothyroidectomy at birth decreased the activity of MAO in the hypothalamus (by 14%), the activity of this deaminating enzyme was significantly enhanced in midbrain (by 14%). However, hypothyroidism failed to exert any appreciable effect on MAO activity of the cortex, brain stem, and striatum. A study of COMT in certain areas of the brain of normal and neonatally thyroidectomized rats demonstrated that, in control animals, whereas the midbrain had the highest activity of COMT, the striatum and hypothalamus showed the lowest activity of this *O*-methylating enzyme. Neonatal thyroidectomy led to significant enhancement in the activity of

COMT in brain stem, striatum, and midbrain, whereas the activity of this enzyme was lowered in the hypothalamic region. By contrast, cerebrocortical COMT activity remained unaffected following neonatal radiothyroidectomy (Rastogi and Singhal, 1975b).

In view of these findings, several mechanisms can be envisaged to explain high levels of 5-HIAA in hypothyroid rats. First, the brains of hypothyroid rats that are underdeveloped both morphologically and biochemically may have inadequate storage mechanism(s) for 5-HT. This would cause a major proportion of the 5-HT to be prematurely deaminated without taking part in neuronal transmission. Second, it is possible that the increased levels of 5-HIAA may be due to increased MAO activity seen in the midbrain of hypothyroid rats. This argument is further strengthened by the fact that the hypothalamus, which showed no significant change in 5-HIAA, had decreased MAO activity in thyroid-deficient rats. That there is a relationship between thyroid and MAO activity was also supported by Trendelenburg (1953) who showed that there was a marked decrease in hepatic MAO activity of rats kept on desiccated thyroid gland. Finally, it is also likely that brains of thyroid-deficient rats may have an impaired efflux mechanism for 5-HIAA. Atack *et al.* (1974) have demonstrated that the process of removal of organic acids in newborns is not quite as efficient as in adults. As a matter of fact, in brains of 4-day-old rats, the elimination of 5-HIAA involving the mechanism of bulk flow in the cerebrospinal fluid system was only 6% of its endogenous rate of formation. The brains of hypothyroid rats that are poorly developed both morphologically and biochemically and are, thus, comparable to brains of very young rats may also have a less developed system for the transport of 5-HIAA.

B. Effect of T_3 Replacement Therapy on Behavioral Activity and Brain NE, DA, and 5-HT

The question as to whether the observed neurochemical changes in central monoamine metabolism following thyroidectomy can be restored by therapy with T_3 was also examined. Data indicate that administration of T_3 produced time- and dose-dependent changes in the levels of NE, DA, 5-HT as well as in the activity of TH and TPH. Treatment with T_3 (10 μg/100 gm) for 10 days, initiated on the twentieth day of age, failed to produce any effect not only on the brain and body weights, but also on NE and TH levels. However, treatment for 20 days (beginning at 10 days of age) and 25 days (beginning at 5 days of age) virtually restored body and brain weights, as well as NE and TH levels (Rastogi and Singhal, 1974b). A 10- or 20-day treatment with T_3 failed to exert any significant effect on brain 5-HT levels, but a 25-day treatment restored this indoleamine to normal. The activity of TPH was markedly increased in hypothyroid rats after T_3 treatment. 5-Hydroxyindoleacetic acid levels, which rose following thyroidectomy, were decreased after T_3 administration for 20 days (Rastogi and Singhal, 1974a).

The changes produced by T_3 treatment were also examined in different regions of the brain after a 25 day treatment with T_3. It was found that there was not only a restoration, but an increase over the control values in NE and DA of cerebellum, hypothalamus, and striatum. A similar rise was seen in 5-HT concentrations of cerebellum, hypothalamus, striatum, striatal TH, and midbrain TPH. The level of 5-HIAA also was restored to normal in midbrain and cerebellum of hypothyroid rats treated with T_3 for 25 days. Although extended treatment of hypothyroid rats with T_3 had no effect on the cerebrocortical MAO, there was a 25% increase in the activity of COMT. Short-term treatment with T_3 (3 consecutive days beginning from the twenty-seventh day of age) revealed that, although a 25-μg/100 gm/day dose of T_3 had no effect, a 100- and 250-μg/gm dose produced a dose-dependent augmentation in NE, DA, and 5-HT levels as well as in the activity of TH and TPH in both radio and chemically thyroidectomized rats. The short-term T_3 treatment, however, had no effect on body and brain weights. Increases in ACh levels in brains of hypothyroid rats were also abolished by short-term T_3 treatment. However, no significant effect of T_3 treatment was observed on the activity of AChE in brains of hypothyroid animals (Hrdina *et al.*, 1975).

C. Effect of Delayed T_3 Treatment on Central Monoamine Metabolism

Whether the observed T_3-stimulated changes brought about in body and brain growth as well as amine metabolism of hypothyroid rats also were related to the age at which T_3 replacement therapy is initiated was examined by delaying the beginning of exogenous thyroid hormone administration. It was observed that, whereas T_3 treatment during early neonatal life (at 5 days of age for 25 days) produced marked changes in body and brain weights, this treatment when begun at the age of 120 days for the same period exerted no appreciable effect. Whereas T_3 treatment started at 5 days of age, significantly enhanced the activities of TH and TPH and the levels of NE, DA, and 5-HT, the hormone produced no appreciable effect on these parameters in several brain regions when the replacement therapy was delayed until adulthood (Rastogi and Singhal, 1974a,b). In point of fact, the level of NE in hypothalamus and that of 5-HT in pons-medulla was even lower than the untreated group. The concentrations of 5-HIAA also remained unaltered in hypothyroid rats when the initiation of T_3 treatment was delayed for 120 days. Because delaying the process of radiothyroidectomy did not interfere with brain biogenic amine metabolism and the T_3 treatment in adult hypothyroid rats failed to manifest any restorative effects, it would appear that a critical period exists in early neonatal life of the animal. The observed neurochemical changes neither arose when thyroid deficiency supervened after cerebral maturation had advanced nor were they reversed by appropriate hormonal therapy. These results may be considered analogous to the human situation in which permanent brain dysfunction can be ameliorated only when T_3 treatment is instituted not later than the third month after birth; initiation of replacement therapy later in life produces little or no remedial effects in cretinous subjects (Smith *et al.*, 1957).

VIII. Thyroid Hormones and Critical Period of Brain Development

During the past decade, there has been increasing interest in investigating the possibility that there may be certain periods of brain development during which even mild interference may produce irreversible alterations in its final form. Earlier studies had shown that thyroid hormone is important during the first 3–6 months of infant's life (Eayrs, 1968). Available data demonstrate that changes caused in brain biochemistry are proportional to the delay in the onset of thyroidectomy. In comparison to the influence of neonatal thyroidectomy, alterations in brain and body weight, appearance, and behavior were less marked if the thyroidectomy was carried out within 5 or 10 days after birth and were almost totally absent when it was performed at 20 days of age. The changes in brain 5-HT and NE levels also were less pronounced if the thyroidectomy was delayed for 5 or 10 days with almost no change in the levels of these neurotransmitters in rats in which thyroidectomy was delayed for 20 days. Similarly, the reduction in the activity of TH and TPH was less if the ^{131}I treatment was delayed for periods up to 20 days (Rastogi and Singhal, 1974a,b). These data suggest that thyroid deficiency at a very early stage of postnatal life markedly affects brain ontogeny. It also seems that, as the morphological and biochemical architecture of the brain starts growing and assumes its final adult profile, there is a concomitant decrease in the influence of thyroid (Singhal *et al.*, 1977).

These findings are in agreement with Eayrs (1968) who showed that the severity of changes in behavioral parameters was related to the onset of thyroid deficiency. The changes related to learning ability and adaptive behavior also were shown to be less marked in rats thyroidectomized at later stages of growth. Similarly, Bradley *et al.* (1960) demonstrated that the EEG of thyroidectomized rats is affected much less if the thyroidectomy is delayed. More recently, Davenport *et al.* (1976) reported that the deficit in "maze-learning" was much more pronounced in rats exposed to antithyroid drug during perinatal life as opposed to those treated only neonatally. These investigators have suggested that the critical period in the life of a rat extends from 1 week before birth to 2 weeks after birth during which thyroid hormone must be present in optimal levels for normal development of brain and behavior.

IX. Combined Use of Tricyclic Antidepressants and Thyroid Hormone: Possible Neurochemical Basis

Kuhn (1957) first reported the therapeutic usefulness of imipramine in the treatment of depression. Later, the similarity between the symptoms of depression and hypothyroidism as well as the pharmacology of imipramine prompted Prange and Lipton (1962) to conduct a systematic study of the relationship between imipramine action and thyroid function. Subsequently, a concept emerged that controlled administration of a thyroid hormone as an adjunct to imipramine therapy might lead to an enhanced antidepressant activity. Later, Prange and associates (1969a,b) reported the therapeutic advantage of combining T_3 and imipramine in both retarded and nonretarded depressed patients. Evidence indicates that the efficacy of imipramine in the treatment of clinically depressed euthyroid patients is enhanced when the drug is administered along with small doses of T_3, suggesting that T_3 may potentiate the sensitivity of NE receptors (Prange *et al.*, 1969b). It was found that T_3 did not enhance the therapeutic efficacy of imipramine by altering the metabolism of this tricyclic antidepressant in brain (Breese *et al.*, 1972). However, it was suggested that T_3 enhanced the sensitivity of adrenergic receptors and that imipramine elevated the effective concentration of this putative neurotransmitter by blocking the neuronal uptake of NE, thus manifesting an additive or synergistic effect in depressed patients. Thyrotropin-releasing hormone (TRH) also has been shown to potentiate the action of tricyclic antidepressants, presumably by releasing thyroid hormone (Prange *et al.*, 1970, 1972a,b). Evidence indicates that surgical thyroidectomy in adult rats results in decreased sensitivity of adrenoceptors in cardiac tissue (Kunos *et al.*, 1974) as well as in the central nervous system (Emlen *et al.*, 1972); this, in turn, may increase the synthesis of NE, probably via a positive servomechanism (Kizer *et al.*, 1974).

A. Thyrotropin-Releasing Hormone: A Potential Antidepressant

Evidence has emerged that in addition to its classical actions on the pituitary, TRH plays an important role in neuronal functioning as well (Yarbrough, 1976; Breese *et al.*, 1975). The widespread distribution of TRH throughout the neuroaxis (Winokur and Utiger, 1974; Hokfelt *et al.*, 1975), coupled with the enhancement of the "dopa–pargyline potentiation test" (Prange *et al.*, 1972b) in both normal and hypophysectomized mice suggests that TRH might serve as an important psychotropic agent. Clinical studies by Itil *et al.* (1975) demonstrated that TRH produced significant effect on human brain function. The computer EEG profile following TRH treatment was similar to that seen after psychostimulant compounds, such as dextroamphetamine, methylphenidate, and isocarboxazid. Behavioral studies indicated that TRH ameliorated the depressive syndrome probably by invoking psychostimulatory effects. Intravenous injection of TRH resulted in increase of interest, desire, and drive for work, food, and sex. It was suggested that TRH might be most effective in patients with psychomotor depression (where the affective disorder may be the result of inhibition of "instinctive" functions) but not in individuals with anxiety, agitation, and restlessness (Itil *et al.*, 1975).

Animal studies by Keller *et al.* (1974) indicated that this polypeptide hormone enhanced the turnover of brain NE as evidenced by increased levels of MOPEG, an effect that was independent of thyroidal axis. Reigle *et al.* (1974) demonstrated increases in normetanephrine-NE-^{3}H levels following intracisternal administration of NE-^{3}H in rats pretreated chronically with TRH. A similar rise in this metabolite level was seen in rats treated with tricyclic antidepressant (Schildkraut *et al.*, 1969c). The histochemical studies of Constantinidis *et al.* (1974) demonstrated that, whereas TRH accentuated the α-methyl-*p*-tyrosine-induced decrease of NE fluorescence, it produced no change in fluorescence of cortical and hypothalamic regions when administered alone. These authors suggested that TRH probably caused an activation of noradrenergic neurons in the brain leading to enhanced synthesis and release of NE and that this might be related to the antidepressant action of TRH in man. Administration of TRH also was found to antagonize the depressant action of ethanol (Breese *et al.*, 1974), pentobarbital (Prange *et al.*, 1974), and α-methyl-*p*-tyrosine (Kulig, 1975). In order to gain deeper insight into the neurochemical mechanisms responsible for the antidepressant action of TRH, studies were designed to examine its influence on NE, DA, and 5-HT metabolism of rat brain.

B. Effect of Thyrotropin-Releasing Hormone on Behavioral Activity and Central Monoamine Metabolism

1. *Increased Locomotor Activity*

Repeated exposure of rats to TRH for 10 days exerted a significant effect on the spontaneous locomotor activity of normal rats (Fig. 15). Whereas injection of 0.4 mg/kg TRH twice a day for 10 days failed to produce any appreciable change, doses of 2 and 4 mg/kg of the hormone led to significant increases in locomotor performance. The highest rise in mobility (264%) was seen in rats receiving an 8-mg/kg dose of TRH twice daily. Our data also show that administration of TRH (4 mg/kg) twice a day resulted in a time-dependent change in this behavioral parameter: there were 48, 103, and 190% increases over the control

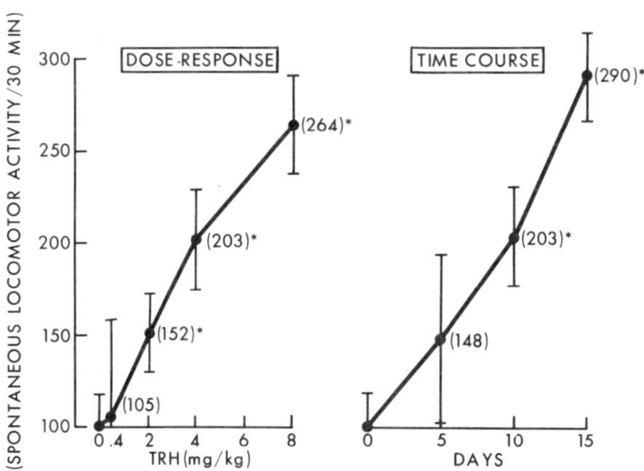

FIG. 15. Influence of various doses of TRH treatment for varying periods of time on spontaneous locomotor activity of rats. Each point represents the mean ± S.E.M. of 6 rats in the group. Thyrotropin-releasing hormone was injected intraperitoneally twice a day with controls receiving physiological saline. Spontaneous locomotor activity was measured 4 hr after the last injection of the hormone or saline. Data are given in percentages taking the control values as 100%. (*) Statistically significant difference when compared with control values ($p < 0.05$).

values in rats injected with this polypeptide for 5, 10, and 15 days, respectively (Agarwal *et al.*, 1977b).

2. *Enhanced Catecholamine and 5-HT Metabolism*

Daily treatment with 20 mg/kg of TRH in two equally divided doses for 10 days significantly increased the synthesis and, presumably, turnover of NE and DA (Rastogi and Singhal, 1977c). This was reflected by enhanced activity of striatal TH and by increased levels of metabolites such as HVA, MOPEG (Fig. 16), and normetanephrine (Reigle *et al.*, 1974). The steady-state levels of NE remained unaltered (Fig. 17), suggesting that its neuronal release probably kept pace with the synthesis of this monoamine. However, DA levels of both hypothalamus and striatum were enhanced, which is in accord with the previous work of Breese *et al.* (1974). The maximal rise in DA was seen in hypothalamus in which a small portion of administered radioactive TRH is also known to be localized (Redding and Schally, 1971). The rise in DA does not seem to be due to increased neuronal uptake, since chronic TRH failed to alter the uptake of NE-^{3}H (Fig. 18). The histochemical and neuro-

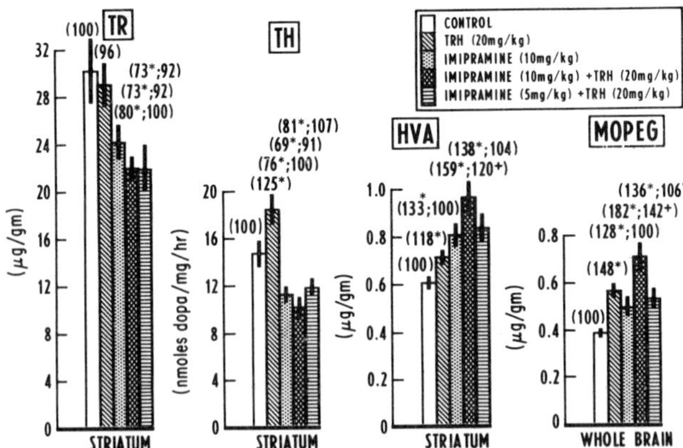

FIG. 16. Effect of imipramine alone and in combination with TRH on TH activity as well as TR, HVA, and MOPEG levels. Each bar represents the mean ± S.E.M. of 6 rats, except the control group that contained 12 animals. The TRH was injected twice a day in two equally divided doses, whereas imipramine was injected once a day by the intraperitoneal route for 10 days. The corresponding controls received an equal volume of the vehicle. The TH activity was assayed in soluble fraction in the presence of cofactor BH_4 according to the procedure of Rastogi *et al.* (1977e), modified from Black (1975). (*) Statistically significant difference when compared with the values of control rats ($p < 0.05$); (†) statistically significant difference when compared with the values of imipramine-treated rats ($p < 0.05$).

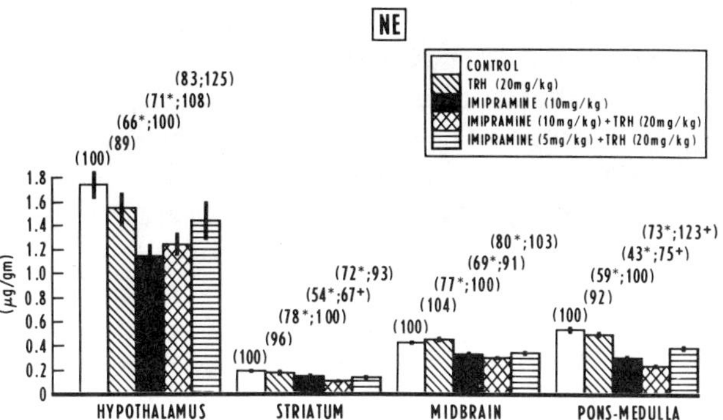

FIG. 17. Effect of imipramine alone and in combination with TRH on NE levels in certain brain regions of rats. (For experimental details, see Fig. 16 caption.) (*) Statistically significant difference when compared with the values of control rats ($p < 0.05$); (†) statistically significant difference when compared with the values of imipramine-treated rats ($p < 0.05$).

chemical studies (Constantinidis *et al.*, 1974; Reigle *et al.*, 1974; Keller *et al.*, 1974) thus provide evidence that TRH treatment activates catecholaminergic neurons in the brain leading to enhanced synthesis of NE and possibly DA.

Segal and Mandell (1974) reported increased motor performance following direct infusion of TRH into the brain. The data support the view that hypermobility in TRH-treated animals might, in fact, be associated with increased functioning of NE- and DA-containing neu-

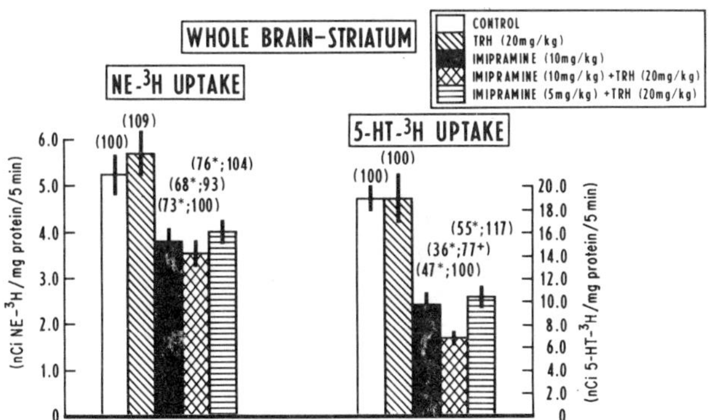

FIG. 18. Effect of imipramine alone and in combination with TRH on synaptosomal uptake of NE-^{3}H and 5-HT-^{3}H. (For experimental details, see Fig. 16 caption.) (*) Statistically significant difference when compared with the values of control rats ($p < 0.05$); (†) statistically significant difference when compared with the values of imipramine-treated rats ($p < 0.05$).

rons in the brain (Agarwal *et al.*, 1976, 1977b). These neuronal changes related to catecholamine metabolism also may underlie the effects of TRH in depressed patients as reported by previous workers (Itil *et al.*, 1975). Repeated injection of TRH for 10 days enhanced TPH activity (Fig. 19) and 5-HT levels in midbrain of rats. The concentration of 5-HIAA was increased only in the hypothalamic region. In view of paucity of information on the effect of TRH on 5-HIAA efflux, it is difficult to state whether TRH treatment actually enhances the release of 5-HT and transport of its metabolite, 5-HIAA, from the brain. It seems possible, however, that TRH may elicit some of its central effects by enhancing 5-HT synthesis and utilization.

C. Effect of Chronic Imipramine on Brain Biogenic Amines

Daily administration of imipramine (10 mg/kg) for 10 days significantly decreased soluble TH activity to 76% in the striatum. The level of striatal TR also was reduced (Fig. 16). The concentrations of NE and DA were significantly reduced in several brain areas, and maximal depletion was seen in hypothalamus and pons-medulla. By contrast, chronic imipramine treatment markedly elevated the concentration of striatal HVA and whole-brain MOPEG by 33% and 28%, respectively (Fig. 16). Data in Fig. 18 demonstrate that this tricyclic antidepressant blocked the synaptosomal uptake of 5-HT-^{3}H and NE-^{3}H. Chronic imipramine treatment decreased midbrain TP levels as well as TPH activity to 81 and 63% of control values, respectively (Fig. 19). The levels of 5-HT and 5-HIAA also were significantly reduced in hypothala-

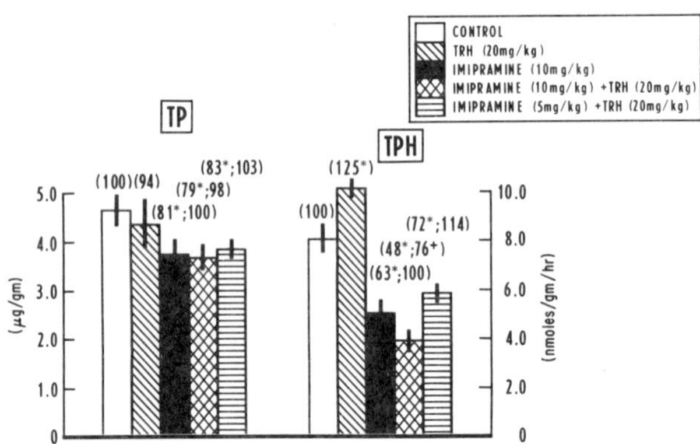

FIG. 19. Effect of imipramine alone and in combination with TRH on midbrain TP and TPH. (For experimental details, see Fig. 16 caption.) (*) Statistically significant difference when compared with the values of control rats ($p < 0.05$); (†) statistically significant difference when compared with the values of imipramine-treated rats ($p < 0.05$).

mus, striatum, and midbrain. Monoamine oxidase activity was decreased (by 13%) after imipramine, although the change was statistically nonsignificant.

It is believed that the uptake into presynaptic neurons is the major mechanism for terminating the biological activity of the released neurotransmitter. A fraction of NE or DA that escapes reuptake subsequently undergoes enzymic inactivation forming extraneuronal metabolites of NE (such as normetanephrine and MOPEG) or of DA (such as HVA). The levels of normetanephrine or HVA may, thus, reflect the amounts of NE or DA present at their respective receptor sites. Administration of lithium, which manifests its antimanic effect by facilitating NE uptake, was found to reduce brain MOPEG levels (Rastogi and Singhal, 1977a). By contrast, imipramine, which invokes its antidepressant effect by increasing the availability of NE in the synaptic gap, lowered endogenous NE (Schildkraut *et al.*, 1971; Tarlov *et al.*, 1973) and enhanced the levels of MOPEG (Fig. 16) and normetanephrine (Schildkraut *et al.*, 1969c). In line with our data, Nielsen *et al.* (1975) reported a 22% rise in HVA-^{3}H levels following acute imipramine treatment in rats pretreated with L-dopa-^{3}H. However, this change was statisically nonsignificant. It is probable that chronic imipramine treatment impairs the uptake of DA into noradrenergic storage granules in which dopamine β-hydroxylase is sequestered, which then results in diminished conversion of DA into NE.

The decreased activity of soluble TH in striata of imipramine-treated animals as observed in our study and reported by Mandell (1975) may be an adaptive change in response to presumably higher synaptic gap concentration of NE, which by receptor-mediated feedback mechanism, could decrease TH. Leonard and Kafoe (1976) found that imipramine treatment decreased the synthesis of brain DA as assessed by the incorporation of tyrosine-^{3}H into this monoamine. Because TR has been shown to play a modulating role in catecholamine formation (Wurtman *et al.*, 1974), the possibility exists that decreased levels of TR (Leonard and Kafoe, 1976), in addition to low TH activity, may, in part, be responsible for reduced synthesis of brain NE. Data from studies on depressed patients treated with various tricyclic antidepressants also have suggested that these drugs may decrease NE biosynthesis (Schildkraut *et al.*, 1965, 1972). Schildkraut *et al.* (1970) also suggested that in spite of relatively low concentrations of NE or reduced presynaptic neuronal activity (as evidenced by decreased TH), chronic imipramine increased the rate of disappearance of NE from brain by blocking its neuronal uptake and, in turn, increasing the levels of extraneuronal metabolites. Our finding that the activity of midbrain COMT, which is a presynaptic enzyme, was increased 27% by imipramine would seem to indicate that the increased levels of MOPEG or normetanephrine (Schildkraut *et al.*, 1970) may, in part, be due to accelerated *O*-methylation of NE. Dunner *et al.* (1971) reported low COMT levels in red cells of depressed patients, particularly those suffering from unipolar depression. However, the situation in brain is not quite clear, and further studies are necessary to delineate the importance of imipramine-stimulated rise in brain COMT activity.

Previous studies have demonstrated that administration of imipramine or chlorimipramine, which are known to block 5-HT uptake, elevated extraneuronal concentrations of 5-HT (Carlsson *et al.*, 1969a,b). The slowed uptake of 5-HT prevents this amine from reaching MAO; this, in turn, results in a decrease of 5-HIAA (Alpers and Himwich, 1971). In line with our data, Bruinvels (1972) reported decreased formation of 5-HT from its precursor TP, in rats given imipramine. However, this tricyclic failed to decrease brain 5-HT synthesis from 5-hydroxytryptophan. The finding that chronic imipramine failed to alter 5-hydroxytryptophan decarboxylase activity (R. B. Rastogi, unpublished data) supports the view that imipramine probably decreases the activity of rate-limiting enzyme, TPH, by a receptor-mediated feedback mechanism.

From these results, consensus seems to emerge that TRH and imipramine elicit their antidepressant effect by enhancing the levels of putative neurotransmitters, NE, DA, and 5-HT, at their corresponding pre- and/or postsynaptic receptor sites. Thyrotropin-releasing hormone primarily increases the synthesis and possible release of NE, DA, and 5-HT, whereas imipramine blocks the neuronal uptake of these putative neurohormones, resulting in a larger fraction of amines available for interaction with receptor sites.

D. Effect of Thyrotropin-Releasing Hormone in Combination with Imipramine

Chronic TRH treatment in doses of 20 mg/kg/day (which by itself failed to produce any significant change in synaptosomal uptake of NE-^{3}H and 5-HT-^{3}H) potentiated the effect of imipramine on the blockade of monoamine uptake, especially that of 5-HT-^{3}H in synaptosomes (Fig. 18). Similarly, more pronounced decreases in the activity of striatal TH as well as in the concentrations of NE, DA, 5-HT, and 5-HIAA were observed in certain brain areas of rats treated with both TRH and imipramine. The combined use of TRH and imipramine also produced synergistic effects on HVA, MOPEG, and TPH (Figs. 16 and 19). Although further studies are needed to elucidate the basis of synergistic action of TRH and imipramine on monoaminergic neurons, it is possible that TRH elicits its effect by increasing the turnover of catecholamines, whereas imipramine blocks their reuptake into presynaptic neurons.

The finding that imipramine in a smaller dose (5 mg/kg) along with TRH produced effects on the aminergic system that were similar to those seen with a larger dose (10 mg/kg) of imipramine alone may be of clinical importance. Several interpretations can be offered for the observed potentiation of imipramine action by TRH. It is probable that imipramine possesses some antithyroid property and that TRH, by acting on pituitary, may rectify it. Fischetti (1962) reported that in the rabbit, small doses of imipramine increased thyroid secretion, whereas larger doses decreased it. However, Prange *et al.* (1969b) failed to observe any change in protein-bound iodine values in patients treated with imipramine for 27 days. The possibility also exists that TRH alters the levels of imipramine in the brain by influencing its metabolism centrally and/or peripherally. Moreover, it is probable that TRH hastens the demethylation of imipramine into desmethylimipramine, which is presumed to be a more potent tricyclic antidepressant than imipramine.

The present data demonstrate that TRH accelerates the action of imipramine on central amine disposition and metabolism. Our data raise the possibility that by inclusion of TRH in the treatment regimen, the doses of imipramine can be significantly reduced. This could be important, particularly in view of a number of side effects on the cardiovascular and the central nervous system exerted by usual therapeutic doses of imipramine (Gauthier *et al.*, 1965; Garrison and Moffitt, 1962; Giles, 1963; Brown *et al.*, 1971; Hishikawa *et al.*, 1965; Hartmann, 1968).

X. Summary and Concluding Remarks

There have been developments over the past decade that have greatly advanced our understanding of the role of hormones, particularly thyroid hormone in the control of mammalian neurogenesis during the critical period of neonatal life. Data demonstrate that depressed behavior and mental deficit seen in thyroid-ablated animals might be associated with decreased synthesis and turnover of brain NE, DA, and 5-HT as well as an increased accumulation of acetylcholine and ratio of ACh to DA. By contrast, behavioral excitability seen in neonatally hyperthyroid rats may be associated with enhanced activity of noradrenergic, dopaminergic, and 5-hydroxytryptaminergic neurons in the brain. Further, cholinergic activity was enhanced contradicting the hypothesis that an increased ratio of DA to ACh is responsible for enhanced motor

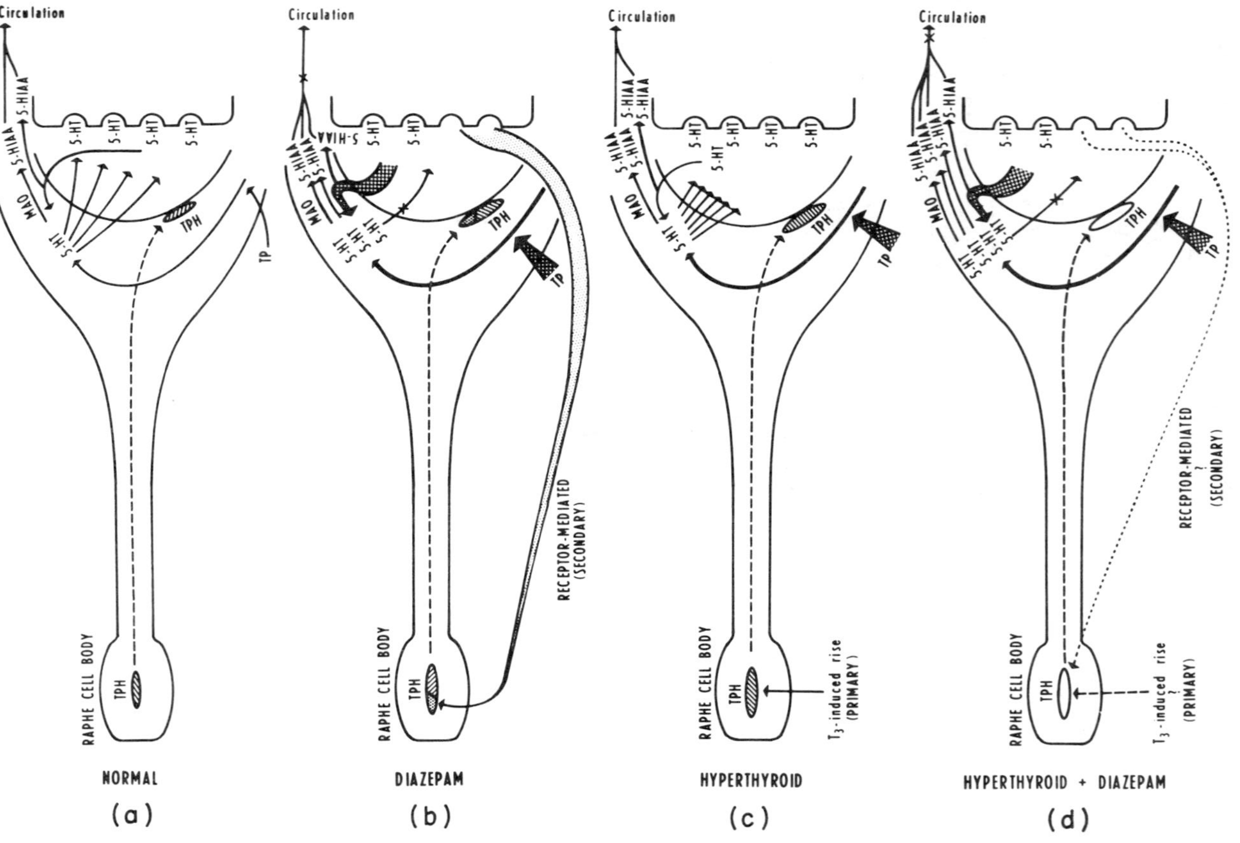
Circulation
5-HIAA
MAO
5-HT
TPH
TP
RECEPTOR-MEDIATED
?
(SECONDARY)
RAPHE CELL BODY
T_3-induced rise
?
(PRIMARY)
NORMAL
(a)
DIAZEPAM
(b)
HYPERTHYROID
(c)
HYPERTHYROID + DIAZEPAM
(d)

activity. Unlike Parkinson's disease or Huntington's chorea, hyperthyroidism is not generally associated with qualitative changes in motor performance, and it is probable that simultaneous increases in cholinergic and dopaminergic functions (without marked alterations in the ratio of these putative neurotransmitters) would only produce quantitative changes in spontaneous locomotion. Thyroid hormone administration in mature animals failed to exert any significant effect on the locomotor activity as well as on TH and TPH enzymes that regulate the biosynthesis of catecholamine and 5-HT, respectively. Caution must therefore be exercised in extrapolating to adult animals the influence of thyroid hormone on central monoamines in neonatal subjects. Furthermore, because neonatal hyperthyroidism seems to share a number of behavioral and neurochemical features common with mania, use of hyperthyroid rats could serve as an adequate experimental model to study the underlying neuronal mechanisms of antimanic drugs.

Whereas chronic lithium treatment in normal rats failed to change spontaneous locomotor activity, this antimanic agent suppressed the hypermobility induced by L-triiodothyronine, amphetamine (Segal *et al.*, 1975), or L-dopa (Smith, 1976). Data have been presented to show that lithium manifests its antimanic effect by suppressing the turnover of DA and NE in brains of hyperthyroid rats, which is in line with the catecholamine hypothesis of mania formulated by previous workers (Messiha *et al.*, 1970; Murphy *et al.*, 1971; Ryback and Schwab, 1971; Bunney *et al.*, 1972). However, the involvement of 5-hydroxytryptaminergic neurons in the mediation of antimanic effect of lithium also needs consideration, particularly in view of the present data as well as those

---

FIG. 20. A hypothetical model illustrating the mechanism of action of diazepam on 5-hydroxytryptaminergic system in normal and hyperthyroid rats. (a) In 5-hydroxytryptaminergic neurons of control rats, tryptophan is taken up into the nerve endings and converted into 5-HT by TPH, which is synthesized in the raphe cell body and transported by axonal transport to nerve endings. The 5-HT thus formed is eventually released and facilitates neural transmission by activating the receptors. A portion of 5-HT (nonfunctional) that never takes part in the transmission process is deaminated by MAO within the presynaptic neurons. (b) Following long-term diazepam treatment, there is a significant decrease in release and rise in the uptake of 5-HT resulting in lowering of the effective levels of this indoleamine in the synaptic cleft. The resulting interactions are described in the text. (c) In hyperthyroid rats, there is a T_3-induced rise in TPH activity (probably because of increased synthesis of the enzyme). The enhanced synthesis and utilization of 5-HT does not produce a change in steady-state level of this indoleamine. (d) In diazepam-treated hyperthyroid animals, even though the synaptosomal uptake of TP seems to be augmented when compared to hyperthyroid or diazepam-treated normal rats, the change in synaptosomal synthesis of 5-HT was not too pronounced. In effect, diazepam treatment reduced the turnover of 5-HT in brains of hyperthyroid animals.

obtained by Kane (1970) and Itil *et al.* (1971). Because hyperthyroid animals also show anxiety (Wheatley, 1972), studies were designed to investigate the neurochemical mechanism of the tranquillizing action of diazepam in L-triiodothyronine-treated rats. Administration of diazepam antagonized the L-triiodothyronine-induced rise in locomotor performance. Like lithium, diazepam also decreased the synaptic gap concentrations of NE and DA in hyperthyroid rats, although the mechanisms involved are apparently different. Lithium seemed to decrease the synthesis and facilitate the uptake of NE and DA, whereas diazepam decreased turnover of these catecholamines.

Previous studies using specific pharmacological tools have demonstrated that, whereas reduced turnover of NE may be associated with the depressant action, the decreased turnover of 5-HT in brain is responsible for the antianxiety action of diazepam (Stein *et al.*, 1975). Figure 20 illustrates a hypothetical model to explain the mode of action of diazepam on 5-hydroxytryptaminergic neurons in brains of normal and hyperthyroid rats. In serotonergic nerve endings of normal rats, chronic diazepam, in addition to impairing the release of 5-HT, facilitates the synaptosomal uptake of this indoleamine, thus producing a deficiency of 5-HT at the vicinity of corresponding receptor sites. This, by a negative feedback mechanism, increases TPH activity in cell bodies of 5-HT-ergic neurons, which are known to be localized in the raphe nucleus. Because intraneuronal TPH is not saturated with its substrate TP, an augmented neuronal transport of this amino acid will result in an increased synthesis of 5-HT. The newly formed unstored 5-HT "spills over" and is, in turn, deaminated by MAO to form increased amounts of 5-HIAA, the efflux of which is also known to be impaired by diazepam (Chase *et al.*, 1970). Figure 20 also illustrates that, like in normal rats, diazepam enhanced the uptake of 5-HT and decreases the presynaptic liberation of this amine in hyperthyroid animals. In brief, diazepam antagonizes the L-triiodothyronine-stimulated rise in 5-HT turnover.

Data also have been presented to compare the neurochemical effects of imipramine with those exerted by TRH, a potential antidepressant drug relatively free of undesirable side effects on the central nervous system. Chronic imipramine treatment augmented the levels of norepinephrine, dopamine, and 5-HT in the synaptic gap by blocking their uptake. By contrast, TRH enhanced the biosynthesis and turnover of these important putative neurohumors. The possibility that TRH potentiates the effects of imipramine on various neuronal components of the monoaminergic system may be of clinical importance and needs to be further explored. Finally, it is important to investigate the effects of a psychotropic drug in an experimental model analogous to psychiatric illness for which the drug is therapeutically employed rather than in normal animals. Indeed, it could be quite presumptuous to hypothesize the biological mechanisms that may underlie the action of a psychotropic agent only on the basis of data obtained from normal laboratory subjects.

Acknowledgments

This work was supported by grant No. 296-70C from the Ontario Mental Health Foundation. Some of the original work reviewed in this article, to which appropriate reference is made in the text, was carried out with our colleagues, Drs. R. A. Agarwal, P. D. Hrdina, and Y. Lapierre. The authors thank Mr. S. Klosevych, Chief of Medical Communication Services of the University of Ottawa, and his staff in the preparation of various illustrations. Finally, we are indebted to Mrs. Diane McNeil for her expert editorial assistance in the assembling of this manuscript.

References

Agarwal, R. A., Rastogi, R. B., and Singhal, R. L. (1976). *Proc. Can. Fed. Biol. Soc.* **19,** 730.

Agarwal, R. A., Lapierre, Y. D., Rastogi, R. B., and Singhal, R. L. (1977a). *Br. J. Pharmacol.* **60,** 3.

Agarwal, R. A., Rastogi, R. B., and Singhal, R. L. (1977b). *Res. Commun. Chem. Pharmacol.* **15,** 743.

Alpers, H. A., and Himwich, H. E. (1972). *J. Pharmacol. Exp. Ther.* **180,** 531.

Anton-Tay, F., and Wurtman, J. (1971). *In* "Frontiers of Neuroendocrinology" (L. Martini and W. F. Ganong, eds.), pp. 45–66. Oxford Univ. Press, London and New York.

Aquiltonius, S. M., and Sjoström, R. (1971). *Life Sci.* **10,** 405.

Atack, C., Bass, N. H., and Lundborg, P. (1974). *Brain Res.* **77,** 111.

Azmitia, E. C., Jr., Algeri, S., and Costa, E. (1970). *Science* **169,** 201.

Baer, L., Kassir, S., and Fieve, R. (1970a). *Psychopharmacologia* **17,** 216.

Baer, L., Durrel, J., Bunney, W. E., Jr., Levy, B. S., Murphy, D. L., Greenspan, K., and Cardon, R. V. (1970b). *Arch. Gen. Psychiatry* **23,** 40.

Balazs, R. (1971). *Cell. Aspects Neural Growth Differ., Proc. Conf., 1969* p. 273.

Balazs, R., Brooksbank, B. W. L., Davison, A. N., Eayrs, J. T., and Wilson, D. A. (1969). *Brain Res.* **15,** 219.

Balazs, R., Kovacks, S., Cocks, W. A., Johnson, A. L., and Eayrs, J. T. (1971). *Brain Res.* **25,** 555.

Barnett, R. J. (1948). Thesis, pp. 59–71. Yale University, School of Medicine, New Haven, Connecticut.

Bartholini, G., Blum, J. E., and Pletscher, A. (1969). *J. Pharm. Pharmacol.* **21,** 297.

Beley, A., Beley, P., and Bralet, J. (1975). *Arch. Int. Physiol. Biochim.* **83,** 471.

Bindler, E. H., Wallach, M. B., and Gershon, S. (1971). *Arch. Int. Pharmacodyn. Ther.* **190,** 150.

Bisanti, L., and Cavallotti, C. (1972). *Prog. Brain Res.* **38,** 327.

Black, I. B. (1975). *Brain Res.* **95,** 170.

Bliss, E. L., and Ailion, J. (1971). *Life Sci.* **10,** 1161.

Bliss, E. L., Migeon, C. J., Branch, C. H. H., and Samuels, L. T. (1956). *Psychosom. Med.* **18,** 56.

Blumblatt, M. J., and Winston, F. (1970). *Lancet* **1,** 832.

Board, F., Wadeson, R., and Persky, H. (1957). *AMA Arch. Neurol. Psychiatry* **78,** 612.

Bradley, P. M., Earys, J. T., and Schmalbach, K. (1960). *Electroencephalogr. Clin. Neurophysiol.* **12,** 467.

Breese, G. R., Traylor, T. D., and Prange, A. J., Jr. (1972). *Psychopharmacology* **25,** 101.

Breese, G. R., Cooper, B. R., Prange, A. J., Cott, J. M., and Lipton, M. A. (1974). *In* "The Thyroid Axis, Drugs and Behaviour" (A. J. Prange, Jr., ed.), p. 115. Raven, New York.

Breese, G. R., Cott, J. M., Cooper, B. R., Prange, A. J., Jr., Lipton, M. A., and Plotnikoff, N. P. (1975). *J. Pharmacol. Exp. Ther.* **193,** 11.

Broitman, S. T., and Donoso, A. O. (1971). *Experientia* **27,** 1308.

Brown, T. C. K., Dwyner, M. E., and Stocks, J. G. (1971). *Med. J. Aust.* **2,** 848.

Bruinvels, J. (1972). *Eur. J. Pharmacol.* **20,** 231.

Bunney, W. E., Davis, J. M., Jr., Weill Malherbe, H., and Smith, E. R. B. (1967). *Arch. Gen. Psychiatry* **16,** 448.

Bunney, W. E., Jr., Goodwin, F. K., Murphy, D. L., House, K. M., and Gordon, F. K. (1972). *Arch. Gen. Psychiatry* **27,** 304.

Bursten, B. (1961). *Arch. Gen. Psychiatry* **4,** 267.

Butcher, L. L., and Engel, J. (1969). *J. Pharmacol. Exp. Ther.* **21,** 614.

Caesar, P. M., Collins, G. G. S., and Sandler, M. (1970). *Biochem. Pharmacol.* **19,** 921.

Carlsson, A., Corrodi, H., Fuxe, K., and Hokfelt, T. (1969a). *Eur. J. Pharmacol.* **5,** 357.

Carlsson, A., Jonason, J., Lindquist, M., and Fuxe, K. (1969b). *Brain Res.* **12,** 456.

Casper, R., Vernadakis, A., and Timiras, P. S. (1967). *Brain Res.* **5,** 524.

Cavallotti, C., and Luigi, B. (1972). *Prog. Brain Res.* **38,** 69.

Chase, T. N., Katz, R. I., and Kopin, I. J. (1970). *Neuropharmacology* **9,** 103.

Cohen, E. L., and Wurtman, R. J. (1976). *Science* **191,** 561.

Colburn, R. W., Goodwin, F. K., Bunney, W. E., Jr., and Davis, J. M. (1967). *Nature (London)* **215,** 1395.

Constantinidis, J., Geissbuhler, F., Gaillard, J. M., Hovaguimian, T. H., and Tissot, R. (1974). *Experientia* **30,** 1182.

Cooper, T. B., and Simpson, G. M. (1969). *Curr. Ther. Res.* **11,** 603.

Coppen, A. (1965). *Br. J. Psychiatry* **111,** 1133.

Cote, M. G., Blovin, A., and Gascon, A. (1970). *J. Pharm. Pharmacol.* **22,** 129.

Coyle, J. T. (1972). *Biochem. Pharmacol.* **21,** 1935.

Crossland, J., and Slater, P. (1968). *Br. J. Pharmacol. Chemother.* **33,** 42.

Curry, J. J., and Heim, L. M. (1966). *Nature (London)* **209,** 915.

Dalton, K. (1971). *Proc. R. Soc. Med.* **64,** 1249.

Davenport, J. W., and Dorcey, T. P. (1972). *Horm. Behav.* **3,** 97.

Davenport, J. W., Gonzalez, L. M., Hennies, R. S., and Hagquist, W. M. (1976). *Horm. Behav.* **7,** 139.

Davis, J. M. (1975). *Res. Publ., Assoc. Res. Nerv. Ment. Dis.* **54,** 134.

Dewhurst, K. E., El Kabir, D. J., and Harris, G. W. (1969). *Br. J. Psychiatry* **115,** 1003.

Dunner, E. L., Cohn, C. K., Gershon, E. S., and Goodwin, F. K. (1971). *Arch. Gen. Psychiatry* **25,** 348.

Eayrs, J. T. (1960). *Br. Med. Bull.* **16,** 122.

Eayrs, J. T. (1961). *J. Neuroendocrinol.* **22,** 409.

Eayrs, J. T. (1964). *Arch. Biol.* **75,** 529.

Eayrs, J. T. (1968). *In* "Endocrinology and Human Behaviour" (R. P. Michael, ed.), p. 239. Oxford Univ. Press, London and New York.

Emlen, W., Segal, D. S., and Mandell, A. J. (1972). *Science* **175,** 79.
Engström, G., Svensson, T. H., and Waldeck, B. (1974). *Brain Res.* **77,** 471.
Ernst, A. M. (1967). *Psychopharmacologia* **10,** 316.
Fernström, J. D., and Wurtman, R. J. (1971). *Science* **173,** 149.
Fieve, R. R., and Platman, S. R. (1968). *Am. J. Psychiatry* **125,** 527.
Fischetti, B. (1962). *Arch. Ital. Sci. Farmacol.* **12,** 33.
Foldes, A., and Costa, E. (1975). *Biochem. Pharmacol.* **24,** 1617.
Freud, S. (1905). "Three Essays on the Theory of Sexuality," Standard ed., Vol. VII. Hogarth Press, London.
Friedman, E., and Gershon, S. (1973). *Nature (London)* **243,** 520.
Frizel, D., Malleson,, A., and Marks, V. (1967). *Lancet* **2,** 1360.
Fuxe, K., Hokfelt, T., and Ungerstedt, V. (1970). *Int. Rev. Neurobiol.* **13,** 93.
Garcia Argiz, C. A., Pasquini, J. M., Kaplun, B., and Gomez, C. J. (1967). *Brain Res.* **6,** 635.
Garrison, H. F., and Moffitt, E. M. (1962). *J. Am. Med. Assoc.* **179,** 456.
Gauthier, M., Boissier, J. R., Gorciex, A., and Simon, P. (1965). *Proc. Eur. Soc. Study Drug Toxic.* **6,** 171.
Geel, S. E., and Timiras, P. S. (1967a). *Brain Res.* **4,** 135.
Geel, S. E., and Timiras, P. S. (1967b). *Endocrinology* **80,** 1069.
Geel, S. E., Valcana, T., and Timiras, P. S. (1967). *Brain Res.* **4,** 143.
Gelber, S., Campbell, P. L., Deibler, G. E., and Sokoloff, L. (1964). *J. Neurochem.* **11,** 221.
Geller, I., and Blum, K. (1970). *Eur. J. Pharmacol.* **9,** 319.
Gershon, S., Baldessarini, R. J., and Weeler, S. C. (1974). *Neuropharmacology* **13,** 987.
Gibbons, J. L. (1964). *Arch. Gen. Psychiatry* **10,** 572.
Gibbons, J. L., and McHugh, P. (1962). *J. Psychiatr. Res.* **1,** 162.
Giles, H. McC. (1963). *Br. Med. J.* **2,** 844.
Glass, G. S., Heninger, G. R., and Lansky, M. (1971). *Am. J. Psychiatry* **128,** 705.
Goodman, L. S., and Gilman, A. (1975). *In* "The Pharmacological Basis of Therapeutics" (L. S. Goodman and A. Gilman, eds.), 5th ed., p. 201. Macmillan, New York.
Goodwin, F. K., and Sack, R. L. (1973). *In* "Frontiers in Catecholamine Research" (E. Usdin and S. Snyder, eds.), p. 1157. Pergamon, Oxford.
Goodwin, F. K., Post, R., Dunner, D., and Goden, E. (1973). *Am. J. Psychiatry* **130,** 73.
Gourdon, J., Clos, J., Coste, L., Dainat, J., and Legrand, J. (1973). *J. Neurochem.* **21,** 861.
Grahame-Smith, D. G., (1971). *J. Neurochem.* **18,** 1053.
Grahame-Smith, D. G., and Parfitt, A. G. (1970). *J. Neurochem.* **17,** 1339.
Grave, G. D., Satterthwaite, S., Kennedy, C., and Sokoloff, L. (1973). *J. Neurochem.* **20,** 495.
Green, A. R., and Kelly, P. H. (1976). *Br. J. Pharmacol.* **57,** 141.
Greenblat, R. B. (1965). *N. Engl. J. Med.* **272,** 305.
Greengrass, P. M., and Tonge, S. R. (1971). *J. Pharm. P armacol.* **23,** 897.
Greengrass, P. M., and Tonge, S. R. (1972). *Br. J. Pharmacol.* **46,** 533.
Greengrass, P. M., and Tonge, S. R. (1973). *Br. J. Pharmacol.* **47,** 660.
Greengrass, P. M., and Tonge, S. R. (1974a). *Arch. Int. Pharmacodyn. Ther.* **210,** 75.
Greengrass, P. M., and Tonge, S. R. (1974b). *Arch. Int. Pharmacodyn. Ther.* **211,** 291.
Greengrass, P. M., and Tonge, S. R. (1974c). *Arch. Int. Pharmacodyn. Ther.* **212,** 48.
Hamburgh, M., and Flexner, L. B. (1957). *J. Neurochem.* **1,** 279.
Hamburgh, M., Mendoza, L. A., Burkhard, J. F., and Weil, F. (1971). *Cell. Aspects Neural Growth Differ., Proc. Conf., 1969* p. 321.
Hamon, M., and Glowinski, J. (1974). *Life Sci.* **15,** 1533.

Hartmann, E. (1968). *Psychopharmacologia* **12,** 346.
Hegarty, A. B. (1955). *Br. Med. J.* **1,** 637.
Hishikawa, Y., Nakai, K., Ida, H., and Kaneko, Z. (1965). *Electroencephalogr. Clin. Neurophysiol.* **19,** 518.
Hokfelt, T., Ffindie, S., and Hellerström, C. (1975). *Acta Endocrinol., Suppl.* **80,** 5.
Hole, K. (1972). *Dev. Psychobiol.* **5,** 157.
Hrdina, P. D., Rastogi, R. B., and Singhal, R. L. (1974). *Int. Congr. Physiol.* [*Proc.*], *26th, 1974* p. 330.
Hrdina, P. D., Ghosh, P. K., Rastogi, R. B., and Singhal, R. L. (1975). *Can. J. Physiol. Pharmacol.* **53,** 709.
Itil, T. M., Polvan, N., and Holden, J. M. C. (1971). *Dis. Nerv. Syst.* **32,** 193.
Itil, T. M., Patterson, C. D., Polvan, M. D., Bigelow, A., and Bergey, B. (1975). *Dis. Nerv. Syst.* **36,** 529.
Jacobson, S. (1963). *J. Comp. Neurol.* **121,** 5.
Janowsky, D. S., El-Yousef, M. K., Davis, J. M., Hubbard, B., and Sekerke, H. J. (1972). *Lancet* **1,** 1236.
Javoy, F., Glowinski, J., and Kordon, C. (1968). *Eur. J. Pharmacol.* **4,** 103.
Jequier, E., Robinson, D. S., Lovenberg, W., and Sjoerdsma, A. (1969). *Biochem. Pharmacol.* **18,** 1071.
Johansson, S., Levi, L., and Lindstedt, S. (1970). "Reports from the Laboratory for Clinical Stress Research," No. 17. Karolinska Institute, Stockholm, Sweden.
Kales, A., Henser, G., Jacobsen, A., Kales, J. D., Hanley, J., Zweizig, J. R., and Paulson, M. J. (1967). *J. Clin. Endocrinol. Metab.* **27,** 1593.
Kane, F. J., Jr. (1968). *Am. J. Obstet. Gynecol.* **102,** 1053.
Kane, F. J., Jr. (1970). *Am. J. Psychiatry* **126,** 1020.
Katz, R. I., and Kopin, I. J. (1969). *Biochem. Pharmacol.* **18,** 1935.
Katz, R. I., Chase, T. N., and Kopin, I. J. (1968). *Science* **162,** 466.
Keller, H. H., Bartholini, G., and Pletscher, A. (1974). *Nature (London)* **248,** 528.
Khanna, N. K., and Pandhi, P. (1972). *Jpn. J. Pharmacol.* **22,** 261.
Kizer, J. S., Palkovits, M., Zivin, J., Brownstein, M., Saavedra, J. M., and Kopin, I. J. (1974). *Endocrinology* **95,** 799.
Klawans, H. L., and Rubowitz, R. (1972). *Neurology* **22,** 107.
Klee, C. B., and Sokoloff, L. (1964). *J. Neurochem.* **11,** 709.
Kleinschmidt, H. J., Waxenberg, S. E., and Cukor, R. (1956). *J. Mt. Sinai. Hosp., N.Y.* **23,** 131.
Knapp, S. (1975). *In* "Neurobiological Mechanisms of Adaptation and Behaviour" (A. J. Mandell, ed.), p. 155. Raven, New York.
Knapp, S., and Mandell, A. J. (1973). *Science* **180,** 645.
Krawiec, L., Garcia Argiz, C. A., Gomez, C. J., and Pasquini, J. M. (1969). *Brain Res.* **15,** 209.
Kuhn, R. (1957). *Schweiz. Med. Wochenschr.* **87,** 1135.
Kulig, B. M. (1975). *Neuropharmacology* **14,** 489.
Kunos, G., Kunos, I. V., and Nickerson, M. (1974). *Nature (London)* **250,** 779.
Lapierre, Y. D., Rastogi, R. B., and Singhal, R. L. (1977). *GWAN Int. Psychiatr. Res. Meet.* (in press).
Laverty, R., and Taylor, K. M. (1968). *Anal. Biochem.* **22,** 269.
Legrand, J. (1967). *Arch. Anat. Microsc. Morphol. Exp.* **56,** 205.
Leonard, B. E., and Kafoe, W. F. (1976). *Biochem. Pharmacol.* **25,** 1939.
Libow, L. S., and Durrell, J. (1965). *Psychosom. Med.* **27,** 377.
Lidz, T., and Whitehorn, J. (1949). *J. Am. Med. Assoc.* **139,** 698.

Luine, V. N., McEwen, B. S., and Black, I. B. (1977). *Brain Res.* **120,** 188.
McClure, D. J. (1966). *J. Psychosom. Res.* **10,** 189.
McGeer, E. G., Gibson, S., and McGeer, P. L. (1967). *Can. J. Biochem.* **45,** 1557.
McMenamy, R. H., and Oncley, J. L. (1958). *J. Biol. Chem.* **233,** 1436.
Maletzky, B., and Blachley, P. (1971). "The Use of Lithium in Psychiatry," p. 47. CRC Press, Cleveland, Ohio.
Mandell, A. J. (1975). *In* "Neurobiological Mechanisms of Adaptation and Behaviour" (A. J. Mandell, ed.), p. 17. Raven, New York.
Mandell, A. J., and Mandell, M. P. (1967). *J. Am. Med. Assoc.* **200,** 792.
Mason, J. W. (1975). *In* "Emotions—Their Parameters and Measurement" (L. Levi, ed.), p. 143. Raven, New York.
Mason, J. W., Hartley, L. H., and Kotchen, T. A. (1973). *J. Clin. Endocrinol. Metab.* **37,** 403.
Merryman, W., Boiman, R., Barnes, L., and Rothchild, J. (1954). *J. Clin. Endocrinol. Metab.* **14,** 1567.
Messiha, F. S., Agallianos, D., and Clower, C. (1970). *Nature (London)* **225,** 868.
Messiha, F. S., Davage, C., Turek, I., and Hanlon, T. (1974). *J. Nerv. Ment. Dis.* **158,** 338.
Moir, A. T. B. (1971). *Br. J. Pharmacol.* **43,** 715.
Morton, J. H., Addition, H., and Addison, R. G. (1953). *Am. J. Obstet. Gynecol.* **65,** 1182.
Murphy, D. L., Brodie, H. K. H., Goodwin, F. K., and Bunney, W. E. J. (1971). *Nature (London)* **229,** 135.
Nicholson, J. L., and Altman, J. (1972). *Brain Res.* **44,** 13.
Nielsen, M., Eplov, L., and Scheel-Kruger, J. (1975). *Psychopharmacology* **41,** 249.
Olson, L., and Fuxe, K. (1971). *Brain Res.* **28,** 165.
Perez-Cruet, J., Tagliamonte, A., Tagliamonte, P., and Gessa, G. L. (1971). *J. Pharmacol. Exp. Ther.* **178,** 325.
Pfenninger, K., Akert, K., Moore, H., and Sandri, C. (1971). *J. Ultrastruct. Res.* **35,** 451.
Poillon, W. N. (1971). *Biochem. Biophys. Res. Commun.* **44,** 64.
Poitou, P., and Bohuon, C. (1975). *J. Neurochem.* **25,** 535.
Poitou, P., Guérinot, F., and Bohuon, C. (1974). *Psychopharmacologia* **38,** 75.
Post, R. M., Kotin, J., Goodwin, F. K., and Gordon, E. K. (1973). *Am. J. Psychiatry* **130,** 67.
Prange, A. J., Jr., and Lipton, M. A. (1962). *Nature (London)* **196,** 588.
Prange, A. J., Jr., McCurdy, R. L., and Cochrane, C. M. (1967). *J. Psychiatr. Res.* **5,** 1.
Prange, A. J., Jr., Wilson, I. C., and Rabon, A. M. (1969a). *Present Status Psychotropic Drugs, Proc. Int. Congr. Coll. Int. Neuro-Psychopharmacol., 6th, 1968* Excerpta Med. Found. Int. Congr. Ser. No. 180, p. 532.
Prange, A. J., Jr., Wilson, I. C., Rabon, M. *et al.* (1969b). *Am. J. Psychiatry* **126,** 457.
Prange, A. J., Jr., Wilson, I. C., Knox, A., McClane, T. S., and Lipton, M. A. (1970). *Am. J. Psychiatry* **127,** 191.
Prange, A. J., Jr., Wilson, I. C., Lara, P. P., Alltop, L. B., and Breese, G. R. (1972a). *Lancet* **2,** 999.
Prange, A. J., Jr., Wilson, I. C., Knox, A. E., McClane, T. K., Breese, G. R., Martin, B. R., Alltop, L. B., and Lipton, M. A. (1972b). *J. Psychiatr. Res.* **9,** 187.
Prange, A. J., Jr., Wilson, I. C., Lara, P. P., and Alltop, L. B. (1974). *In* "The Thyroid Axis, Drug and Behaviour" (A. J. Prange, Jr., ed.), p. 135. Raven, New York.
Randrup, A., and Munkvad, I. (1968). *Neuro-Psychopharmacologie* **1,** 18.
Rastogi, R. B. (1975). Ph.D. Thesis, p. 80. University of Ottawa, School of Medicine.
Rastogi, R. B., and Singhal, R. L. (1974a). *J. Pharmacol. Exp. Ther.* **191,** 72.

Rastogi, R. B., and Singhal, R. L. (1974b). *Brain Res.* **81,** 253.
Rastogi, R. B., and Singhal, R. L. (1974c). *Endocr. Res. Commun.* **1,** 261.
Rastogi, R. B., and Singhal, R. L. (1975a). *Fed. Proc., Fed. Am. Soc. Exp. Biol.* **34,** 3140.
Rastogi, R. B., and Singhal, R. L. (1975b). *J. Cell Biol.* **67,** 354.
Rastogi, R. B., and Singhal, R. L. (1976a). *Life Sci.* **18,** 851.
Rastogi, R. B., and Singhal, R. L. (1976b). *J. Pharmacol. Exp. Ther.* **198,** 609.
Rastogi, R. B., and Singhal, R. L. (1977a). *J. Pharmacol. Exp. Ther.* **201,** 92.
Rastogi, R. B., and Singhal, R. L. (1977b). *Can. J. Physiol. Pharmacol.* **55,** 490.
Rastogi, R. B., and Singhal, R. L. (1977c). *Fed. Proc., Fed. Am. Soc. Exp. Biol.* **36,** 951.
Rastogi, R. B., and Singhal, R. L., and Hrdina, P. D. (1975). *Neuropharmacology* **4,** 747.
Rastogi, R. B., Lapierre, Y. D., and Singhal, R. L. (1976a). *Coll. Int. Neuropsychopharmacol., 10th Congress,* p. 199.
Rastogi, R. B., Lapierre, Y. D., and Singhal, R. L. (1976b). *J. Neurochem.* **26,** 443.
Rastogi, R. B., Merali, Z., and Singhal, R. L. (1977a). *J. Neurochem.* **28,** 789.
Rastogi, R. B., Hrdina, P. D., Dubas, T., and Singhal, R. L. (1977b). *Brain Res.* **123,** 188.
Rastogi, R. B., Lapierre, Y. D., and Singhal, R. L. (1977c). *J. Psychiatr. Res.* **13,** 65.
Rastogi, R. B., Lapierre, Y. D., and Singhal, R. L. (1977d). *Can. J. Physiol. Pharmacol.* (in press).
Rastogi, R. B., Agarwal, R. A., Lapierre, Y. D., and Singhal, R. L. (1977e). *Eur. J. Pharmacol.* **43,** 91.
Rawson, R. W. (1953). *Am. J. Med. Sci.* **226,** 405.
Redding, T. W., and Schally, A. V. (1971). *Fed. Proc., Fed. Am. Soc. Exp. Biol.* **30,** 23.
Rees, L. (1953). *J. Ment. Sci.* **99,** 62.
Reigle, T. G., Avni, J., Platz, P. A., Schildkraut, J. J., and Plotnikoff, N. P. (1974). *Psychopharmacology* **37,** 1.
Reis, D. J., and Fuxe, K. (1969). *Proc. Natl. Acad. Sci. U.S.A.* **64,** 108.
Reis, D. J., Moorhead, D. T., and Merlino, N. (1970). *Arch. Neurol. (Chicago)* **22,** 31.
Richardson, D., Scudder, C. L., and Karczmar, A. G. (1970). *Pharmacologist* **12,** 227.
Richter, D., and Crossland, J. (1949). *Am. J. Physiol.* **159,** 247.
Rizzo, N. D., Fox, H. M., Laidlaw, J. C., and Thorn, G. W. (1954). *Ann. Intern. Med.* **41,** 798.
Robichaud, R. C., and Sledge, K. L. (1969). *Life Sci.* **8,** 965.
Rose, D. P. (1969). *Lancet* **1,** 321.
Rubin, R., and Mandell, A. (1966). *Am. J. Psychiatry* **123,** 387.
Ryback, R. S., and Schwab, R. S. (1971). *N. Engl. J. Med.* **285,** 788.
Sachar, E. J. (1975). *In* "Topics in Psychoendocrinology" (E. J. Sachar, ed.), p. 135. Grune & Stratton, New York.
Schanberg, S. M., Schildkraut, J. J., and Kopin, I. J. (1967). *Biochem. Pharmacol.* **16,** 393.
Schapiro, S. (1966). *Endocrinology* **78,** 527.
Schildkraut, J. J., Gordon, E. K., and Durell, J. (1965). *J. Psychiatr. Res.* **3,** 213.
Schildkraut, J. J., Schanberg, S. M., and Kopin, I. J. (1966). *Life Sci.* **5,** 1479.
Schildkraut, J. J., Dodge, G. A., and Logue, M. A. (1969a). *Dis. Nerve Syst.* **30,** suppl., 44.
Schildkraut, J. J., Schanberg, S. M., Breese, G. R., and Kopin, I. J. (1969b). *Biochem. Pharmacol.* **18,** 1971.
Schildkraut, J. J., Dodge, G. A., and Logue, M. A. (1969c). *J. Psychiatr. Res.* **7,** 29.
Schildkraut, J. J., Winokur, A., and Applegate, C. W. (1970). *Science* **168,** 867.
Schildkraut, J. J., Winokur, A., Draskoczy, P. R., and Hensle, J. H. (1971). *Am. J. Psychiatry* **127,** 1032.

Schildkraut, J. J., Draskoczy, P. R., Gershon, E. S., Reich, P., and Grab, E. L. (1972). *J. Psychiatr. Res.* **9,** 173.
Schneckloth, R. E., Kurland, G. S., and Freedberg, A. S. (1953). *Metab. Clin. Exp.* **2,** 546.
Schubert, J. (1973). *Psychopharmacologia* **32,** 301.
Segal, D. S., and Mandell, A. I. (1974). *In* "Thyroid Axis, Drugs and Behaviour" (A. J. Prange, Jr., ed.), p. 129. Raven, New York.
Segal, D. S., Callaghan, M., and Mandell, A. J. (1975). *Nature (London)* **254,** 58.
Shen, J. T., and Ganong, W. F. (1976). *J. Pharmacol. Exp. Ther.* **199,** 639.
Shopsin, B., Blum, M., and Gershon, S. (1969). *Compt. Psychiatry* **10,** 215.
Siegel, M. R., and Sisler, H. D. (1964). *Nature (London)* **200,** 675.
Singhal, R. L., Rastogi, R. B., and Hrdina, P. D. (1975). *Life Sci.* **17,** 1617.
Singhal, R. L., Rastogi, R. B., and Hrdina, P. D. (1976). *In* "Drugs and Central Synaptic Transmission" (P. B. Bradley and B. N. Dhawan, eds.), p. 359. Macmillan, New York.
Singhal, R. L., Rastogi, R. B., and Agarwal, R. A. (1977). *In* "Hormones and Developing Brain" (S. Kumar, ed.). Pergamon, Oxford (in press).
Smith, D. F. (1976). *Pharmacol. Res. Commun.* **8,** 575.
Smith, D. W., Blizzard, R. M., and Wilkins, L. (1957). *Pediatrics* **19,** 1011.
Smith, S. L. (1975). *In* "Topics in Psychoendocrinology" (E. J. Sachar, ed.), p. 19, Grune & Stratton, New York.
Sobrian, S. K., Pappas, B. A., Edson, N., Rastogi, R. B., and Singhal, R. L. (1976). *Res. Commun. Psychol., Psychiatry Behav.* **1,** 419.
Sokoloff, L. (1970). *In* "Protein Metabolism of the Nervous System" (A. Lajtha, ed.), p. 367. Plenum, New York.
Spano, P. F., and Neff, N. H. (1971). *Anal. Biochem.* **42,** 113.
Stein, L., Wise, C. D., and Berger, B. D. (1973). *In* "Benzodiazepines" (S. Garattini, ed.), p. 299. Raven, New York.
Stein, L., Wise, C. D., and Belluzzi, J. D. (1975). *In* "Mechanism of Action of Benzodiazepines" (E. Costa and P. Greengard, eds.), p. 29. Raven, New York.
Taber, E. (1963). *Anat. Res.* **145,** 291.
Tarlov, S. R., Schildkraut, J. J., and Draskoczy, P. R. (1973). *Biochem. Pharmacol.* **22,** 2923.
Tata, J. R., Ernster, L., Lindberg, O., Arrhenims, E., Pedersen, S., and Hedman, R. (1963). *Biochem. J.* **86,** 408.
Timiras, P. S. (1971). *Proc. Int. Soc. Psychoneuroendocrinol., 1970,* p. 242.
Toth, S., and Csaba, B. (1966). *Experientia* **22,** 755.
Trendelenberg, U. (1953). *Br. J. Pharmacol. Chemother.* **8,** 454.
Valcana, T. (1971). *Proc. Int. Soc. Psychoneuroendocrinol., 1970* p. 174.
Valcana, T., Vernadakis, A., and Timiras, P. S. (1967). *Neuroendocrinology* **2,** 326.
Walravens, P., and Chase, H. P. (1969). *J. Neurochem.* **16,** 1477.
Weichsel, M. E., Jr. (1974). *Brain Res.* **78,** 455.
Weichsel, M. E., Jr., and Dawson, L. (1976). *J. Neurochem.* **26,** 675.
Wheatley, D. (1972). *Arch. Gen. Psychiatry* **26,** 229.
Whybrow, P. C., and Ferrell, R. (1974) *In* "The Thyroid Axis, Drugs and Behaviour" (A. J. Prange, Jr., ed.), p. 5. Raven, New York.
Whybrow, P. C., Prange, A. J., Jr., and Treadway, C. R. (1969). *Arch. Gen. Psychiatry* **20,** 48.
Wilson, I. C., Prange, A. J., Jr., McClane, T. K. *et al.* (1970). *N. Engl. J. Med.* **282,** 1063.
Winokur, A., and Utiger, R. D. (1974). *Science* **185,** 265.
Wise, C. D., Berger, B. D., and Stein, L. (1972). *Science* **171,** 180.

Wiswell, J. G., Hurwitz, G. E., Coronho, V., Bing, O. H. L., and Child, D. L. (1963). *J. Clin. Endocrinol. Metab.* **23,** 1102.

Wurtman, R. J., Larin, F., Mostafapour, S., and Fernström, J. D. (1974). *Science* **185,** 183.

Yalmon, I. Lunde, D., Moos, R., and Hamburgh, D. A. (1968). *Arch. Gen. Psychiatry* **18,** 16.

Yamaguchi, K., Shimoyama, M., and Gholson, R. K. (1967). *Biochim. Biophys. Acta* **146,** 102.

Yarbrough, G. G. (1976). *Nature (London)* **263,** 523.

Immune Modulation and Cancer Control

Stanislaw M. Mikulski,* Michael A. Chirigos,†
and Franco M. Muggia*

I. Introduction

Recent reports on the conflicting results of cancer immunotherapy have stimulated us to review certain aspects of tumor immunology, particularly those that could be exploited for cancer treatment. Because we do not know whether the manipulation of the immune system reactivity has a beneficial effect inhibiting growth of cancer, we prefer to replace the term "immunotherapy" by "immune modulation." We would like to concentrate on the host–tumor interrelationship in terms of the meaningful immunological evaluation of the effective host's tumor immunity and on how this effective immunity could be augmented by external factors or manipulations referred to as "extrinsic immune modulators." Particular emphasis will be placed on the cellular components of the immune system involved in the host's response against his tumor and on the possible value of testing for cytotoxic and noncytotoxic tumor-specific and nonspecific reactivity, as well as for factors that may interfere with the effective tumor immunity.

Four major items will be discussed, namely, the components of the immune system with the most important features of various immune

* Cancer Therapy Evaluation Program, National Cancer Institute, National Institutes of Health, Bethesda, Maryland.

† Viral Oncology Program, National Cancer Institute, National Institutes of Health, Bethesda, Maryland.

effectors and also modulatory elements capable of regulating the function of the immune system (Section II), interfering factors (Section III), immunological testing (Section IV), and suggestions for improvement of immunotherapy trials (Section V).

This is not intended to be an exhaustive review nor a prescription for treatment of any particular kind of cancer. We have tried to simplify maximally present concepts of tumor immunology to make them clear and understandable to investigators who employ "immunotherapy" but are not necessarily immunologists. We hope this review will reflect the basic information regarding the great complexity of the immune interactions between the host and his tumor.

II. Components of the Immune System

Figure 1 represents several types of cells that are known to be involved in the complex immune reaction against the tumor.

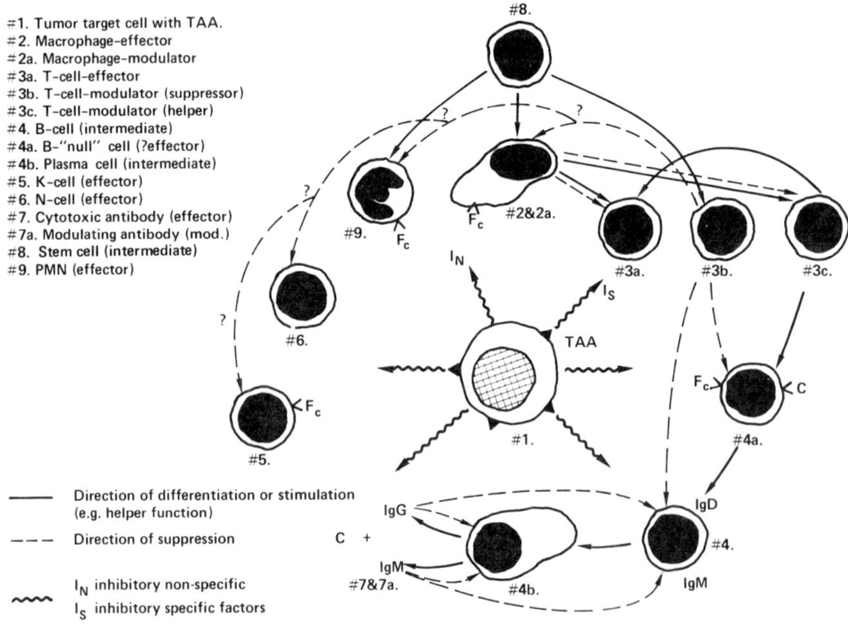

FIG. 1. Schematic representation of a tumor target cell with its cell-surface tumor-associated antigens (TAA) and the most important effector and modulator cells participating in the complex reaction against the tumor.

A. Tumor Cell Targets

A tumor cell (Fig. 1, #1) with its tumor-associated antigens (TAA) (Klein, 1966; Hellström *et al.*, 1973; Hellström and Hellström, 1969) on the cell surface is shown in the center of the diagram. As Medawar and Hunt pointed out (Medawar and Hunt, 1976), the TAA could be a neoantigen(s) synthesized as a result of modification of a normal major histocompatibility complex (MHC) product. Because MHC product in animals and man is a complex set of tissue histocompatibility antigens and other products, including the products of the autosomal dominant immune response (*Ir*) genes closely linked to MHC (Shevach, 1976; Bach and Van Rood, 1976), any modification of this region of the host's genome could result not only in the great diversity of TAAs but also could influence the immune response against autologous tumor. The TAA-specific immunity has been demonstrated in patients with cancer including even those with advanced disease (Hellström and Hellström, 1969).

B. Immune Effectors

1. *Macrophage*

The macrophage (Fig. 1, #2) is a potent phagocytic cell, the activity of which can be stimulated with various agents such as Bacille Calmette Guérin (BCG), methanol extraction residue of BCG (MER), *Corynebacterium parvum,* pyran copolymer, and glucan (Gallily *et al.*, 1976; Gery *et al.*, 1974; Baldwin, 1976; Chassoux and Salomon, 1975; Pimm and Baldwin, 1975; Fisher *et al.*, 1974; Fisher and Wolmark, 1976; Schultz *et al.*, 1976). The activation of macrophages may be reflected by an increased production of lysozyme, the level of which can be measured in serum and be of some predictive value (Yagel *et al.*, 1975; Currie and Eccles, 1976; Currie, 1976).

Macrophages can kill the tumor cell nonspecifically (Schultz *et al.*, 1976; Herberman *et al.*, 1976; Editorial, 1976) in an "innocent bystander" mechanism (Prehn, 1973) or specifically (Schultz *et al.*, 1976; Evans and Alexander, 1972; Van Loveren and Den Otter, 1974b) when they act through the bridge of the fragment crystalline (Fc)-receptor-bound (see Section II,B,5) antibody or specific macrophage-arming factor (SMAF), the identity of which is still poorly defined (Editorial, 1976; Van Loveren and Den Otter, 1974a).

Independent of the mechanism, specific or nonspecific, macrophages must be in close contact with the tumor cells in order to exert their cytotoxic effect (Baldwin, 1976; Evans and Alexander, 1972; Evans, 1972). This might be reflected by the correlation of the response to BCG or MER immune modulation with the macrophage content of the tumor (Baldwin, 1976). The reported shrinkage of pulmonary tumor deposits after intravenous injection of macrophages that are retained in the lungs may reflect this requirement for the close contact between macrophages and tumor cells (Hopper and Pimm, 1976). Macrophages are known to infiltrate tumors to a varying degree, sometimes accounting for over 50% of the tumor mass (Evans, 1972). The macrophage migration into the tumor has been shown to be stimulated by agents preferentially stimulating macrophage system in animals, e.g., pyran copolymer (pyran-3,4-dicarboxylicanhydride tetrahydro-2-methyl-6-(tetrahydro-2,5-dioxo-3-furyl) polymer (Schultz *et al.*, 1977). Other agents, such as levamisole [2,3,5,6-tetrahydro-6-phenylimidazo(2,1-*b*)thiazole hydrochloride], have been shown to stimulate macrophage chemotaxis (Pike and Snyderman, 1976).

Although it has been shown that intralesional or local administration of bacterial modulators rather than systemic administration often seems to be more effective (Krown *et al.*, 1976; Yamamura, 1976; McKneally *et al.*, 1976), there are agents, e.g. pyran copolymer, that are active when administered systemically even as a single dose (Schultz *et al.*, 1977).

It has been shown that the access of macrophages to the tumor may be inhibited by a humoral factor named "macrophage chemotaxis-inhibitory factor," as identified by Snyderman and Pike (1976). This agent is present in cancer-bearing individuals and may interfere with the effective antitumor response. According to some authors (Editorial, 1968, 1976) the capacity of a macrophage-mediated tumor cell kill is limited although the macrophages appear to be able to discriminate between neoplastic and nonneoplastic cell targets (Currie and Basham, 1975; Hibbs *et al.*, 1972). Other components of the immune system such as specifically sensitized lymphocytes or sensitized lymphocyte-derived soluble factors such as SMAF may have to collaborate with the macrophage system in order to ensure the most optimal response against the tumor (Gery *et al.*, 1974; Schultz *et al.*, 1976; Van Loveren and Den Otter, 1974a; Unanue, 1972; Simon and Sheagren, 1971). It should be pointed out that macrophages when activated may also exert a suppressive effect on the other components of the immune system, e.g., T-cell function, especially in viral-induced tumor systems (Kirchner *et al.*, 1974, 1975a,b). Conversely, stimulated macrophages can release a factor(s) that enhances the T-lymphocyte response to various stimuli (Oppenheim *et al.*, 1976).

2. *T Cell*

This is a thymus-derived lymphoid cell (Fig. 1, #3) characterized by its ability to form direct rosettes with sheep red blood cells (SRBC) in man and known to possess specific antigenic cell-surface markers (Bach *et al.*, 1971). There are several functional subpopulations of T cells, such as antigen-sensitive cells, that seem to collaborate very closely with the macrophage system in the recognitive phase of immune response (Shevach, 1976), memory cells, helper cells, suppressor cells, cytotoxic cells, etc. (Brent and Holborow, 1974). The T cells are primarily responsible for transplant rejection (Wagner *et al.*, 1973), graft-versus-host reaction (Segal *et al.*, 1972; Mage and McHugh, 1973), as well as many regulatory processes of other non-T- as well as T-cell functions, e.g., helper and suppressor functions (Katz, 1972) (see Sections II,C,1 and 2).

It has been recognized for several years that T cells are principally involved in the mediation of resistance against most viruses, certain parasites, fungi, and bacteria. Most of the functional regulatory processes as well as certain cytotoxic reactions are mediated through T-cell-derived humoral substances called *lymphokines* (Brent and Holborow, 1974). Some of them may affect macrophage function, e.g., macrophage migration inhibition factor (MIF) (Chess *et al.*, 1974); some may stimulate blastogenic response, i.e., morphologic and biochemical lymphoblastic transformation of lymphocytes mediating the reaction induced by allogeneic cells or mitogens (Geha and Merler, 1974); some may exert direct cytotoxic effects against various target cells after appropriate sensitization (Podleski, 1976); and still others mediate suppressor cell function (Tada *et al.*, 1975) and helper cell function (Taussig and Munro, 1976), the latter enhancing the B-lymphoid cell function and differentiation (see Section, II,C,2). Their function in tumor surveillance is less well-established.

A *cytotoxic T cell* (Fig. 1, #3a) is a cell with T-cell characteristics capable of specifically killing the target cell (Mage and McHugh, 1973; Cerottini *et al.*, 1970). Antigen-specific cell-surface receptors are present on these cells and are capable of reacting against the antigenic determinants present on the surface of target cells and in case of tumor target cells, the TAA antigenic determinants.

3. *B-Lymphoid Cell*

A bursa of Fabricius-equivalent or bone marrow-derived lymphoid cell, the B cell (Fig. 1, #4) is characterized by the presence of surface membrane immunoglobulins. These immunoglobulins are thought to be identical with antigen-specific B-cell surface receptors (Rowe *et al.*,

1973). According to the present concepts, one cell synthesizes only one class and subclass of heavy chain and only one type of light chain of the immunoglobulin molecule, although there is some evidence suggesting that one cell can produce two types of heavy chains at one time (Rowe *et al.*, 1973; Knapp *et al.*, 1973). The best reflection of the view that one cell produces one type of heavy and one type of light chain is the fact that, in monoclonal proliferation of antibody-producing plasma cells, there is only one type of heavy and one type of light chain produced most of the time. It has recently been shown that Hodgkin's disease cells and lacunar cells of nodular sclerosis histology may contain both kappa and lambda light chains within their cytoplasm (Anagnostou *et al.*, 1977). However, normal B-lymphoid cells, which are precursors of plasma cells, possess mainly IgD and IgM classes of immunoglobulins on the cell surface and there is evidence that one cell may synthesize IgD class (delta) and IgM (micron) heavy chains and the same type of light chain that they share (Rowe *et al.*, 1973; Knapp *et al.*, 1973). The final distribution of immunoglobulin synthesis seems to parallel the differentiation of B cells into antibody-producing cells.

Under normal conditions, humoral antibody inhibits, by a negative feedback mechanism, the further proliferation of B cells (Uhr and Moller, 1968; Schwartz, 1972). The impairment of this feedback has been postulated as a basis for an excessive proliferation of B cells in lymphoma and other B-cell proliferative diseases (Schwartz, 1972; Sahiar and Schwartz, 1965, 1966).

It has been shown that IgG may be adsorbed to the B-cell surface Fc receptors secondarily and not necessarily be reflective of the synthesis of this class of immunoglobulin by the cell bearing it (Winchester *et al.*, 1975). Some B cells have Fc and complement (C3) receptors on their surfaces and also receptors for the Epstein-Barr virus (Jondal and Klein, 1973), although it is not certain whether Fc- and C-receptor-positive cells are true B cells, i.e., synthesizing surface membrane immunoglobulins cells, or a "third" population of cells (non-T and non-B cells) as named by Winchester *et al.* (1975). The nature and function of Fc receptors (Mikulski and Billing, 1977) will be discussed below in association with antibody-dependent cellular cytotoxicity (ADCC).

4. *"Null" Cell*

Cells having no T- or B-cell markers are called "null" cells and a portion of this population appears to differentiate into B cells (Chess *et al.*, 1975) (Fig. 1, #4a). The other null cells may differentiate into T cells and possibly other cells as well (Horowitz and Hong, 1977). It has been shown (Chess *et al.*, 1974, 1975) that null cells have functionally active Fc receptors and they may be active as effectors in ADCC. The B cells differentiate into plasma cells, that is, antibody-producing cells (Fig. 1, #4b).

5. *K Cell*

This type of cell (Fig. 1, #5) has been defined as a non-T killer cell, i.e., a lymphocyte without the T- nor B-cell characteristics but active as an effector in ADCC (Perlmann and MacLennan, 1974). This cell has properties very similar to those of a B-null cell (null cell that differentiates into B cell), but it does not seem to differentiate into B cells. Due to the presence of a functionally active Fc receptor for the fragment crystalline of an IgG molecule, these cells are the principal mediators of ADCC. This cytotoxic reactivity is characterized by the fact that humoral IgG antibody determines the specificity of the reaction and forms a bridge connecting the target, e.g., tumor cell, with the effector cell, i.e., K cell. The IgG antibody is the only class of immunoglobulin capable of participating in this kind of cytotoxicity. The sensitivity of this reaction is very high and concentrations as low as 10^{-12} of the IgG antibody have been reported to be able to mediate this cytotoxicity (Perlmann *et al.*, 1972). The cytotoxic function of the effector cells in ADCC system has been reported to be decreased in various cancer patients (Ting and Terasaki, 1974) and also to be decreased in the milieu of cancer patients sera (Mikulski *et al.*, 1977).

6. *N Cell*

This cell is still poorly defined (Fig. 1, #6). The N cell has a lymphoid cell appearance, and, since it has none of the characteristics of the previously mentioned kinds of cells, it may be functionally important in certain genetically determined immune reactions called "natural" cytotoxicity, i.e., not induced by a known immunization (Kiessling *et al.*, 1975a,b; Herberman *et al.*, 1975). The role of these cells remains to be established. They do demonstrate the antitumor cytotoxic activity in several strains of mice including athymic nude mice (Herberman *et al.*, 1975).

7. *Cytotoxic Humoral Antibody*

This is an antibody able to bind complement after reaction with antigen (Fig. 1, #7). Basically two classes of immunoglobulins are involved in the activation of the classic pathway of complement, the most efficient being IgM and the other IgG (with the exception of the IgG4 subclass). Immunoglobulin A can activate an alternate complement pathway.

8. *Stem Cell*

This is a multipotential bone marrow stem cell (Fig. 1, #8) capable of differentiating into all kinds of immunologically competent cells.

9. *Polymorphonuclear Leukocytes (PMN)*

These cells (Fig. 1, #9) are able to participate as effectors in certain ADCC systems (Gale and Zighelboim, 1975). The direct phagocytic activity of these cells seems to be less potent as compared to macrophages. Their role as effectors in ADCC against tumor cells is unknown and remains to be established.

C. Intrinsic Immune Modulators

1. *Suppressor T Cell*

The principal role of this type of T cells (Fig. 1, #3b) is to restrain an excessive humoral antibody production by the B-cell line of lymphoid cells that eventually differentiate into antibody-producing plasma cells (Tada, 1974). Also these cells and perhaps others (e.g., activated macrophages) may suppress other functions of T and non-T cells, e.g., cytotoxic activity (see Fig. 1) (Kirchner *et al.*, 1975a; Katz, 1972; Nachtigal *et al.*, 1975; Peavy and Pierce, 1974; Zembala and Asherson, 1973). One of the dangers of nonspecific immune modulation may be the activation of suppressor cell function that could lead to a general impairment of immune reactivity. This could be dependent on the dose and schedule of the extrinsic immune modulator (Sampson and Lui, 1976), as well as on the original status of patient's immune competence (Churchill and David, 1973; Hooper *et al.*, 1975; Perk *et al.*, 1975; Patt, 1977). Preliminary results from the M. D. Anderson Hospital indicate that, instead of inhibiting tumor growth, thymosin (bovine thymus extract, thymosin Fraction V) may accelerate it when administered to patients with relatively normal T-cell function (Patt, 1977). This could be a result of activation of T suppressor cell function. In certain tumor systems, the augmentation of T-cell system function might be of no benefit or even could be harmful resulting in acceleration of the rate of tumor growth (Gillette and Fox, 1975; Carnaud *et al.*, 1974; Martinez, 1964; Yunis *et al.*, 1969).

Agents such as levamisole and thymosin, acting through similar intracellular mechanisms involving the cyclic nucleotide metabolism [cyclic adenosine monophosphate (cAMP) and cyclic guanosine monophosphate (cGMP)] (Hadden *et al.*, 1975; Bach *et al.*, 1975), appear to have a beneficial effect in cases of decreased T-cell function as measured by either skin delayed hypersensitivity testing (Hirshaut *et al.*, 1973; Levo *et al.*, 1975; Tripodi *et al.*, 1973) or tests such as E-rosette formation (human T lymphocytes forming direct rosettes with SRBC) (Ramot *et al.*, 1976) or lymphokine production (Whitcomb *et al.*, 1976).

In view of the present concepts that the TAA may be related to a normal major histocompatibility complex product, and that the tolerance to self-antigens may be dependent on specifically balanced, suppressor cell-mediated function (Nachtigal *et al.*, 1975; Allison *et al.*, 1971), effective antitumor response may require some degree of desuppression.

2. *Helper T Cell*

This cell (Fig. 1, #3c) enhances the synthesis of humoral antibodies by the B line of cells primarily directed against the so-called T-cell-dependent antigens as opposed to the so-called T-cell-independent polymeric antigens, e.g., lipopolysaccharide, capable of stimulating B cells directly (Basten and Howard, 1973; Coutinho and Moller, 1973). The helper cell stimulates also the differentiation of B cells into antibody-producing plasma cells. Another kind of helper cell may amplify other cellular reactions, e.g., a mixed lymphocyte reaction and lymphocyte cytotoxicity (Bach *et al.*, 1974).

The specific macrophage-arming factor (SMAF) enhancing the cytotoxic activity of macrophages seems to be produced by a specific variety of T cells (Van Loveren and Den Otter, 1974a; Simon and Sheagren, 1971).

3. *Macrophage*

It has been shown that macrophages (Fig. 1, #2a) may exert both immunosuppressive as well as immunostimulatory effect on T cells (Gery *et al.*, 1974; Kirchner *et al.*, 1975a; Oppenheim *et al.*, 1976; Peavy and Pierce, 1974).

4. *Humoral Antibody*

Humoral antibody (Fig. 1, #7a) may also induce antigenic modulation, which may be effected either by shedding of surface antigens or by modification of conformational arrangements of the cell surface (Old *et al.*, 1968; Alexander, 1974). Under normal conditions, it also exerts an inhibitory feedback effect on B-cell proliferation (Uhr and Moller, 1968; Schwartz, 1972). Thus humoral antibody may be viewed in fact as a modulator of a humoral and cellular immune response. For the immunologically specific killing of the tumor to occur, the tumor has to be antigenic, recognition of the TAA(s) has to take place, and the effector activity has to be generated. Finally, the effectors must have access to the tumor cells and the tumor cells have to be susceptible to immune lysis, which is not always the case (MacLennan *et al.*, 1975; Alexander, 1974).

III. Interfering Factors

Cytotoxic responses may be prevented at several levels of the immune reaction (Figs. 1 and 2). If the tumor is non- or only weakly antigenic, the immunologically specific response may be absent or too weak to be effective, particularly in the presence of immunosuppressive factors. Assuming that the tumor is antigenic and that specific tumor-directed immunity is present, it is still not enough to draw any conclusions as to the effective killing of the tumor cells. The most conclusive proof for effective *in vivo* killing of the tumor cells may require the demonstration of cytotoxic reactivity using the patient's own serum and tumor cells or patient's lymphoid or other effectors and tumor cells. The correlation between *in vitro* cytotoxicity and *in vivo* effect at a particular time may not be precise or may be absent because of other factors contributing to

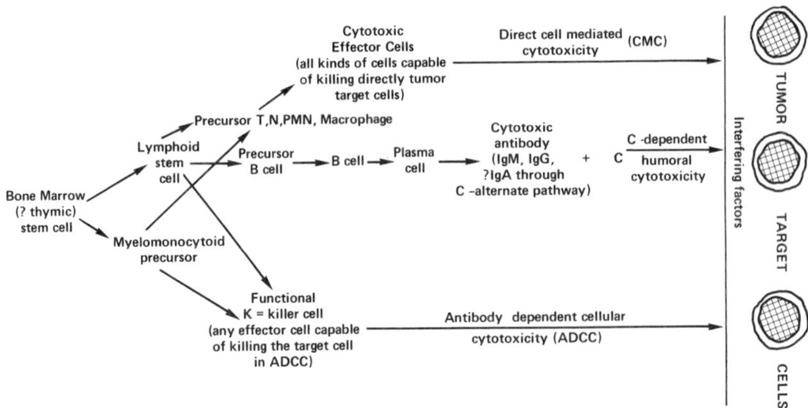

FIG. 2. Schematic representation of the three major cytotoxic effector pathways and factors interfering with the effector tumor cell kill.

tumor regression (e.g., chemotherapy, other treatments), and also due to the time lag between either tumor regression and the disappearance of blocking factors from the serum (or other body fluid) or between the occurrence of blocking factors and tumor progression as estimated clinically. Correlation between the result of cytotoxic tests and the clinical regression may thus require repeated tests. Conversely, increased inhibitory activity might precede the clinical progression of the tumor. There are reports suggesting that cytotoxic reactivity can correlate with the activity of the disease (disappearing of cytotoxic activity with the progression of the disease) (Jerry, 1977) and also that cytotoxic reactivity may be present when other tests, such as mixed lymphocyte reaction is negative (Huntington and Davey, 1976). Many cytotoxic tests should be performed at the same time, namely, direct cell-mediated cytotoxicity, ADCC, and C-dependent cytotoxicity (Fig. 2). In view of the presence of different kinds of inhibitory factors of tumor-directed immunity, such as free TAA and TAA–anti-TAA immune complexes, as well as nonspecific but tumor-associated factors in the extracellular environment of cancer patients, it is imperative to perform these cytotoxic tests in the milieu of autologous sera or other body fluids.

Free TAA and soluble, circulating immune complexes of TAA and anti-TAA antibody are found in the sera of cancer-bearing individuals (Baldwin *et al.*, 1973a; Thomson *et al.*, 1973; Hellström and Hellström, 1970; Tamerius *et al.*, 1976; Amlot *et al.*, 1976; Theofilopoulos *et al.*, 1976; Rossen *et al.*, 1976; Proctor *et al.*, 1973; Heimer and Klein, 1976; Bowen *et al.*, 1975). These are thought to inhibit the effective interaction between the cytotoxic effector cell and the tumor target cell (Hellström and Hellström, 1970; Tamerius *et al.*, 1976; Bowen *et al.*, 1975; Prather and Lausch, 1976; Matthews *et al.*, 1976; Baldwin *et al.*, 1974). Inhibition under these circumstances has an immunologically specific character in all kinds of cytotoxicity except ADCC, in which case it is either nonspecific due to the lack of specificity of the Fc receptor or, more often, tumor-specific if inhibition takes place at the target cell level and immune complexes block with their antigenic component the TAA-specific ADCC antibody-combining sites.

Inhibition may vary depending on the biology of the tumor, e.g., shedding of the surface TAA from the tumor cells (Alexander, 1974), and the type and degree of the humoral immune response against the tumor. A decreased production of a humoral antibody in face of a constantly and inexorably growing tumor may result in a formation of soluble, blocking, TAA–anti-TAA immune complexes at antigen (TAA) excess conditions that are being favored under such circumstances (Lewis, 1974). This deserves more exploration to define a more precise mechanism. The equilibrium of the circulating free TAA and humoral anti-TAA antibody may be affected in several ways. Instead of the formation of *insoluble* complexes in the range of *antibody* excess, which may be easily removable by the reticuloendothelial system (RES), *soluble* complexes having a tendency to circulate may be formed in the range of *antigen* excess (Dixon *et al.*, 1961). Also the quality of antibody response can affect the rate of immune complex elimination by the RES. Antibodies with low avidity (or binding capacity) are much less efficient in this regard (Pincus *et al.*, 1968).

The immunosuppressive effect of tumor-associated inhibitory factors and/or cytoreductive therapy itself (Hersh and Oppenheim, 1967) may interfere not only with the cellular immunity but also may decrease humoral anti-TAA antibody production. In addition, because of unknown reasons, the production of so-called anti-idiotypic antibodies may occur in cancer patients as a reflection of deranged regulatory processes. These antibodies react against the variable portion of anti-TAA antibodies (Jerry, 1977). This may be an additional mechanism of changing antigen–antibody equilibrium in the direction of antigen excess. The growing tumor is potentially the most important source of a constantly increasing amount of free TAA. This creates a situation of a TAA excess that is known to favor the formation of soluble complexes (Matthews *et al.*, 1975; Poskitt *et al.*, 1974). The solubility of these complexes interferes with the effective clearance of them by the RES and, therefore, soluble complexes have the tendency to remain in the circulation as well as the rest of the extracellular compartment. The final result of this disturbed equilibrium may be reflected by an "autoimmune" type of disorder resembling the other so-called immune complex diseases, e.g., nephrotic syndrome secondary to the deposition of TAA–anti-TAA immune complexes in the glomeruli of the kidney (Lewis, 1974; Heaton *et al.*, 1975; Kerkoven *et al.*, 1973; Lokich *et al.*, 1973; Costanza *et al.*, 1973).

In addition there are several humoral nonspecific inhibitory factors recognized in the sera of cancer-bearing individuals, such as the lymphocyte-depressive factor (Field and Caspary, 1972), anergy peptide (Glasgow *et al.*, 1974), macrophage chemotaxis inhibitory factor (Snyderman and Pike, 1976), and other less well-defined factors (Mikulski *et al.*, 1977; Gainor *et al.*, 1976; Hersey *et al.*, 1976; Embleton, 1976; Whitehead *et al.*, 1976a,b; Mortensen *et al.*, 1975; Murgita and Tomasi, 1975; Edwards *et al.*, 1973; Beling and Weksler, 1974; Browne *et al.*, 1976; Israel *et al.*, 1976).

Several cell-mediated immune functions have been shown to be depressed in cancer patients including the ability to form E-rosettes

(Ramot *et al.*, 1976; Whitehead *et al.*, 1976a) and cytotoxic reactivity (Ting and Terasaki, 1974). There have recently been several reports on the beneficial effect of plasmapheresis on various cell-mediated immunity functions including cytotoxic reactivity (Hersey *et al.*, 1976; Browne *et al.*, 1976; Whitehead *et al.*, 1976b) and clinical response of neoplastic lesions in cancer patients (Israel *et al.*, 1976). Specific enhancement by 200 to 500% of the cytotoxic activity of peripheral blood non-T lymphocytes isolated from patients with the metastatic renal cell carcinoma after pretreatment of effectors with the *Vibrio cholerae* neuraminidase (S. M. Mikulski *et al.*, unpublished results) confirms the findings of others (Whitehead *et al.*, 1976a,b; Browne *et al.*, 1976) that in certain kinds of neoplasia in man the effector cells are coated with the more-or-less "detachable" material (?sialomucoprotein) that may interfere with the effective tumor cell killing.

IV. Immunological Testing

Various immunological tests have been used in the evaluation of cancer patients. Delayed-type hypersensitivity (DTH) skin tests using various recall antigens, including tumor-specific antigens (Char *et al.*, 1973, 1974; Baker *et al.*, 1974; Bluming *et al.*, 1971) and agents such as dinitrochlorobenzene (DNCB) the reaction against which reflects a T-cell-mediated contact hypersensitivity and ability to develop primary immune response. They may be very useful in detecting decreased immune competence, but several factors, including the therapy of cancer itself, may affect the interpretation of the tests. Treatment with cyclophosphamide, for example, may be associated with a decrease of the DTH skin reactivity due to immunosuppression (Mullins *et al.*, 1975). Conversely, enhancement of DTH skin reactivity after cyclophosphamide occasionally may occur from inhibition of suppressor cell activity in both human and animal systems (Mullins *et al.*, 1975; Mitsuoka *et al.*, 1976; Parker *et al.*, 1975).

Results from noncytotoxic *in vitro* tests may not correlate with cytotoxic response against the tumor (Bach *et al.*, 1974; Huntington and Davey, 1976). Therefore evaluation of tumor-specific effective immunity should not solely depend on noncytotoxic tests that do not by themselves necessarily reflect the actual host's tumor-killing potential. One reason is that an immune response to cellular antigens appears to be a two-stage phenomenon, the first being a recognitive phase and the second, an effector or destructive phase. The demonstration of the presence of recognitive capacity (e.g., blastogenic transformation and mixed lymphocyte–tumor cell reaction) does not necessarily mean that the second phase, i.e., effective killing response will develop (Bach *et al.*, 1973, 1974; McCoy *et al.*, 1975; Cohen and Howe, 1973). In fact two different antigen systems may be involved—one system that primarily stimulates the recognitive phase of lymphocyte response and the other system against which the cytotoxic reactivity is directed (Bach *et al.*, 1973, 1974). We feel that only cytotoxic testing may give a clue as to the possibilities of *in vivo* tumor cell kill as a direct measure of a second, i.e., destructive phase of immune response, provided that these tests are performed in an autologous system and under the conditions outlined in Table I. In these tests the use of allogeneic or cultured tumor cell-line targets may introduce additional problems of heterogeneity and possibilities of cross-reactivity with other non-TAA antigens. Positive results of a tumor-specific noncytotoxic tests may be reflective of the presence of tumor-specific immunity (sensitization) that parallels the presence of the tumor. Removal of the tumor may result in disappearance of or decrease of this immunity. Therefore, in certain diseases, e.g., osteosarcoma, the presence of positive noncytotoxic results may indicate the persistence of the disease rather and not necessarily the existence of a favorable state of immunity capable of eliminating the tumor cells (Gainor *et al.*, 1976). Also depending on the test, the result may vary, meaning that not only the cell reactivity but also the quality of the stimulus used determines the final result (Holm *et al.*, 1976). Table I summarizes our considerations regarding the usefulness of various immune tests and the kind of information that may be obtained from these tests.

V. Suggestions for Improvement of Immunotherapy Trials

Immune modulation differs from chemotherapy in one major respect: it acts *indirectly* through the host's endogenous immune cellular system. There is usually no dose–effect relationship, i.e., higher doses of immune modulators may be more effective within certain limits but further increases will result most of the time in an immunosuppressive rather than immunostimulatory effect that, in fact, may be a result of stimulation of suppressor cell function (Sampson and Lui, 1976). Also immune modulation will fail if the tumor cannot be reached by the effector mechanism due to the presence of interfering factors (Fig. 2) or if the target tumor cell is resistant to immune lysis (MacLennan *et al.*, 1975; Alexander, 1974). Even when the tumor is nonantigenic or very weakly antigenic, it may still be destroyed by immunologically nonspecific effector mechanisms (see Section, II,B,1), although the efficiency

TABLE I

Immunological Tests Used for Evaluating Cancer Patients

Test[a]	Information obtained
Skin tests with recall antigens, DNCB, and tumor-specific antigens (1–4).	General status of immune competence; ability to develop primary immune response (DNCB); status of tumor-specific immunity by DTH; no direct information regarding actual tumor-killing potential; possibility of obtaining a misleading information, e.g., after treatment with cyclophosphamide or other agents.
Noncytotoxic in vitro *tests:*	
a. Tumor nonspecific, e.g., blastogenic response to nonspecific mitogens, mixed lymphocyte reaction, E-rosette-positive cell enumeration, level of immunoglobulins and complement.	General status of immune competence.
b. Tumor-specific, e.g., specific blastogenic response (5), macrophage or leukocyte migration inhibition tests (6), macrophage chemotaxis inhibition (7). (All tests performed with and without the milieu of autologous body fluid.)	Existence of tumor-specific immunity in terms of tumor recognition but no direct information regarding the actual killing potential. The demonstrable tumor immunity may be reflective of the persistence of the disease and not necessarily the existence of the favorable status of the immune reactivity capable of killing the tumor. Several of these tests may be used to evaluate the inhibitory activity of body fluids.
Cytotoxic tests:	
a. Direct cellular cytotoxicity mediated by T (8, 9) as well as non-T cells (macrophages, ?N cells, etc.) (8, 10, 11). *b*. Antibody-dependent cellular cytotoxicity (ADCC) (12–14). *c*. C-dependent cytotoxicity (15). (All tests performed with and without the milieu of autologous body fluid and before and after "deblocking" treatment of effectors.)	Existence of the killing effector capacity and the immune effector pathway along which it takes place; whether there is a resistance of otherwise immunogenic (as tested by other tests) tumor cells to immune lysis; whether there are cytotoxicity-inhibiting factors and of what nature (employing more sophisticated methods of isolation and fractionation); nature of the decreased cytotoxicity (if present), e.g., is it due to (*a*)lack of specifically immunized effector killer cells or cytotoxic antibodies, (*b*) inhibition by a humoral inhibitory factors, (*c*) inhibition by an increased suppressor cell activity, etc.

[a] Key to references cited: (1) Char *et al.*, 1973; (2) Char *et al.*, 1974; (3) Baker *et al.*, 1974; (4) Bluming *et al.*, 1971; (5) Gainor *et al.*, 1976; (6) McCoy *et al.*, 1975; (7) Snyderman and Pike, 1976; (8) Herberman *et al.*, 1976; (9) Cerottini *et al.*, 1970; (10) Kiessling *et al.*, 1975a; (11) Herberman *et al.*, 1975; (12) Ting and Terasaki, 1974; (13) Mikulski *et al.*, 1977; (14) O'Toole *et al.*, 1973; (15) Huntington and Davey, 1976.

of this seems to be limited. It seems to us that several requirements have to be satisfied in order for immune modulation to have a chance to be effective. The appropriate evaluation of the patient's immune system status cannot be overemphasized. This could allow for the use of an appropriate immune modulator in appropriate dose, route, schedule, and relation to other modalities of cancer treatment. The major items to be considered include the following:

1. Immunologically responsive cells capable of being stimulated by extrinsic immune modulators have to be present and evaluation of their function performed.
   a. Total pool of bone marrow precursor cells and stem cells could, perhaps, be estimated by evaluation of the colony-forming capacity (CFC); a separate pool of stem and precursor cells may be present within the thymus gland (Ford *et al.*, 1966; Kadish and Basch, 1976).
   b. Qualitative and quantitative evaluation of T-cell system, which would involve evaluation of separate functions if possible, e.g., cytotoxic activity, helper activity, and suppressor activity. In view of the reportedly increased susceptibility of T-deficient animals to DNA (Allison *et al.*, 1974; Stutman, 1975) as well as RNA (Collavo *et al.*, 1976) viral-induced oncogenesis, this approach could be valuable in evaluation of patients suspected of having tumor of putative viral etiology or co-etiology (Levine *et al.*, 1976) and in all cases suggestive of disturbed regulatory immune functions, e.g., inadequate suppression of B-lymphoid cell proliferation in lymphoproliferative disorders.
   c. Evaluation of B-cell function, and, particularly, whether or not there is an adequate production of specific anti-TAA antibody. The latter may be essential for the establishment of equilibrium preventing the formation of soluble immune complexes capable of blocking effective antitumor cytotoxic response and also of antibodies capable of feedback inhibiting of B-cell proliferation (anti-idiotypic antibodies).
   d. Evaluation of the macrophage function, e.g., measurement of the tissue or serum level of lysozyme, as pointed out earlier, and chemotaxis that could be reflective of the macrophage ability to penetrate the tumor.
2. Testing of the tumor-specific cytotoxic reactivity as means of determining the presence of effective antitumor response and the efficacy of immune modulation employed.

3. Evaluation of patients for the presence of inhibitory factors interfering with the effective antitumor cytotoxic response using both cytotoxic and noncytotoxic tests. If such factors are demonstrable, then reevaluation should be performed after "deblocking" procedures, e.g., plasmapheresis. Evaluation should also include testing for lymphocyte or other effector-directed antibodies that may interfere with the effector receptor function and, therfore, affect effector activity (Mikulski *et al.*, 1977).

For example, if intensive chemotherapy or other cytoreductive therapy markedly diminishes the bone marrow and other, for instance thymic, stem cells and precursors of the future immunocompetent cells (Ford *et al.*, 1966; Kadish and Basch, 1976; Kenady *et al.*, 1977) (Fig. 1, #8), we cannot expect immune modulation to be effective at all. However, the use of immune modulators, such as thymosin, after immunosuppression has already taken place, may significantly improve the immune status and may be reflected by improvement of clinical status and trend toward a lower mortality rate (P. B. Chretien, personal communication). This effect could be due to the induction of maturation of preexistent precursors into immunocompetent cells (Kenady *et al.*, 1977), but it might be insufficient if further generation of precursor cells from stem cells would be required in face of a deficient pool of the latter.

Although increased tolerance to chemotherapy has been reported after treatment with levamisole (Lods *et al.*, 1976), it is still unclear whether other immune modulators could be of use in this regard. It should be pointed out that modulators such as *Corynebacterium parvum* and other bacterial modulators may increase the bone marrow colony-forming capacity (Fisher and Wolmark, 1976; Dimitrov *et al.*, 1975) but, at the same time, the activation of cellular proliferation may be associated with increased susceptibility of marrow to cell-cycle-specific chemotherapeutic agents (Greenberg *et al.*, 1974) as well as acute irradiation (Gordon *et al.*, 1977). Therefore it seems to us that timing of immune modulation and other modalities of treatment may be of great importance in influencing the final result. The observations that CFC of the bone marrow may correlate with response to treatment and survival in human acute leukemia (Granstrom and Gahrton, 1974) suggest that the cellular reserve is critical. It would be interesting to look more closely at possible correlations of marrow CFC and the response to immune modulation in man.

In patients where only intolerable myelosuppressive doses of chemotherapy have to be used to achieve therapeutic effect, the transplantation of the *a priori* stored autologous marrow could be considered. It would be particularly applicable to patients with solid tumors without bone marrow involvement and possibly, even in acute leukemias during complete remission. Results of Epstein *et al.* (1969) and Storb *et al.* (1974) in dogs and preliminary trials in man (Buckner *et al.*, 1972; Kurnick, 1962; Tobias *et al.*, 1977) suggest that autotransplantation of the marrow may be an alternative approach for allowing use of higher doses of chemotherapy when required and where myelosuppression is a dose-limiting toxicity (Storb *et al.*, 1974).

The question of a correlation between the *in vitro* cytotoxicity and *in vivo* killing response has been discussed earlier as well as the necessity of performing the tests, including cytotoxic, in the milieu of autologous serum or other body fluid.

The choice of an immune modulator depends on the total immune evaluation and the biology of malignancy. Specifically, levamisole and/or thymosin could be of use, e.g., in cases with demonstrable decrease in T-cell function; BCG could be most active when administered locally or regionally or in some cases systemically; and *Corynebacterium parvum* would be able to activate macrophage system of several organs after systemic administration.

Tumors derived from cells normally forming the immune system and particularly hematologic malignancies deserve a separate comment. Immune modulation of these malignancies may be associated with specific problems, e.g., lack of the immunoresponsive precursor cells in acute leukemia, even before any therapy has been instituted, may be present. In lymphoproliferative malignancies, there may be an excessive proliferation of B lymphocytes due to either the loss of suppressor cell function or of feedback inhibition by humoral antibody (Uhr and Moller, 1968; Schwartz, 1972). Excessive immune stimulation may be associated with an increased risk of activation of latent oncogenic viruses (Hirsch, 1974; Schwartz *et al.*, 1973) and, perhaps, this may be related to the early relapses after nonspecific immune modulation with BCG in some cases of lymphoma (Magrath and Ziegler, 1976). In multiple myeloma, it is conceivable that we are dealing with the reverse of the phenomenon seen in lymphoma, i.e., excessive negative feedback inhibition of normal B-cell proliferation by the monoclonal antibody or its fragments. It has recently been shown that decreased normal immunoglobulin production in myeloma seems to be induced at least in some cases by a distinct subpopulation of adherent cells having no characteristics of T cells (monocyte?) (Broder *et al.*, 1975; Waldmann *et al.*, 1976), suggesting some kind of a suppressor mechanism.

The General Approach to Immunotherapy

It has been previously suggested that combining tumor-specific with nonspecific immune modulation may prevent the development of the immunological enhancement of tumor growth (Jacobs and Kripke, 1974) that may occur when nonspecific immune modulator is administered alone (Jacobs and Kripke, 1974; Lokich, 1975). Also the administration of the tumor-specific antigen alone may result in abrogation of the preexistent tumor-directed immunity (Baldwin *et al.*, 1973b; Thomson *et al.*, 1973) particularly when the soluble tumor antigen is used (Embleton, 1976b). This effect seems to be due to an increase of blocking activity by either free TAA or when it is complexed with antibody. There are more reports suggesting that the combination of tumor-specific vaccine with nonspecific immune modulator is more effective than either component administered alone (Browder, 1977; Mohr, 1977). And, finally, we would like to reemphasize that the success of immune modulation is critically dependent on adequate cytoreduction of the tumor. In view of that, the use of immune modulation in an advanced disease remains very problematic in terms of direct antineoplastic activity. Deliberately we have decided not to focus on any particular type of immune modulation and this is because we believe all kinds of modulation can be influenced to a greater or lesser degree by the factors discussed in the foregoing. Adoptive and passive transfer of tumor-specific immunity are undergoing several trials at present. It remains to be seen whether this therapeutic approach will be influenced by interfering factors.

In summary, it appears that the clinical immune modulation of cancer could be based on a more rational basis of the knowledge of tumor immunology. We recognize several limitations of performing the more sophisticated immunologic tests on a widespread basis, but we feel that an attempt in this direction should be made. Then immune modulation could be tailored to an individual patient with a particular tumor and could, hopefully, become a more effective therapeutic modality. It would also allow for immunological stratification in a more meaningful way of patients entering immunotherapy trials.

VI. Summary

In our evaluation of the present status of tumor immunology, we have focused on those aspects that could be helpful for improvement of efficacy of immune modulation as one of the modalities of cancer treatment. Particular emphasis has been placed on cellular components of the immune system, factors that are known to interfere with tumor-directed immunity, and the quality of immunological testing as a means of evaluating the existence of antitumor immune reactivity and the effect of immune modulation employed. On the basis of the information presented, it appears that, in order for immune modulation to be effective, three major requirements have to be fulfilled: (*1*) immunoresponsive cells capable of being stimulated and of mediating the effect of extrinsic immune modulators have to be present; (*2*) effector cytotoxic immune reactivity and tumor cell target susceptibility to immune lysis have to be present; and (*3*) interfering factors capable of blocking an effective antitumor response have to be looked for and, if found, they should be eliminated whenever feasible. Proper immunological evaluation of the cancer patient should allow for an appropriate choice of immune modulator or a combination thereof for a particular disease. Two phases of therapeutic immune modulation could be envisaged: first, immunological evaluation and, second, proper immune modulation consisting of reconstitution of deficient immune competence, if present, and stimulatory immune modulation using various extrinsic modulators augmenting the host antitumor response.

References

Alexander, P. (1974). *Cancer Res.* **34,** 2077.

Allison, A. C., Denman, A. M., and Barnes, R. D. (1971). *Lancet* **2,** 135.

Allison, A. C., Monga, J. N., and Hammond, V. (1974). *Nature (London)* **252,** 746.

Amlot, P. L., Slaney, J. M., and Williams, B. D. (1976). *Lancet* **1,** 449.

Anagnostou, D., Parker, J. W., Taylor, C. R., Chir, B., Phil, D., Tindle, B. H., and Lukes, R. J. (1977). *Cancer* **39,** 1032.

Bach, F. H., Segall, M., Zier, K. S., Sondel, P. M., Alter, B. J., and Bach, M. L. (1973). *Science* **180,** 403.

Bach, F. H., Schendel, D. J., Widmer, M. B., Alter, B. J., and Bach, M. L. (1974). *Adv. Biosci.* **12,** 63.

Bach, J.-F., Dardenne, M., Goldstein, A. L., Guha, A., and White, A. (1971). *Proc. Natl. Acad. Sci. U.S.A.* **68,** 2734.

Bach, M. A., Fournier, C., and Bach, J.-F. (1975). *Ann. N.Y. Acad. Sci.* **249,** 316.

Baker, M. A., Taub, R. N., Brown, S. M., and Ramachandar, K. (1974). *Br. J. Haematol.* **27,** 627.

Baldwin, R. W. (1976). *Transplant. Rev.* **28,** 62.

Baldwin, R. W., Price, M. R., and Robins, R. A. (1973a). *Br. J. Cancer* **28,** Suppl. I, 37.

Baldwin, R. W., Embleton, M. J., and Price, M. R. (1973b). *Int. J. Cancer* **12,** 84.

Baldwin, R. W., Embleton, M. J., Price, M. R., and Robins, A. (1974). *Cancer* **34,** Suppl. 4, 1452.

Basten, A., and Howard, J. G. (1973). *In* "Thymus Dependency" (A. J. S. Davies and R. L. Carter, eds.), p. 265. Plenum, New York.

Beling, C. G., and Weksler, M. E. (1974). *Clin. Exp. Immunol.* **18,** 537.

Bluming, A. Z., Ziegler, J. L., Fass, L., and Herberman, R. B. (1971). *Clin. Exp. Immunol.* **9,** 713.

Bowen, J. G., Robins, R. A., and Baldwin, R. W. (1975). *Int. J. Cancer* **15,** 640.

Brent, L., and Holborow, J. (1974). *Prog. Immunol., Int. Congr. Immunol., 2nd, 1974* Vol. 3.

Broder, S., Humphrey, R., Durm, M., Blackman, M., Meade, B., Goldman, C., Strober, W., and Waldmann, T. (1975). *N. Engl. J. Med.* **293,** 887.

Browder, W. (1977). *Prog. Cancer Res. Ther.* **5,** (in press).

Browne, O., Bell, J., Holland, P. D. J., and Thornes, R. D. (1976). *Lancet* **2,** 96.

Buckner, C. D., Rudolph, R. H., Fefer, A., Clift, R. A., Epstein, R. B., Funk, D. D., Neiman, P. E., Slichter, S. J., Storb, R., and Thomas, E. D. (1972). *Cancer* **29,** 357.

Carnaud, C., Ilfeld, D., Levo, Y., and Trainin, N. (1974). *Int. J. Cancer* **14,** 168.

Cerottini, J. C., Nordin, A. A., and Brunner, K. T. (1970). *Nature (London)* **228,** 1308.

Char, D. H., Lepourhiet, A., Leventhal, B. G., and Herberman, R. B. (1973). *Int. J. Cancer* **12,** 409.

Char, D. H., Hollinshead, A., Cogan, D. G., Ballintine, E. J., Hogan, M. J., and Herberman, R. B. (1974). *N. Engl. J. Med.* **291,** 274.

Chassoux, D., and Salomon, J.-C. (1975). *Int. J. Cancer* **16,** 515.

Chess, L., MacDermott, R. P., Sondel, P. M., and Schlossman, S. F. (1974). *Prog. Immunol., Int. Congr. Immunol., 2nd, 1974* Vol. 3, p. 125.

Chess, L., Levine, H., MacDermott, R. P., and Schlossman, S. F. (1975). *Fed. Proc., Fed. Am. Soc. Exp. Biol.* **34,** 1031.

Churchill, W. H., and David, J. R. (1973). *N. Engl. J. Med.* **289,** 375.

Cohen, L., and Howe, M. L. (1973). *Proc. Natl. Acad. Sci. U.S.A.* **70,** 2707.

Collavo, D., Colombatti, A., Biasi, G., Chieco-Bianchi, L., and Davies, A. J. S. (1976). *J. Natl. Cancer Inst.* **56,** 603.

Costanza, M. E., Pinn, V., Schwartz, R. S., and Nathanson, L. (1973). *N. Engl. J. Med.* **289,** 520.

Coutinho, A., and Moller, G. (1973). *Nature (London), New Biol.* **245,** 12.

Currie, G. A. (1976). *Br. J. Cancer* **33,** 593.

Currie, G. A., and Basham, C. (1975). *J. Exp. Med.* **142,** 1600.

Currie, G. A., and Eccles, S. A. (1976). *Br. J. Cancer* **33,** 51.

Dimitrov, N. V., Andre, S., Eliopoulos, G., and Halpern, B. (1975). *Proc. Soc. Exp. Biol. Med.* **148,** 440.

Dixon, F. J., Feldman, J. D., and Vasquez, J. J. (1961). *J. Exp. Med.* **113,** 899.

Editorial. (1968). *Lancet* **1,** 185.

Editorial. (1976). *Lancet* **2,** 27.

Edwards, A. J., Rowland, G. F., and Lee, M. R. (1973). *Lancet* **1,** 687.

Embleton, M. J. (1976a). *Br. J. Cancer* **33,** 584.

Embleton, M. J. (1976b). *Int. J. Cancer* **18,** 622.

Epstein, R. B., Storb, R., Clift, R. A., and Thomas, E. D. (1969). *Cancer Res.* **29,** 1072.

Evans, R. (1972). *Transplantation* **14,** 468.

Evans, R., and Alexander, P. (1972). *Nature (London)* **236,** 168.

Field, E. J., and Caspary, E. A. (1972). *Br. J. Cancer* **26,** 164.

Fisher, B., and Wolmark, N. (1976). *Cancer Res.* **36,** 2241.

Fisher, B., Wolmark, N., and Fisher, E. (1974). *In* "Neoplasm Immunity: Theory and Application" (R. G. Crispen, ed.), p. 1. ITR.

Ford, C. E., Micklem, H. S., Evans, E. P., Gray, J. G., and Ogden, D. A. (1966). *Ann. N.Y. Acad. Sci.* **129,** 283.

Gainor, B. J., Forbes, J. T., Enneking, W. F., and Smith, R. T. (1976). *Cancer* **37,** 743.

Gale, R. P., and Zighelboim, J. (1975). *J. Immunol.* **114,** 1047.

Gallily, R., Yagel, S., and Weiss, D. W. (1976). *Adv. Exp. Med. Biol.* **73,** 351.

Geha, R. S., and Merler, E. (1974). *Cell. Immunol.* **10,** 86.

Gery, I., Baer, A., Stupp, Y., and Weiss, D. W. (1974). *Isr. J. Med. Sci.* **10,** 984.

Gillette, R. W., and Fox, A. (1975). *Cell. Immunol.* **19,** 328.
Glasgow, A. H., Nimberg, R. B., Menzoian, J. O., Saporoschetz, I., Cooperband, S. R., Schmid, K., and Mannick, J. A. (1974). *N. Engl. J. Med.* **291,** 1263.
Gordon, M. Y., Aguado, M., and Blackett, N. M. (1977). *Eur. J. Cancer* **13,** 229.
Granstrom, M., and Gahrton, G. (1974). *Acta Med. Scand.* **196,** 221.
Greenberg, P., Bax, I., Mara, B., and Schrier, S. (1974). *Blood* **44,** 375.
Hadden, J. W., Coffey, R. G., Hadden, B. M., Lopez-Corrales, E., and Sunshine, G. H. (1975). *Cell. Immunol.* **20,** 98.
Heaton, J. M., Menzin, M. A., and Carney, D. N. (1975). *J. Clin. Pathol.* **28,** 944.
Heimer, R., and Klein, G. (1976). *Int. J. Cancer* **18,** 310.
Hellström, I., Warner, G. A., Hellström, K. E., and Sjögren, H. O. (1973). *Int. J. Cancer* **11,** 280.
Hellström, K. E., and Hellström, I. (1969). *Adv. Cancer Res.* **12,** 167.
Hellström, K. E., and Hellström, I. (1970). *Annu. Rev. Microbiol.* **24,** 373.
Herberman, R. B., Nunn, M. E., Holden, H. T., and Lavrin, D. H. (1975). *Int. J. Cancer* **16,** 230.
Herberman, R. B., Holden, H. T., Ting, C. C., Lavrin, D. H., and Kirchner, H. (1976). *Cancer Res.* **36,** 615.
Hersey, P., Isbister, J., Edwards, A., Murray, E., Adams, E., Biggs, J., and Milton, G. W. (1976). *Lancet* **1,** 825.
Hersh, E. M., and Oppenheim, J. J. (1967). *Cancer Res.* **27,** 98.
Hibbs, J. B., Jr., Lambert, L. H., Jr., and Remington, J. S. (1972). *Nature (London) New Biol.* **235,** 48.
Hirsch, M. S. (1974). *Johns Hopkins Med. J.,* Suppl. **3,** 177.
Hirshaut, Y., Pinsky, C., Marquardt, H., and Oettgen, H. F. (1973). *Cancer Res.* **14,** 109.
Holm, G., Mellstedt, H., Bjorkholm, M., Johansson, B., Killander, D., Sundblad, R., and Soderberg, G. (1976). *Cancer* **37,** 751.
Hooper, J. A., McDaniel, M. C., Thurman, G. B., Cohen, G. H., Schulof, R. S., and Goldstein, A. L. (1975). *Ann. N.Y. Acad. Sci.* **249,** 125.
Hopper, D. G., and Pimm, M. V. (1976). *Lancet* **2,** 255.
Horowitz, S., and Hong, R. (1977). *Prog. Cancer Res. Ther.* **5,** (in press).
Huntington, S. J., and Davey, F. R. (1976). *Fed. Proc., Fed. Am. Soc. Exp. Biol.* **35,** 414.
Israel, L., Edelstein, R., Mannoni, P., and Radot, E. (1976). *Lancet* **2,** 642.
Jacobs, D. M., and Kripke, M. L. (1974). *J. Natl. Cancer Inst.* **52,** 219.
Jerry, L. M. (1977). *Prog. Cancer Res. Ther.* **5,** (in press).
Jondal, M., and Klein, G. (1973). *J. Exp. Med.* **138,** 1365.
Kadish, J. L., and Basch, R. S. (1976). *J. Exp. Med.* **143,** 1082.
Katz, D. H. (1972). *Transplant. Rev.* **12,** 141.
Kenady, D. E., Chrétien, P. B., Potvin, C., Simon, R. M., Alexander, J. C., and Goldstein, A. L. (1977). *Cancer* (in press).
Kerkoven, P., Briner, J., and Blumberg, A. (1973). *Schweiz. Med. Wochenschr.* **103,** 1706.
Kiessling, R., Klein, E., and Wigzell, H. (1975a). *Eur. J. Immunol.* **5,** 112.
Kiessling, R., Klein, E., Pross, H., and Wigzell, H. (1975b). *Eur. J. Immunol.* **5,** 117.
Kirchner, H., Chused, T. M., Herberman, R. B., Holden, H. T., and Lavrin, D. H. (1974). *J. Exp. Med.* **139,** 1473.
Kirchner, H., Glaser, M., and Herberman, R. B. (1975a). *Nature (London)* **257,** 396.
Kirchner, H., Fernbach, B. R., Holden, H. T., and Herberman, R. B. (1975b). *Z. Immunitaetsforsch.* **150,** 213.
Klein, G. (1966). *Annu. Rev. Microbiol.* **20,** 223.

Knapp, W., Bolhuis, R. L. H., Radl, J., and Hijmans, W. (1973). *J. Immunol.* **111,** 1295.
Krown, S. E., Pinsky, C. M., Hirshaut, Y., and Oettgen, H. F. (1976). *Clin. Res.* **24,** 377A.
Kurnick, N. B. (1962). *Transfusion* **2,** 178.
Levine, P. H., Pearson, G. R., Herberman, R. B., Rabson, A. S., and Burton, G. J. (1976). *Cancer Res.* **36,** Part II, 565.
Levo, Y., Rotter, V., and Ramot, B. (1975). *Biomedicine* **23,** 198.
Lewis, M. G. (1974). *J. Clin. Pathol.* **27,** 83.
Lods, J. C., Dujardin, P., and Halpern, G. M. (1976). *Lancet* **1,** 548.
Lokich, J. J. (1975). *Lancet* **1,** 331.
Lokich, J. L., Galvanek, E. G., and Moloney, W. C. (1973). *Arch. Intern. Med.* **132,** 597.
McCoy, J. L., Jerome, L. F., Dean, J. H., Perlin, E., Oldham, R. K., Char, D. H., Cohen, M. H., Felix, E. L., and Herberman, R. B. (1975). *J. Natl. Cancer Inst.* **55,** 19.
McKneally, M. F., Maver, C., Kausel, H. W., and Alley, R. D. (1976). *J. Thorac. Cardiovasc. Surg.* **72,** 333.
MacLennan, I. C. M., Gale, D. G. L., and Wood, J. (1975). *Int. J. Cancer* **15,** 995.
Mage, G. M., and McHugh, L. L. (1973). *J. Immunol.* **111,** 652.
Magrath, I. T., and Ziegler, J. L. (1976). *Br. Med. J.* **1,** 615.
Martinez, C. (1964). *Nature (London)* **203,** 1188.
Matthews, N., De Kretser, T., and Nairn, R. C. (1975). *Immunology* **28,** 1081.
Matthews, N., Chalmers, P. J., Flannery, G. R., and Nairn, R. C. (1976). *Br. J. Cancer* **33,** 279.
Medawar, P., and Hunt, R. (1976). *Cancer Res.* **36,** 3453.
Mikulski, S. M., and Billing, R. (1977). *Cell. Immunol.* **28,** 69.
Mikulski, S. M., Billing, R., and Terasaki, P. I. (1977). *J. Natl. Cancer Inst.* (in press).
Mitsuoka, A., Baba, M., and Morikawa, S. (1976). *Nature (London)* **262,** 77.
Mohr, S. J. (1977). *Prog. Cancer Res. Ther.* **5,** (in press).
Mortensen, R. F., Osmand, A. P., and Gewurz, H. (1975). *J. Exp. Med.* **141,** 821.
Mullins, G. M., Anderson, P. N., and Santos, G. W. (1975). *Cancer* **36,** 1950.
Murgita, R. A., and Tomasi, T. B., Jr. (1975). *J. Exp. Med.* **141,** 269.
Nachtigal, D., Zan-Bar, I., and Feldman, M. (1975). *Transplant. Rev.* **26,** 87.
Old, L. J., Stockert, E., Boyse, E. A., and Hokim, J. (1968). *J. Exp. Med.* **127,** 523.
Oppenheim, J. J., Shneyour, A., and Kook, A. I. (1976). *Fed. Proc., Fed. Am. Soc. Exp. Biol.* **35,** 390.
O'Toole, C., Perlmann, P., Wigzell, H., Unsgaard, B., and Zetterlund, C. G. (1973). *Lancet* **1,** 1085.
Parker, D., Katz, S. I., and Turk, J. L. (1975). *Int. Arch. Allergy Appl. Immunol.* **49,** 276.
Patt, Y. Z. (1977). *Prog. Cancer Res. Ther.* **5,** (in press).
Peavy, D. L., and Pierce, C. W. (1974). *J. Exp. Med.* **140,** 356.
Perk, K., Chirigos, M. A., Fuhrman, F., and Pettigrew, H. (1975). *J. Natl. Cancer Inst.* **54,** 253.
Perlmann, P., and MacLennan, I. C. M. (1974). *Prog. Immunol., Int. Congr. Immunol., 2nd, 1974* Vol. 3, p. 347.
Perlmann, P., Perlmann, H., and Wigzell, H. (1972). *Transplant. Rev.* **13,** 91.
Pike, M. C., and Snyderman, R. (1976). *Nature (London)***261,** 136.
Pimm, M. V., and Baldwin, R. W. (1975). *Nature (London)* **254,** 77.
Pincus, T., Haberkern, R., and Christian, C. L. (1968). *J. Exp. Med.* **127,** 819.
Podleski, W. K. (1976). *Am. J. Med.* **61,** 1.
Poskitt, P. K., Poskitt, T. R., and Wallace, J. H. (1974). *J. Exp. Med.* **140,** 410.

Prather, S. O., and Lausch, R. N. (1976). *Fed. Proc., Fed. Am. Soc. Exp. Biol.* **35,** 826.
Prehn, R. T. (1973). *In* "Immunological Parameters of Host-Tumor Relationships" (D. W. Weiss, ed.), Vol. 2, p. 171. Academic Press, New York.
Proctor, J., Rudenstam, C. M., and Alexander, P. (1973). *Biomedicine* **19,** 248.
Ramot, B., Biniaminov, M., Shoham, C., and Rosenthal, E. (1976). *N. Engl. J. Med.* **294,** 809.
Rossen, R. D., Reisberg, M. A., Hersh, E. M., and Gutterman, J. U. (1976). *Fed. Proc., Fed. Am. Soc. Exp. Biol.* **35,** 758.
Rowe, D. S., Hug, K., Forni, L., and Pernis, B. (1973). *J. Exp. Med.* **138,** 965.
Sahiar, K., and Schwartz, R. S. (1965). *J. Immunol.* **95,** 345.
Sahiar, K., and Schwartz, R. S. (1966). *Int. Arch. Allergy* **29,** 52.
Sampson, D., and Lui, A. (1976). *Cancer Res.* **36,** 952.
Schultz, R. M., Papamatheakis, J. D., Stylos, W. A., and Chirigos, M. A. (1976). *Cell. Immunol.* **25,** 309.
Schultz, R. M., Papamatheakis, J. D., Luetzeler, J., Ruiz, P., and Chirigos, M. A. (1977). *Cancer Res.* **37,** 358.
Schwartz, J. A., Schwartz, R. S., Hirsch, M. S., Phillips, S. M., and Black, P. H. (1973). *J. Natl. Cancer Inst.* **51,** 507.
Schwartz, R. S. (1972). *Lancet* **1,** 1266.
Segal, S., Cohen, I. R., and Feldman, M. (1972). *Science* **175,** 1126.
Shevach, E. M. (1976). *Fed. Proc., Fed. Am. Soc. Exp. Biol.* **35,** 2048.
Simon, H. B., and Sheagren, J. N. (1971). *J. Exp. Med.* **133,** 1377.
Snyderman, R., and Pike, M. C. (1976). *Science* **192,** 370.
Storb, R., Epstein, R. B., Graham, T. C., Kolb, H. J., Kolb, H., and Thomas, E. D. (1974). *Transplantation* **18,** 357.
Stutman, O. (1975). *J. Immunol.* **114,** 1213.
Tada, T. (1974). *In* "Immunological Tolerance: Mechanisms and Potential Therapeutic Applications" (D. H. Katz and B. Benacerraf, eds.). Academic Press, New York.
Tada, T., Taniguchi, M., and Takemori, T. (1975). *Transplant. Rev.* **26,** 106.
Tamerius, J., Nepom, J., Hellström, I., and Hellström, K. E. (1976). *J. Immunol.* **116,** 724.
Taussig, M. J., and Munro, A. J. (1976). *Fed. Proc., Fed. Am. Soc. Exp. Biol.* **35,** 2061.
Theofilopoulos, A. N., Wilson, C. B., and Dixon, F. J. (1976). *J. Clin. Invest.* **57,** 169.
Thomson, D. M. P., Eccles, S., and Alexander, P. (1973). *Br. J. Cancer* **28,** 6.
Ting, A., and Terasaki, P. I. (1974). *Cancer Res.* **34,** 2694.
Tobias, J. S., Weiner, R. S., Griffiths, C. T., Richman, C. M., Parker, L. M., and Yankee, R. A. (1977). *Eur. J. Cancer* **13,** 269.
Tripodi, D., Parks, L. C., and Brugmans, J. (1973). *N. Engl. J. Med.* **289,** 354.
Uhr, J. W., and Moller, G. (1968). *Adv. Immunol.* **8,** 81.
Unanue, E. (1972). *Adv. Immunol.* **15,** 95.
Van Loveren, H., and Den Otter, W. (1974a). *J. Natl. Cancer Inst.* **52,** 1917.
Van Loveren, H., and Den Otter, W. (1974b). *J. Natl. Cancer Inst.* **53,** 1057.
Wagner, H., Rollinghoff, M., and Nossal, G. J. V. (1973). *Transplant. Rev.* **17,** 3.
Waldmann, T. A., Broder, S., Krakauer, R., MacDermott, R. P., Durm, M., Goldman, C., and Meade, B. (1976). *Fed. Proc., Fed. Am. Soc. Exp. Biol.* **35,** 2067.
Whitcomb, M. E., Merluzzi, V. J., and Cooperband, S. R. (1976). *Cell. Immunol.* **21,** 272.
Whitehead, R. H., Thatcher, J., Teasdale, C., Roberts, G. P., and Hughes, L. E. (1976a). *Lancet* **1,** 330.
Whitehead, R. H., Teasdale, C., and Hughes, L. E. (1976b). *Lancet* **2,** 748.
Winchester, R. J., Fu, S. M., Hoffman, T., and Kunkel, H. G. (1975). *J. Immunol.* **114,** 1210.

Yagel, S., Gallily, R., and Weiss, D. W. (1975). *Cell. Immunol.* **19,** 381.
Yamamura, Y. (1976). International Conference on Immunotherapy of Cancer: Present Status of Trials in Man.'' Natl. Cancer Inst., Bethesda, Maryland.
Yunis, E. J., Martinez, C., Smith, J., Stutman, O., and Good, R. A. (1969). *Cancer Res.* **29,** 174.
Zembala, M., and Asherson, G. L. (1973). *Nature (London)* **244,** 227.

Suramin: With Special Reference to Onchocerciasis

F. HAWKING

The Commonwealth Institute of Helminthology
St. Albans, England

I. Introduction

Suramin was introduced by the Bayer workers in 1920 after more than 8 years of research on ureas of the aminonaphthalene-sulfonic type, starting from the trypanocidal activity of trypan red (discovered by Ehrlich and Shiga, 1904), of trypan blue (Mesnil and Nicolle, 1906), and of Afridol violet discovered in 1906 (for details, see Findlay, 1930, p. 259). It was tested on a few patients in Europe (1921–1922), and then extensive therapeutic trials were carried out in Africa by Kleine and Fischer (1923). The compound was found to be very valuable for the treatment of human trypanosomiasis, especially of the East African type, which could be cured by no other drug. During recent years it has been supplanted to some extent by melarsoprol, and in the future it may be further supplanted by Berenil for human trypanosomiasis. During experiments on trypanosomiasis in volunteers in 1945, Van Hoof *et al.* (1947) discovered that it also acted upon onchocerciasis (see also Wanson, 1950) and since then it has been widely used for the treatment of this filarial infection.

Trypanosomes and onchocercal worms are very different organisms, yet the action of suramin on each of them is so remarkable that it seems that it must depend on the same active part of the suramin molecule. For experimental and historical reasons, much more is known about the action of suramin on trypanosomes than on *Onchocerca*. Accordingly, knowledge about the action on trypanosomes is cited in the following so that it may be used to illuminate the action on *Onchocerca*.

II. Chemistry

Suramin* is a trisodium salt of 8,8′-(3″,3‴-ureylenebis(3⁗-benzamido-4⁗-methylbenzamido))bis-1,3,5-naphthalenetrisulfonic acid:

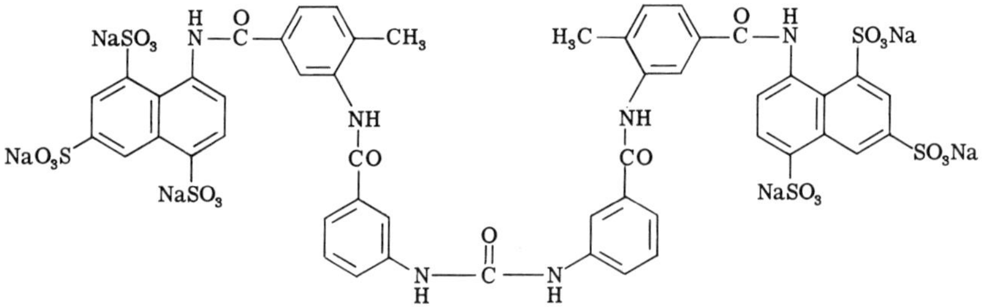

A. Physical Characteristics

Suramin is a pinkish white flocculent powder, with high solubility in water (more than 10% w/v); its solutions are stable to boiling. Suramin is hygroscopic and absorbs moisture from the atmosphere unless kept in a desiccator; the presence of this unsuspected water may cause error in quantitative experiments. It should be stored in the dark and under dry conditions.

* Synonyms: Antrypol, Germanin, Bayer 205, Fourneau 309, belganyl. Naphuride, and Naganol

B. Methods of Estimation

It can be estimated in body fluid by various methods. Following the method of Dangerfield *et al.* (1938), the suramin is hydrolyzed by boiling with hydrochloric acid for 6 hours, and the products are diazotized and coupled with methyl-α-naphthylamine to produce a purple color. This method detects concentrations down to about 5 mg/liter, which is the level where serum itself gives a blank value. A later method that depends on the action of suramin in bleaching 2-*p*-dimethylaminostyryl-6-acetamidoquinolinemethochloride was described by Gage *et al.* (1948); it is effective in the range 0.5–150 mg/liter. Another method was described by Vierthaler and Boselli (1939). More recently, a method for pharmaceutical estimation was reported by Thoma *et al.* (1967); it is based on precipitation with 2-ethoxy-6,9 diaminoacridin lactate and back titration of the excess precipitate by flocculation analysis.

C. Relation of Structure and Activity

The slightest deviation from the formula given in the preceding is accompanied by diminution of trypanocidal activity; even change of position of the sulfonic acid groups has this effect (Fourneau *et al.*, 1924; Findlay, 1930, p. 261; Findlay, 1950, p. 406). The capacity of suramin to combine with the plasma proteins depends on the naphthylamine-trisulfonic groups (Spinks, 1948). Many of the pharmacological properties of suramin, e.g., its binding to serum proteins are due to its general structure as a large molecule with many sulfonic acid groups. Many other large molecules with sulfonic acid groups have similar pharmacological properties, which need not necessarily be related to the specific action of suramin on *Onchocerca* and on trypanosomes.

III. Absorption and Distribution

When given by mouth, suramin is absorbed from the intestine only to a limited extent. When given by subcutaneous or intramuscular injection it causes intense local irritation. Consequently, it is practically always administered by intravenous injection.

After intravenous injection suramin combines with the serum proteins and much of it circulates in the blood. Some of it (probably combined with protein) is taken up by the cells of the reticuloendothelial system. In the bloodstream it persists for long periods (up to 6 months in man) and its excretion in the urine is very slow; both the persistence and the slow excretion are due to a combination of suramin with the blood proteins. In the plasma of treated rabbits, 70–90% of the suramin is bound to plasma proteins and this serves to protect the enzymes against it. The combination is usually about 0.6 mole suramin to 1 mole protein, but it may be 2 moles suramin to 1 mole protein. Suramin combines with proteins of all kinds: serum globulins (including euglobulin and pseudoglobulin) egg albumin, casein, fibrinogen, gelatin, histones, etc. This combination with protein takes place very quickly (within a few minutes). It depends on different structures from those of the trypanocidal action, and many other large molecules with terminal napthylaminesulfonic acid groups and chondroitin sulfate combine in the same way (Spinks, 1948). The combination presumably takes place with basic groups on the protein, probably by electrostatic forces, but blockage of free amino groups by di-2-chloroethyl sulfone does not prevent combination with suramin (Wilson and Wormall, 1949). The thiol groups of proteins are not involved. Suramin does not diffuse into red blood corpuscles or into the cerebrospinal fluid except in small amounts.

The extent of the accumulation in the blood varies considerably in different subjects, with corresponding variation in the toxic and therapeutic effects (Hawking, 1940). Four days after an intravenous injection of 4.5 mg/kg into rabbits, the plasma concentration was 14 mg/liter, i.e., 11% of the dose in the plasma and 89% in tissues or elsewhere (Vierthaler and Boselli, 1939). In other rabbits, 4 days after 28 mg/kg, 36 mg/liter or 4.6% of the dose was reported in the plasma and 95% elsewhere (Dangerfield *et al.*, 1938).

Man retains the compound in the plasma less well than rabbits. In man, 1 day after 1 gm per patient intravenously the plasma concentration was 25–60 (mean 40) mg/liter, i.e., only 10% of the dose was still in the plasma (Hawking, 1940). After 5 days the plasma concentration was 8–20 mg/liter and after 10 days, 8 mg/liter. After four doses of 1 gm given over a period of a few days, the plasma concentration 1 day after the last dose is often 150 mg/liter and in 1 patient it was as high as 340 mg/liter. After three to four doses, a level of about 5 mg/liter may still be detected 150–200 days later.

According to chemical estimations (Boursnell *et al.*, 1939), no depot of suramin is formed in any tissue; but, by histological methods, suramin can be shown to be taken up as granules by cells of the reticuloendothelial system and by the epithelium of the proximal convoluted tubules of the kidney where it can be demonstrated by staining with neutral red or with Giemsa's stain (von Jancso and Jancso-Gabor, 1952). The cells of the reticuloendothelial system include those of the liver spleen and bone marrow and also the histiocytes of connective tissue all over the body.

The suramin is first bound to serum protein and then it is taken up by the phagocytic cells. It can be found as granules in the connective tissue histiocytes more than 12 days after its injection. More recent work has shown that these granules are really lysosomes in which suramin has accumulated (see Section III,C,3).

A. Excretion

Small amounts are excreted in the urine during the first few days after administration but most of the compound administered cannot be recovered. Traces have been demonstrated by biological tests in the milk of goats treated with suramin (Mayer and Zeiss, 1922).

B. Metabolism

Apparently suramin is relatively resistant to catabolism in the body, as is shown by its long persistence in the blood. Spinks (1948) could not obtain any evidence that suramin is hydrolyzed *in vivo*; and products of suramin produced by acid hydrolysis are rapidly eliminated (Dewey and Wormall, 1946). Apparently, suramin is not hydrolyzed *in vivo* or, if so, only very slowly. There is no evidence for conversion into an active metabolite, and it seems almost certain that the chemotherapeutic activity of suramin is due to the intact molecule.

(A more detailed review of suramin distribution, etc., is given by Findlay, 1950, p. 404.)

IV. Biochemistry and Pharmacology

A. Combination with Proteins and Other Large Molecules

Suramin combines well with serum proteins and with other proteins (see Section III). The combination of suramin with serum proteins may displace other drugs, e.g., chlorpromazine or sulfonamides, or anticogulants such as phenprocoumon (Huethwohl and Jahnchen, 1971).

The toxic action of crystal violet on various organisms (e.g., paramecia, miracidia, perfused toad's heart) is antagonized by suramin and by other large molecules such as Chlorazol fast pink; this action is probably another example of nonspecific combination (Riedel and El-Dakhakhny, 1964). Suramin also forms complexes with large molecules such as terephthalanilides, e.g., HSC 57133 (a compound developed to treat leukemia), and this complex formation has been used to delay the toxicity and to enhance the excretion of such anticancer agents (Yesaiv *et al.*, 1968). Suramin further forms complexes with basic trypanocidal compounds such as pentamidine and homidium (see the following and Section VII,A,3).

B. Action on Enzymes

Suramin may destroy or inhibit many different enzymes. The most sensitive enzymes examined seem to be hyaluronidase (inhibited at 10^{-5}–10^{-6} *M*), fumarase (at 10^{-7} *M*), urease at pH 5 (at 10^{-4} *M*), hexokinase (at 10^{-4}–10^{-5} *M*) and RNA polymerase (10^{-5} *M*). In general, the strong affinity of suramin for protein suggests that it inhibits enzymes by binding to free cationic amino acid residues in the area of the active center (Williamson, 1970). This action on enzymes seems to be of two kinds: (*1*) specific action on enzymes concerned with DNA and RNA metabolism, which may be the basis of its antiparasitic action (discussed in Section VI); and (*2*) nonspecific action on enzymes of all types, probably due to its tendency to combine with proteins and large molecules. Typical examples are given by the enzymes trypsin and fumarase. Similar action is shown by many polysulfuric acid compounds, e.g., on succinic dehydrogenase (Stoppani and Brignone, 1957; Hill and Hutner, 1968). Suramin and similar compounds inhibit the calcification of rats' epiphyses *in vitro* (Harris *et al.*, 1969) and the transport of calcium in sarcoplastic reticulum, together with the ATPase enzyme related to calcium transport (Layton and Azzi, 1974).

Suramin inhibits various other ATPases (especially in membrane preparations) and enzymes requiring ATP (Fortes *et al.*, 1973). It also inhibits various enzymes concerned with phosphorylation and dephosphorylation (Rodnight, 1970). Smeesters and Jaques (1968) found that, in rat liver cells, suramin treatment markedly decreased the activities of the lysosomal enzymes β-glycerophosphatase, β-*N*-acetylaminodeoxyglucosidase, and β-glucuronidase but not of β-galactosidase, acid maltase, or the protease cathepsin D.

Suramin inhibits mitochondrial oxidative enzymes obtained from *Crithidia fasciculata* (Bacchi *et al.*, 1968), but it is not clear that this action is a specific one.

Jaffe *et al.* (1972) extracted reductases from various filarial adult worms and from schistosomes and found them to be somewhat more sensitive to the inhibitory action of suramin than mammalian reductases; on the other hand, other compounds, such as methotrexate and a related diaminoquinazoline, were more active in inhibition, and the reaction probably has little to do with the antifilarial action.

Although suramin combines with many enzymes, it is not a *general* enzyme poison. In the body, most enzymes are protected against suramin by the strong combination that it forms with plasma proteins. Wills and Wormall (1949) distinguish two classes of enzymes affected probably in different ways: Group A is not inhibited by suramin at pH 7.0 but is inhibited at acid pH, e.g., urease (suramin probably does not combine with the active center of these enzymes but bridges over it); Group B is strongly inhibited by suramin at pH 7.0 and not so dependent on pH, e.g., hexokinase and succinic dehydrogenase (suramin probably combines with the active center of these enzymes).

C. Lysosomes

Suramin forms complexes with serum proteins and is then taken up into lysosomes where it accumulates, just as acidic vital dyes do. This accumulation occurs in the reticuloendothelial cells all over the body but particularly in the Kupffer cells of the liver and in the cells of the convoluted tubules of the kidney.

1. *Liver*

In the liver, suramin has been studied recently by Buys *et al.* (1973). With rats, about 2% of the dose injected could be found in the Kupffer cells. It stabilizes the membranes of the lysosomes. Suramin and the other compounds act on the enzymes of the lysosomes, inhibiting the acid phosphatase of the hepatocytes and the cathepsin D of the Kupffer cells. Probably this action on the enzymes involves irreversible denaturation (Davies *et al.*, 1971).

2. *Kidneys*

Suramin is filtered (in small amounts) through the capillary walls of the glomeruli and is reabsorbed by the cells of the proximal convoluted tubules where it accumulates as granules. These granules can be demonstrated by staining with neutral red or Giemsa (von Jancso and Jancso-Gabor, 1952). The effects of suramin have been studied in detail with histochemical methods by Wesolowski *et al.* (1972). They treated mice with 400 mg/kg—a high dose but one that does not cause necrosis of the tubules—and they examined the kidney 24 and 72 hours later. They found (*a*) a fall in acid phosphatase activity in the cytoplasm of the convoluted tubules and an appearance of this enzyme in the brush border; (*b*) an increase in alkaline phosphatase, ATPase, and 5-nucleotidase in the brush border of the convoluted tubules and in the endothelium of the capillaries of the glomeruli; (*c*) an increase in granules of succinic dehydrogenase and cytochrome oxidase in cells of the proximal convoluted tubules and in the thick segments of Henle's loop. They interpret these changes as follows.

Suramin behaves like many other electronegative large molecules, such as trypan blue or horseradish peroxidase, i.e., it joins in a complex with the serum proteins, it is filtered through the renal glomeruli, and it is reabsorbed in the proximal convoluted tubules by the process of endocytosis. In the first phase of endocytosis, these substances are adsorbed to the surface of the tubule cells in conjunction with mucopolysaccharides. In the second stage of endocytosis, the proteins behave as activators; and the cell membrane (plus the accumulated substance) is invaginated to form phagosomes in the cell cytoplasm. Energy for this reaction is supplied by the enzymes of the cell membrane (alkaline phosphatase, ATPase, and 5-nucleotidase) all of which are increased after suramin treatment. Because these enzymes are also increased in the glomerulus, it may be that passage of suramin through the glomerulus is an active rather than a passive process. As succinic dehydrogenase and cytochrome oxidase become more abundant after suramin in the cells of the proximal convoluted tubules and of the thick segment of Henle's loop, it appears that the metabolism of these cells is increased during endocytosis. Later the phagosomes fuse with the primary lysosomes (rich in hydrolytic enzymes) producing secondary lysosomes. As already stated, acid vital dyes and similar compounds such as suramin stabilize lysosomal membranes and inhibit the proteolytic enzymes in them, especially acid phosphatase (thus contributing to the long persistence of suramin). In all this suramin behaves like acidic vital dyes, independent of its specific antitrypanosomal or antifilarial action.

If the accumulation of suramin in the kidney cells is too great, then they degenerate producing albuminuria and all the lesions seen by conventional histological methods. After toxic doses of suramin in animals, histological examination shows profound degeneration of the convoluted tubules with hydropic changes and sloughing of the epithelium; later, in animals that do not die, there is regenerative hyperplasia (Humphreys and Donaldson, 1941). Hyaline casts are found in the tubules; throughout the cortex there may be a few necrotic foci, minute hemorrhages, and perivascular round cell infiltration (Duncan and Manson-Bahr, 1923).

3. *Placenta*

In the same way, when suramin or trypan blue are injected into pregnant rats they are concentrated in the lysosomes of the phagocytic epithelial cells of the yolk sac but they do not penetrate into the embryo itself. In the yolk sac they probably interfere with metabolites required by the embryo and this may well explain the teratogenic action of both these compounds (see Section V,A,1) (Lloyd and Beck, 1969).

4. *Intracellular Bacilli*

The concentration of suramin in lysosomes probably explains its action in increasing the growth of tubercle bacilli or of *Mycobacterium lepraemurium* in phagocytes, since these bacilli grow in lysosomes (Hart, 1968; Wong and Ma, 1963). This action is nonspecific since it is also shown by dextrans and by macromolecules, such as polyvinylpyrrolidone. In peritoneal macrophages cultured *in vitro*, suramin prevents phagosomes (which contain digestive enzymes) from fusing with lysosomes (which may contain foreign bodies, such as tubercle bacilli) and, thus, the digestion of the tubercle bacilli is inhibited (Hart and Young, 1975).

D. Blood Clotting and Complement

As already stated, suramin inhibits numerous enzymes including proteases, chymotrypsin, and papain. As a result of this enzyme inhibition, it interferes with the formation and hemolytic action of complement and with blood clotting. The findings vary somewhat according to the method of experimentation. In particular, at 70 μg/ml it inhibits the activation of component C1 to C1 esterase and also the activity of the C1 esterase (Eisen and Loveday, 1973). Suramin inhibits the reactions of sheep RBC with C1, C1 and 4, C14 and C2, C14 and C3–9 (Fong and Good, 1972). In connection with blood clotting, at 0.2–1.0 mg/ml (much above therapeutic concentrations), it inhibits the action of thrombin on fibrinogen, and in fibrinolysis, it inhibits the action of plasminogen. It also interferes with the formation of kinin (Eisen and Loveday, 1973). All these actions may be nonspecific due to its general tendency to bind to proteins.

1. *Hereditary Angioneurotic Edema (Quinke's Disease)*

This is a rare disease due to hereditary lack of C1-esterase inhibitors, so that in these patients the complement system is too active, leading to the release of substances that increase the permeability of capillaries. Because suramin is an inhibitor of complement and C1-esterase, it has been used, often with success, in the treatment of this condition (Brackertz, 1974; Schultz, 1974) (see Section VII,C,1).

E. Other Nonspecific Actions of Suramin

Suramin and other anionic substances, such as trypan blue, sulfobromophthalein, and lithium carmine, suppress the accumulation of iodine in the thyroid gland of rats; cationic substances do not act in this way (D'Addabbo *et al.*, 1961; Kallee and Hartenstein, 1960).

Naphthalene sulfonic acids (including suramin) dissolve fibrin clots at low concentration; this effect depends on the presence of several acidic sulfonic groups (Kaulla, 1963).

When dilute solutions of suramin (acidic) and pentamidine (basic) are mixed, a precipitate that removes part of the pentamidine from the system develops. This probably explains the observations of Guimaraes and Lourie (1951) that a previous dose of suramin inhibited some of the toxic actions of pentamidine, especially the dangerous fall in blood pressure; it also inhibited some of the actions of histamine. (It would be valuable to investigate a combination of suramin and Berenil, given simultaneously or successively for the treatment of trypanosomiasis, ultimately in man. Would the suramin diminish the dangerous action of Berenil on the blood pressure while potentiating its trypanocidal action? Or would it neutralize the trypanocidal effect?).

In summary, it is probable that most of these reactions of suramin (except those on RNA/DNA or cell division) have nothing to do with the antitrypanosomal or antifilarial actions of suramin, but they may explain some of the toxic results or nonspecific treatments such as of angioneurotic edema.

V. Toxicity

A. In Animals

The acute toxic dose (LD_{50}) for mice by intravenous injection is about 620 mg/kg. The chief toxic effect in animals is on the kidney where it causes degeneration of the convoluted tubules; there may be minute hemorrhages and degenerative changes also in the liver, lungs, and central nervous system. In some of the animals *(Mastomys natalensis)* that were treated by Lämmler *et al.* (1975) with suramin, 40 mg/kg, s.c., for 5 days, i.e., one-third of the maximum tolerated dose, edema of the nose and front feet developed 3 weeks later. These parts may have a lower temperature than the rest of the body. This happened both in uninfected animals and in those infected with *Litomosoides carinii*, and presumably it was due to a direct toxic action of the drug. It is curious that there was a delay of 16 days after the last dose of drug before these ill effects became apparent.

1. *Toxicity in a Chimpanzee*

The toxic effects of suramin have recently been studied by Gibson *et al.* (1977) in a chimpanzee which was given the excessive total dosage of 152 mg/kg during 36 days. The animal became emaciated and developed hemorrhages, chronic diarrhea, anemia, lymphocytopenia, and albuminuria. At autopsy the primary lesions were found in the intestine, kidney, spleen, and peripheral blood. The intestines were hyperemic and swollen with petechiae and ecchymoses; in the colon there was extensive ulceration and atrophy of the mucosa, and in the jejunum there was acute suppurative enteritis. The kidney tubules were degenerating. The spleen and the femoral and mesenteric lymph nodes were atrophic with few lymphocytes. There was no degeneration of the adrenal cortex. It is possible that the ulceration in the colon and the atrophy of the spleen and lymph nodes were due to the susceptibility of tissues with a high rate of cell division to an inhibitory action of suramin on DNA replication.

2. *Suramin during Pregnancy*

Suramin does not pass through the placenta into the embryo (at least in rats and mice), but it accumulates in the lysosomes of the phagocytic epithelial cells of the umbilical vesicle (which develops from the yolk sac), interfering with the nutrition of the embryo and, thus, producing ill effects (see also Section IV,C,3). Trypan blue has the same action. Rat embryos are susceptible to suramin and trypan blue only at a very restricted period before the embryo is surrounded by the yolk sac (Lloyd and Beck, 1969). The ill effects on the embryos of mice and rats have been studied by Tuchman-Duplessis and Mercier-Parot (1973) and by Mercier-Parot and Tuchman-Duplessis (1973). The action is different in mice from that in rats. Furthermore, the results obtained in these rodents cannot be assumed to occur in other animals or in humans.

a. Rats. Suramin is very toxic for pregnant rats, and 30 mg/kg (little more than the human therapeutic dose) daily from day 1 to day 12 killed 8% of the mother rats, and 75 mg/kg daily killed 14%. On the other hand, the fetuses were not affected by doses of 30 to 75 mg/kg, but they were killed and absorbed after large doses of 100 to 170 mg/kg. In rats, suramin is essentially an abortive drug and does *not* cause malformation.

b. Mice. Fetuses are most susceptible to suramin given during the middle third of pregnancy, especially on days 9–11. At this time, 25 mg/kg is tolerated, but 40–65 mg causes a 64% mortality among the fetuses; many of those which are born, die within 3 days; after that the survivors live and develop well, although some of them suffer from necroses and amputations of limbs. In fetuses that are affected but not killed, there are developmental abnormalities, namely, cleft palate, harelip, cataracts, and abnormalities of the limbs. Those fetuses which are born may suffer from necroses of the limbs, nose, and tail which necroses later proceed to amputations.

It is fortunate that the human therapeutic use of suramin had become well-established before the thalidomide disaster, otherwise it would probably never have been permitted to proceed as far as clinical trial. Actually, suramin has now been given to many women for over 45 years and no case of infant malformation has been reported and no abortifacient action has been described. Anderson *et al.* (1976) mention a woman who must have conceived 1–2 weeks before the first of four weekly injections of 1 gm suramin and who later gave birth to a normal child. The development of the placenta in humans is different from that of rodents and the experimental results in the latter are not directly applicable to humans. Nevertheless, it is probably wise to regard pregnancy as a counterindication to suramin treatment for a chronic nonfatal condition such as onchocerciasis but not for a potentially fatal infection such as trypanosomiasis.

B. In Man

In man the toxic reactions due to suramin have been studied mostly in patients treated for trypanosomiasis. Reactions are more common in poorly nourished patients. The toxicity is cumulative owing to accumulation of the compound in the blood following repeated doses.

1. *Immediate Reactions*

1. Nausea and sometimes vomiting. This is much reduced if the intravenous injection is given very slowly; with this precaution, vomiting is rare and of little importance.

2. Collapse with nausea, vomiting, shock, sweating, and loss of consciousness. The collapse may be preceded by a short period of motor excitement and congestion of the face and body. [Fain (1942) found this occurred in 12 out of 4500 patients treated. Apted (1970) estimated it might occur in 1 in 2000–4500 cases.] It is best avoided by giving only 0.1–0.2 gm as the first dose. It is probably nonspecific, being due to the injection of a large polyanionic molecule.

3. Colic occurs rarely. There may be slight rise of temperature within half an hour, and various urticarial skin eruptions have been seen in 0.2% of patients (Harding and Hutchinson, 1948).

2. *Late Reactions (after 3 to 24 Hours)*

1. Fever may appear 2–3 hours after injection and may reach 40°C. This might be nonspecific and due to pyrogens, etc. It is probably not due to death of trypanosomes, since trypanosomes do not die until after 12 to 36 hours.

2. Intense photophobia and lachrymation, sometimes with palpebral edema have been noted after 24 hours (this must be rare).

3. Abdominal distension and constipation.

4. Cutaneous hyperesthesia of the soles or palms. The pain begins 24–48 hours after injection and may persist for a week or much longer and the skin may desquamate. In some groups of patients, this has been common (10%), e.g., Kissi people of Sierra Leone and in Venezuela, whereas in Tanzania it has been rare. Its explanation is unclear.

3. *Delayed Late Reactions (after Some Days)*

1. Irritation of the kidney is the commonest toxic reaction after suramin. Before each dose of suramin, the urine should be tested for albumin. A slight cloud can be disregarded. If it is assumed that some protein is normally filtered through the glomerulus and reabsorbed in the tubules, a slight albuminuria might be due to inhibition by suramin of reabsorption in the tubules, rather than to irritation and destruction of kidney cells. If, however, there is a heavy deposit and casts or red blood cells, further treatment with suramin should be postponed or abandoned. (For detailed description of the action on the kidney, see Section IV,C,2). Polyuria and thirst may also occur (? due to action in the kidney). It has been reported by Kennedy and Terry (1972) that 3 patients who were treated with suramin for onchocerciasis developed generalized aminoaciduria; 8 months later 1 patient still had persistent aminoaciduria, but in all 3 patients the urinary protein was normal. Apparently, the state of their urines before suramin is not known, and the significance of this report is difficult to evaluate.

2. Exfoliative dermatitis is usually a late manifestation. It is rare, but dangerous. In Venezuela, Gonzalez-Guerra *et al.* (1964) saw 2 nonfatal cases in 2037 patients; in North Cameroon, Fuglsang and Anderson (1974) saw 1 nonfatal case among 100 heavily infected patients.

3. Stomatitis may be an early complication; it may be severe and extend to the bronchi. Fuglsang and Anderson (1974) saw 1 case in 100 patients.

4. Jaundice is rare but dangerous. Jaundice may also be due to syringe transmission of virus hepatitis.

5. A certain amount of debility and weakness is common during suramin treatment. Sometimes this develops to severe prostration, which may be accompanied by chronic diarrhea and which occasionally terminates fatally after some weeks or months (Fuglsang and Anderson, 1974). The exact pathogenesis of this important and distressing syndrome is unknown. Possibly suramin interferes with the multiplication of cells with a naturally high rate of division, e.g., the epithelium of the intestine and lymphocytes. Compare the chimpanzee above (see Section V,A,1.)

Late toxic reactions to suramin seem to be more common among people who have lived on a starvation diet. In addition to those systemic reactions, there may be aggravation of ocular lesions, especially anterior uveitis, which is probably caused by the slow death of the microfilariae within the eye. In their series of 100 heavily infected patients, Fuglsang and Anderson (1974) saw posterior synechiae in 3, heavy flare or fresh keratic precipitates in 13, and fine flare or cells in 25.

4. *Allergic Reactions*

In the treatment of onchocerciasis, there may be additional reactions due to the death of adult worms and microfilariae. These come on usually after the fourth or fifth dose. They include the following:

Mild manifestations: (1) urticaria and swelling of the affected limb; (2) tenderness and swelling around nodules or impalpable worms; and (3) itching, swelling, and inflammation of the skin with papular or vesicular eruptions and desquamation (due to death of microfilariae).

More severe reactions: (1) deep abscesses around worms dying deep between muscles; and (2) painful immobilization of the hip joint due to death of worms near the hip joint capsule (Duke and Anderson, 1972).

Such severe reactions following the administration of suramin for onchocerciasis can usually be controlled by stopping the drug and giving betamethasone, 1 mg, 3 times a day, for a few days.

5. *Clinical Experiences*

Satti and Kirk (1957), working in the early days of suramin treatment for onchocerciasis, gave much too high doses, e.g., 10 gm in 19 days, and observed 4 deaths among 20 patients. The toxic reactions were those just listed as well as gingivitis leading to ulceration of the gums and mouth and persistent severe headache. These reactions were undoubtedly due to the excessively high dosage. Gonzalez-Guerra *et al.* (1964) in Venezuela gave 6.5 gm during 7 weeks to 2037 persons infected with *Onchocerca*; 1253 (66%) had no reactions. The others (in descending order of frequency) had edema, pruritus, albuminuria, fever, headache, urticaria, and conjunctivitis. Many of those with edema and pruritus had burning pains on the soles and the feet. There was 1 death (a woman aged 40) from cerebral vascular accident probably not related to treatment, and 2 nonfatal cases of exfoliative dermatitis who recovered after some months. One man had severe prostration and great pain in the hips (? due to death of worms). These authors considered that the side effects, although rarely grave, were undoubtedly a nuisance. In a later report, Convit (1974) states that 26,963 patients had been treated in the field in Venezuela with doses of 5 to 6 gm during 5 to 6 weeks and there had been no deaths due to suramin.

Apted (1970), who has had great experience with the treatment of trypanosomiasis, concludes that, although there is a formidable list of possible reactions, none of these reactions is common except kidney damage, usually mild, and that suramin is really one of the safest drugs in use (for trypanosomiasis). It is important that the compound should be stored dry and in the dark and that the solution should be made (with pyrogen-free water) immediately before the injection and that the intravenous injection should be given slowly. The first dose should not be more than 0.2 gm for an adult to test for possible idiosyncrasy. Suramin should not be given to patients in poor general condition, or with evidence of allergy or of kidney or liver disease, or to pregnant women (especially those in early pregnancy).

Severe reactions due to onchocerciasis, as described in the foregoing, and chronic diarrhea are indications for stopping treatment and so are ulceration of the mouth and tongue. There are suggestions (Rodger, 1958; Nnochiri, 1964) that some batches of drug may cause more reactions than others. Reactions are also more severe in some countries than in others, especially in areas of intense onchocerciasis in the West African savanna. (See also Section VII,B,2.)

6. *Toxicity of Suramin for Adrenal Glands*

It was reported by Wells *et al.* (1937) and by Tomlinson and Cameron (1938) that 2 patients treated for pemphigus with large doses of suramin (16 gm in 10 months) had died and had shown degenerative changes in the cortex of the adrenal glands. Also Mahoney and Barrie (1950) described a woman who was treated for pemphigus with suramin in doses of 1 gm every 2 days for 10 doses. Five weeks later she died with acute adrenal necrosis, but it was not clear whether the necrosis was due to the suramin or to the pemphigus. In view of the earlier deaths, investigations were made in animals by Humphreys and Donaldson

(1941). They treated 100 guinea pigs and some other animals with 1–30 subtoxic doses of suramin so that 23 of the guinea pigs died and 64 out of the total had lesions in the adrenals. Histologically degenerative changes were found in the cortex, often as bands; with repeated doses there was also general atrophy of the cortex caused by disappearance of cells. On the other hand, Frisch and Gardner (1958) could find no harmful effects of suramin on the adrenals of rats given 40 mg/kg every other day for 21 days, even though 6 out of 18 died during this treatment. Moreover, Talbott *et al.* (1940) question the importance of suramin in the aforementioned human cases, since they found changes of the blood suggesting adrenal insufficiency even in untreated cases of pemphigus. Also Goldzieher (1945) reported 6 cases of death from pemphigus with histological signs of severe organic damage in the adrenal cortex, but none of these patients had received suramin.

It will be noticed that all the workers just cited were concerned with pemphigus treated with high doses of suramin and that the much more numerous workers with trypanosomiasis and onchocerciasis have not reported adrenal lesions. Consequently, it seems unlikely that toxic damage to the adrenals is a serious risk during properly conducted suramin treatment. However, Anderson *et al.* (1976) mention that 4 out of 76 patients treated with four doses of 1 gm suramin for savanna onchocerciasis died 1–2 months later with nonspecific symptoms, especially pain on swallowing. If postmortem examinations could be obtained in such cases, it might be well to pay special attention to the adrenal glands.

VI. Antiparasitic Action

The lethal effect of suramin on filariae and on trypanosomes probably depends fundamentally on a similar intracellular reaction, but for historical and experimental reasons almost all of the investigations have been made on the antitrypanosomal action.

A. Action on Trypanosomes

The mode of action of suramin on trypanosomes is still obscure. It has been reviewed by Hawking (1963a), Williamson (1970), and Williamson *et al.* (1975). Briefly, suramin is not trypanocidal *in vitro* except in unbiological concentrations of 1 mg/ml at 37°C for 24 hours (Hawking, 1939). The growth *in vitro* of *Crithidia* or *Trypanosoma rhodesiense* at 26°C was prevented by concentrations greater than 0.1 mg/ml (Hawking, 1963b). On the other hand, a minute dose of 0.03 mg/100 gm is very effective in mice after a delay of more than 24 hours. The action is probably due to the unchanged suramin itself and not to any active metabolite. When trypanosomes are exposed to suramin *in vitro* or *in vivo*, only small (but significant) amounts of drug can subsequently be extracted from them; nevertheless, some fixation of drug must occur, because exposure of trypanosomes to suramin greatly reduces their power to infect other mice, i.e., further multiplication of the trypanosomes is diminished or abolished. Probably, suramin is initially bound to a primary site on the trypanosome from which it can be washed off up to 1 hour (reversing the loss of infectivity) and then, later, it is more firmly bound to a secondary site from which it cannot be washed and where it produced its main action (Hawking, 1939). If mice infected with *Trypanosoma evansi* are given a minimal effective dose of suramin i.p. (0.03 mg/100 mg), the trypanosomes may continue to divide 7 times during the next 35 hours; then their number remains stationary for perhaps 30 hours, after which their number rapidly diminishes to zero (Hawking and Sen, 1960). During the stationary phase, the chief morphological changes are (*a*) the percentage of dividing forms is diminished, (*b*) there are many large multinuclear forms suggesting that division of the cytoplasm has been inhibited more than that of the nucleus, and (*c*) the cytoplasm contains many basophilic inclusion bodies (which presumably are the same as the vacuolated lysosomes seen with the electron microscope, as described in Section VI,A,3).

This delayed action of suramin might be explained in general terms by an hypothesis that somehow suramin interferes slightly with the RNA–DNA replication mechanism and that each replication becomes more imperfect until the mechanism is brought to a halt by the accumulation of errors. The same delayed inhibition of cell multiplication is produced by homidium and by quinapyramine, but the site of interference with the RNA–DNA system might well be different.

It has been suggested by von Jancsó and von Jancsó (1934) that, besides its direct action, suramin also acts like an opsonin so that slightly damaged trypanosomes are removed from the circulation by the phagocytes of the reticuloendothelial system. This may well occur to some extent, but there is still a latent period of over 24 hours before phagocytosis begins; this latent period would not occur with an opsonin for bacteria.

1. *Biochemistry of RNA and DNA*

If it is explained in simple terms, the genetics of cells are determined by DNA that stores the codified information, and this information is transferred to the rest of the cell (to make enzymes, proteins, etc.) via RNA of which these are various forms (soluble RNA, ribosome RNA, transfer RNA, messenger RNA, etc.). Ribonucleic acid is synthesized from nucleotide triphosphates, such as AMP and ATP, by enzymes (RNA polymerase) that are dependent on DNA as a template to organize the sequence in which the different nucleotides are built into the chain. The DNA can come either from the nucleus or from the kinetoplast of the trypanosome. These enzymes, polymerases, are specifically inhibited by certain trypanocidal compounds, such as homidium, suramin, and quinapyramine, that act by *preventing multiplication* of trypanosomes rather than by directly *killing* them as arsenicals do. Suramin and homidium are particularly powerful against RNA polymerases. Homidium, which has a small basic molecule, probably acts by combining with the DNA template and thus destroying its pattern for synthesis of RNA. Suramin with a large acidic molecule probably acts on the enzyme itself, perhaps combining with or covering over the "active center" (Hill and Bonilla, 1974).

2. *Experimental Evidence*

In support of the foregoing hypothesis, various pieces of experimental evidence can be quoted.

A simple biochemical system in the ribosomes of *Crithidia fasciculata* has been described by Kahan *et al.* (1968) and Lantz *et al.* (1968) who studied the incorporation of leucine-^{14}C into protein. The system required a soluble enzyme (leucyl–sRNA synthetase, M.W. 105,000) together with ATP, a regenerating system, and guanosine triphosphate. This system was inhibited by suramin, quinapyramine, and pentamidine in concentrations of 0.25 to 0.5 m*M*. (All these drugs inhibit the multiplication of trypanosomes.) They inhibited both leucyl–sRNA synthetase (pentamidine most active) and the incorporation of leucyl-^{14}C–sRNA into protein (suramin most active), i.e., they inhibited both the charging system and the transfer system. Kahan *et al.* concluded that the loss of functional activity produced by the drugs resulted from alterations in the secondary structure of the transfer RNAs.

3. *Morphology by Electron Microscope*

The early morphological changes in trypanosomes produced within 5 to 6 hours by suramin and other trypanocidal drugs have been studied with the electron microscope by Macadam and Williamson (1974). (This period may have been too short for the delayed action of suramin to manifest itself.) During the first 6 hours, suramin produced no visible change in the nucleus, nucleolus, or kinetoplast. The main changes were in the ribosomes and the lysosomes.

a. Ribosomes. The ribosomes (which consist mostly of RNA) were reduced in number both generally and focally; in some parts they were aggregated together; and their normal aspect and normal polysomal configuration were lost. The same changes were also produced by arsenicals.

Suramin is known to inhibit RNA polymerase in high dilution, $10^{-5}\,M$ (Waring, 1965; Hill and Bonilla, 1974). The disruption of ribosomes (seen by electron microscopy) suggests that (*a*) ribosomal synthesis of protein must be inactivated and (*b*) this inactivation may be due to impaired synthesis of ribosomal RNA by inhibition of RNA polymerase.

Because there is no alteration of the nucleolus (which is composed largely of RNA) and no microgranules are produced during the 6-hour observation period, the ribosomal lesions may be due to suramin blocking the site on ribosomes that combines with messenger RNA. [This site for mRNA is blocked in cell-free preparations of *Escherichia coli* by large polyanionic molecules such as polyvinyl sulfate, which is analogous in many ways to the polysulfonic acid structure of suramin (Shinozawa *et al.*, 1968).] Trypanosomes made resistant to suramin become hypersensitive to puromycin, which acts on the anabolism of nucleotides, and this also suggests that a prime action of suramin is on ribosomes (Williamson, 1965).

The biochemical evidence about suramin seems to be more plentiful for RNA enzymes than for DNA ones, but this may partly be due to RNA enzymes being easier to investigate than DNA ones. The biological evidence (namely, slowing down of cell division after a latent period of up to seven divisions) points rather to DNA as the fundamental site of lesion. In any case, suramin may well interfere with the DNA–RNA system at many different places, and the demonstration of interference at one particular place does not prove that there may not be interference at other, even more important places.

b. Lysosomes. Suramin also produced large numbers of vacuolated lysosomes. Suramin is known to bind strongly to protein, and thus pinocytosis and localization in lysosomes would be facilitated. Suramin is also known to inactivate the enzymes of lysosomes, and this inactivation would explain the vacuolated lysosomes seen by electron microscopy. On the other hand, most of the compounds studied by Macadam and Williamson (1974) produced vacuolated lysosomes in trypanosomes, so this lysosome phenomenon may well be a general one with little specific significance for suramin.

4. *Note about Cell Division*

Because light microscopy shows many multinucleated trypanosomes, the inhibition by suramin of cell multiplication may act more powerfully or earlier on the cytoplasm than on the nucleus. If streptococci or clostridia are cultivated in the presence of suramin, they grow in long chains instead of breaking up into separate organisms. This happens because the subdivision of the chains into separate organisms depends on an enzyme resembling lysozyme and this enzyme (like many others) is inhibited by suramin (Lominski *et al.*, 1958; Shaikh and Lominski, 1975). It may be that division of the cytoplasm of trypanosomes is also partially dependent on a similar enzyme (liable to be inhibited by suramin). In that case, failure of cell division after suramin would be a side effect, not closely related to the specific action on the RNA and DNA metabolism leading to the death of the parasite.

5. *Other Evidence*

Further examples of suramin interfering with cell division are provided by seedlings of *Vicia faba* and by sea urchin eggs. If young roots of *V. faba* are exposed for 6 hours to 0.5% suramin they cease to show cell division, but they recover if the suramin is washed out of them. The chromosome patterns are distorted showing chromosome bridges and fragmentation, and the cells show multiple nuclei and abnormal mitotic figures (Milovidov, 1961). If sea urchin eggs, *Paracentrotus lividus* or *Sphaerechinus granularis*, are exposed to suramin at a concentration of 1/1000 just before or just after fertilization with sperms, many multipolar mitoses develop so that the eggs contain many nuclei but there is no division into single blastomeres; later the eggs die (Jirovec, 1943a,b). (If ripe eggs are mixed with sperms in seawater containing suramin 1/50–1/5000, the sperms cluster round the eggs but no fertilization occurs; this may be due to suramin stabilizing the outer cell membranes.) In both these examples, the concentrations of suramin is very high; nevertheless, they are interesting as further illustrations of suramin interfering with cell division.

By contrast, another action of suramin on *Paracentrotus* eggs is probably nonspecific, as it is stronger with dyes containing sulfonic acid groups. If fertilized eggs are soaked in suramin 1/100–1/1000, the development of ectoderm is favored against that of mesoentoderm and hatching is delayed. But this action is shown 10–100 times more strongly by Chlorazol sky blue and by Evans blue, respectively (and also by zinc). It is probably due to the polysulfonic acid structure and not to the specifically trypanocidal one (Lallier, 1958).

B. Action on Filariae

1. *Adult Worms*

a. Litomosoides carinii. It has usually been reported that suramin had no action upon *L. carinii* in cotton rats, but this conclusion was due to the period of observation being only 2 weeks, which is too short. Lämmler *et al.* (1971b) showed that, if 40 mg/kg, s.c., was given on five successive days to infected *Mastomys natalensis*, all the adult worms were killed, provided the animals were observed for 6 weeks. (The same result was achieved with double this dose in cotton rats; Lämmler and Herzog, 1974.) The worms started to die after 5 weeks, and they were all dead by 6 weeks from the beginning of treatment. In the first 28 days, squash preparations showed no change in the embryos or microfilariae of the uterus, but after this time the production of microfilariae ceased and the embryos were deformed and degenerated. After 42 days the dead worms were embedded in masses of fibrin. The antifilarial reaction of suramin is remarkable in that, although the treatment ceased after 5 days, the worms did not begin to die until 4 to 5 weeks later.

b. Onchocerca volvulus. Suramin kills the adult worms, as was first discovered by Van Hoof *et al.* (1947), this being the first indication of the antifilarial activity of the compound. When suramin is given in the usual dosage of 1 gm per week, the worms begin to die after the fourth or fifth dose at which time allergic reactions begin to appear, as described in the following. This delay of death until 5 weeks after the beginning of treatment is similar to what happens with *L. carinii*. The lethal action is exerted first on the female worms, whereas the male worms stay alive and motile much longer. This sex difference is not specific for suramin, but occurs with most antifilarial drugs, probably because male worms have a less active metabolism than females. Apparently, a plasma concentration of suramin greater than 10 mg/100 ml should be maintained for about 2 weeks in order to ensure the death of all the adult female worms (Duke, 1968a). The death of the worms is accompanied by general and local inflammatory reactions, which is discussed in detail in the following. Ashburn *et al.* (1949) made histological examinations of 34 nodules from 21 patients who had been treated with suramin in a total dose of 0.14 gm/kg or more. In nodules that were removed 60 days after treatment, the contents of the uteri had undergone necrosis or there were only normal or degenerating ova with no microfilariae. In nodules excised after longer periods, the degeneration was more complete.

c. Wuchereria bancrofti. In Tahiti, Thooris (1956) treated 20 patients and found that 1 year later the number of microfilariae was reduced to 5% of its original number; so apparently suramin kills the adult worms and the microfilariae gradually die out (see Section VII,B,3).

d. Other Filariae. The action of suramin on *Loa loa, Dipetalonema perstans*, or *Dirofilaria immitis* is not known. It would be valuable to make observations when opportunity occurred. In particular observations should be made on patients treated with suramin for onchocerciasis who may also be infected with *Dipetalonema perstans. Dipetalonema witeae* is usually supposed to be insensitive, but I have found no actual references, and the period of observation might have been too short.

2. *Microfilariae*

Suramin seems to have little action on microfilariae of *Onchocerca* or other filariae, and, after 6 weeks of treatment, when the adult worms have been killed, great numbers of microfilariae remain. The natural life of *Onchocerca* is probably well over 10 months, so that even when their replenishment is cut off, it takes up to 18 months for them to dwindle and disappear. On the other hand, there is considerable evidence that, after suramin treatment, many of the microfilariae are killed much earlier than this, especially round about the sixth week after the beginning of treatment. The pronounced dermatological reactions (pruritus, urticaria, etc.) suggest that many of the microfilariae in the skin have died as a result of treatment. Duke (1968a) calculated that 2 weeks after a total dose of 9.5 gm given during 10 weeks, 92% of the microfilariae in the skin had been removed. According to the hypothesis developed in Section VI,B,5 that suramin acts by interference with cell division, such death of microfilariae would be difficult to explain, since microfilariae have no dividing cells. It may be that when suramin kills the adult worms, it provokes such a strong antifilarial immunological reaction that many of the microfilariae are also attacked by antibodies, etc., even though they have not been directly affected by the compound.

3. *Immature Worms*

a. Litomosoides carinii. Suramin has a pronounced action upon all immature stages of *L. carinii* in *M. natalensis* (Lämmler and Hertzog, 1974; Lämmler and Wolf, 1977). When given subcutaneously at 40 mg/kg/day for 5 days, beginning on the seventh, fourteenth, or twenty-eighth day after infection, it completely prevented the development of infection. A good but incomplete prophylactic action was exerted if the treatment was given for 5 days directly after the infection. Lower doses were not effective. These findings were confirmed by Wolf (1976); as often happens, female worms were more susceptible than males. The least susceptible period was 2–6 days after infection, i.e., the third stage of the larvae.

b. Onchocerca volvulus. In 2 human volunteers, studied earlier by Duke (1968c), the results were less encouraging. The men were given 1 gm weekly for 7 or 5 weeks prior to inoculation and the suramin blood concentration at the time of inoculating infective larvae would be more than 15 mg/100 ml. Thirty-five or 50 infective larvae were inoculated intradermally, and 4–5 days later biopsies were taken at the site of inoculation. In one man, 2 live and 1 dead parasites were found (? slight prophylaxis) and in the other man, no larvae were found; apparently all the larvae had moved away and it was assumed that no prophylaxis had occurred. It may be noted that Wolf (1976) has found that after inoculation of *L. carinii* larvae the first 2–6 days are the times of least susceptibility; furthermore, since suramin acts so slowly on adult worms (6 weeks), the observation period of 4 to 5 days was too short to be significant.

In chimpanzees, however, which could be studied more exhaustively, suramin prevented the development of infection. Duke (1974) inoculated 2 chimpanzees with 750–860 infective larvae during a 12-month period. Treatment was started 2 weeks after the last inoculation and was given as 17 or 21 mg/kg, respectively, weekly for 8 weeks. In one chimpanzee, no microfilariae could be found in the skin during a 30-month period; the other chimpanzee was autopsied 4 weeks after the last treatment, and contained only two bundles of dead worms.

4. *Microfilariae Developing in Vectors*

The action of suramin on *L. carinii* developing in mites has apparently not been investigated. With *O. volvulus,* Duke (1968b) found that when *Simulium* was fed on patients with serum concentrations of 10 to 14 mg suramin per 100 ml, development of the microfilariae was not prevented. Later after the fifth to seventh dose of suramin, although some microfilariae were ingested by the vectors, they did not develop in them. Apparently, the action of suramin was exerted on the microfilariae in the man rather than in the *Simulium*.

5. *Mode of Action on Filariae*

Our knowledge of the action of suramin is incomplete, and experimentation with *Onchocerca* is difficult. Its effect is exerted only on the adult worms or on the immature forms developing in the vertebrate host. The most remarkable feature of its action is its extreme slowness. During a course of treatment for onchocerciasis, the worms do not begin to die until after 4 to 5 weeks; and when *L. carinii* is exposed to suramin for 5 days *in vivo*, the worms do not die until 5 weeks after the end of treatment. This long delay before the death of filarial worms forms a remarkable analogy with the long delay (of seven cell divisions) before the death of trypanosomes takes place. With such a complicated chemical structure as suramin, it seems most likely that the antitrypanosomal and the antifilarial actions both depend on the same chemical configuration and, ultimately, on interference with the same biochemical processes in the parasites. Accordingly the following hypothetical account of the probable mode of antifilarial action is put forward.

1. Suramin combines with the filarial worm. Some combination is essential for any drug action. In view of the large molecular size, suramin probably penetrates by mouth and intestine rather than through the cuticle. The amount of drug fixed in this way is probably limited. It should be investigated using radioactive suramin and *L. carinii* in *Mastomys*. Estimations should be made of the concentration of drug inside the female and male worms compared with that in the plasma of the host; and radioautography should be employed to determine which part of the worm contains the most drug. It is anticipated that it will be located in the gonads.

2. By analogy with trypanosomes, suramin probably acts by interference with cell multiplication. In adult nematodes, most of the body cells do not multiply—it is only the gonad cells that continue active multiplication. Therefore special morphological study should be made of the developing oocytes and of the corresponding male cells at weekly intervals after the first day of treatment (*L. carinii* in *Mastomys*). For this purpose the technique of examination of flattened living cells by phase contrast, as described by Taylor and Terry (1960), would be advantageous. It is postulated that suramin progressively deranges the multiplication of these cells (? by inhibition of RNA or DNA polymerase) so that after a delay the cells of the gonads are killed.

3. It would be interesting to investigate whether the action of suramin on *L. carinii* in *Mastomys* is potentiated by puromycin (see action of puromycin on drug-resistant trypanosomes, Section VI,A,3,a). If this were so, a combination of suramin plus puromycin might be valuable for human onchocerciasis.

6. *Possible Antifilarial Action of Homidium and Similar Compounds*

As described above, suramin is a very effective compound for killing the adult worms of *Onchocerca* and of *Litomosoides,* but its lethal action is not manifested until 5 weeks after the beginning of treatment. Further, suramin is also effective in killing trypanosomes but again its lethal action is not manifested until after a latent period of seven trypanosome divisions. It seems to act not by directly killing the trypanosomes but by disrupting and ultimately preventing cell division. It may, therefore, be pointed out that certain other trypanocidal compounds, namely, phenanthridinium compounds (e.g., homidium) and quinapyramine, also have the same type of action on trypanosomes, that is, inhibition of cell division. Homidium is also known to be as active as suramin in inhibiting enzymes concerned with RNA and DNA metabolism (see Section VI,A,1). In view of all this, it is strongly recommended that further investigations should be actively undertaken on the antifilarial action of phenanthridiums (especially homidium), of quinapyramine, and of similar compounds. For the properties of these substances, see Hawking (1963a) and Williamson (1970). Two phenanthridinium compounds, namely dimidium and 7-amino-9-*p*-aminophenyl-10-methylphenanthridinium were found by Sewell and Hawking (1950) to be active on *Litomosoides*; in fact, they were much more active than suramin according to the technique used by these workers, which involved only 2 weeks of observation. Recently, preliminary experiments (not yet published) have been carried out by Dr. M. J. Worms and the author on *Litomosoides* in cotton rats: the compound is given by injection on 5 consecutive days and the rats are killed for examination after 40 to 60 days. In these circumstances, homidium, 5 mg/kg, killed all or many of the female worms but not the male ones; 10 mg/kg killed practically all the female worms but, in 1 of the 2 rats at this dose, the male worms survived. These results on the female worms are almost as good as those obtained with suramin at 40 mg/kg. Preliminary results with isometamidium (2 mg/kg, i.m.) and Berenil (20 mg/kg, s.c.) were disappointing: no antifilarial action was found. Quinapyramine, 5 mg/kg s.c., had no action in one rat but, in another, it killed 20 out of 22 female worms. Further investigation of homidium (and possibly of quinapyramine) is urgently needed.

VII. Therapeutic Use

A. Against Trypanosomes

1. *Clinical and Veterinary Use*

Clinically, suramin was long (1925–1950) the only effective treatment for Rhodesian sleeping sickness, and it is still the standard remedy although it has been supplemented by the arsenical, melarsoprol. It is very effective in curing patients before the nervous system is involved; but after this has happened it cannot produce a permanent cure because it does not penetrate into the brain. It is used extensively for the early stages of *gambiense* sleeping sickness (in combination with arsenicals and other compounds). The course of treatment recommended by Apted (1970) for Rhodesian sleeping sickness in Tanzania is 0.2 gm, i.v., as an initial test dose and then 1 gm, i.v., on days 1, 3, 6, 14, and 21. This course quickly builds up a high concentration in the blood and enables the treatment to be completed in 3 weeks. About 10% of patients fail to maintain a high concentration in the blood, with resultant poor therapeutic results. It is desirable to check the blood concentrations by chemical estimation, when this is possible.

In veterinary practice, suramin has been used extensively for *Trypanosoma brucei* infections in horses and other animals and for *T. evansi* in camels (Sudan) or cattle.

2. *Suramin Drug Resistance of Trypanosomes*

In clinical practice, drug resistance to suramin is unknown. In the laboratory, trypanosomes can be made suramin-resistant, but the process takes much longer than with arsenicals. On repeated passage through mice, the resistance is gradually lost in about 6 months. Trypanosomes made resistant to suramin may become hypersensitive to puromycin and to the aminonucleoside of puromycin (Williamson, 1965) that interfere with nucleic acids or nucleoprotein synthesis.

3. *Suramin Complexes*

Suramin (which has six acidic groups) combines with basic compounds such as pentamidine and homidium to give insoluble complexes that are less toxic than the parent compound. They are deposited at the site of injection and are slowly absorbed, producing prophylaxis against trypanosomes over long periods. These complexes were introduced by Williamson and Desowitz (1956) and Desowitz (1957) for the prevention of infection with *Trypanosoma congolense* and *Trypanosoma vivax* in cattle. Thus, when 10 mg/kg homidium content was injected, intramuscularly, homidium suraminate gave protection for 13 months. In principle, these compounds were promising, but in actual practice they proved to have disadvantages because they caused irritation and local toxicity at the site of intramuscular injection; if sloughing occurred, the depot of drug and its protective action were lost.

B. Against Onchocerciasis

Accounts of the use of suramin for the treatment of onchocerciasis have been given by Ashburn *et al.* (1949), Burch (1949), Wanson (1950), Burch and Ashburn (1951), Sarkies (1952), Nelson (1955), Satti and Kirk (1957), and many other authors quoted below.

The problem differs according to whether it concerns individual patients under close medical supervision or whether it concerns large numbers of subjects under field conditions.

The clinical results in each case may be considered from three aspects: (1) the effect on the worms (it usually kills the adult worms but leaves many microfilariae alive); (2) the direct toxic effects of suramin on the host (these have been considered in Section V); and (3) the inflammatory reactions provoked the death of the filariae (these may be pronounced, especially in North Cameroon).

The reactions to suramin are similar to those provoked by diethylcarbamazine, but they are much later in appearing (usually about the sixth week) and they are more prolonged and less severe (in keeping with the more gradual liberation of filarial protein). After the fifth weekly dose or sometimes after the fourth dose, there may be erythematous and pruritic eruptions; there may be violent prurigo of parts of the skin that harbor microfilariae; there may be conjunctivitis and photophobia. There may be fever for a few days to 2 weeks, during which the temperature may rise to 39°–40°C. There may be pains in the joints; violent pain and stiffness sometimes develop in the hip joints, suggesting death of worms localized there (see also Sections V,B,4 and 5 and VII,B,2). One of the earliest complications is iritis, which sometimes appears after the second or third dose.

1. *Treatment of Individual Patients*

Duke and Anderson (1972) recommend an initial dose of 0.1 to 0.2 gm to test for a rare idiosyncrasy which may produce sudden collapse; then 1 gm intravenously weekly per adult of 60 kg weight to a total dose of 6 gm. Before each dose the urine should be tested for albuminuria. Light albuminuria can be disregarded, but heavy albuminuria with many casts and/or an ill-looking patient indicate postponement or cessation of treatment. Severe reactions can usually be controlled by stopping the drug and giving betamethasone, 1 mg 3 times a day, for several days and then tailing off.

At the end of this suramin treatment the adult female worms should be moribund, but there will still be microfilariae in the skin. Three weeks after the last dose of suramin, a 3-day course of diethylcarbamazine (200 mg twice daily) should be given to destroy them. Usually this produces a mild onchocercal reaction, in which case, it should be repeated every 3 weeks until no reaction occurs.

Relation of Dosage to Effect and Toxicity. Duke (1968a) investigated the relations among the dosage schedule, the therapeutic effect, and the toxicity. Briefly, a dose of 1 gm/week, totalling 5–6 gm suramin, was sufficient to kill all the adult worms, and total doses of 7.5, 8.5, or 9.5 gm offered no therapeutic advantages, and might be more toxic. Doses totalling 4.1 gm were on the border line of effectiveness, but in some patients they did not kill all the worms. Doses of 0.5 gm/week for 7 to 8 weeks were less effective in killing all the worms, and the clinical complications were not reduced in proportion to the dose, so that this course was not recommended. Doses of 0.5 gm given daily to a total of 2.7 gm during 5 days were effective but were very poorly tolerated and could not be recommended for general use. Doses of 0.25 gm weekly for 8 weeks had very little action on the worms. Apparently, it is necessary to maintain a plasma concentration of at least 10 mg/100 ml for 1 to 2 weeks in order to kill all the adult worms.

These findings are very valuable, but it would be desirable to make further investigations to determine more closely the dosage schedule that gives the optimum ratio between therapeutic response and toxicity. For a fatal infection such as trypanosomiasis, the therapeutic response must be complete (i.e., every trypanosome must be killed); and to achieve this result, the risk of a few deaths from toxicity can be tolerated. For a nonfatal infection, such as onchocerciasis, the toxicity must be low with no risk of death but an incomplete therapeutic response (i.e. the survival of a few worms) can be tolerated. Because patients vary in the extent to which they retain suramin in their plasma, it would be desirable to supplement such investigations by estimations of the plasma concentrations. The optimum dosage schedule might well differ from one geographical area to another, according to the intensity of infection and the severity of the reactions.

Further, investigations should also be made on the optimum ratio between the intensity of treatment and its duration. The lower the intensity the less would be the toxicity. On the other hand, Duke (1968a) showed that a total dosage of 2.7 gm suramin, given in daily doses over 5 days, to patients infected with *Onchocerca* produced a more marked effect on the parasite than when the same total dose was given at weekly intervals over 5 weeks. Likewise 8 weekly doses of 0.25 gm in adult males produced little or no detectable effect on the worms.

2. *Large-Scale Treatment*

The employment of suramin on a wide scale in heavily infected areas is controversial. In Mexico it is considered too dangerous and it is not used at all. On the other hand, in Venezuela (Rivas *et al.*, 1965), Ghana (Conran and Waddy, 1959), and Uganda (Cherry, 1960), it has been used widely and successfully without significant numbers of dangerous ill effects. A pilot trial by Picq *et al.* (1974, p. 192) also gave good results with no ill effects.

In Venezuela, where onchocercal infection may be relatively light, Gonzalez Guerra *et al.* (1964) and Rivas *et al.* (1965) treated 3719 patients, mostly with a total dose of 4.5 gm (given as 0.5 gm and then 1 gm weekly per 50 kg body weight). They excluded patients with persistent albuminuria, hypertension, general bad condition, or marked anemia. Twelve to twenty-four months later, no microfilariae could be found in the skin of 96 to 100% of those patients who had received over 4.5 gm suramin. There were three grave nonfatal accidents (2 exfoliative dermatitis and 1 generalized long-lasting prostration) and one death due to cerebrovascular accident and not due to suramin. On the other hand, 34% of the patients experienced minor reactions (especially pruritus, urticaria, palmar-plantar edema, fever, headache, and pains in the joints) which were most numerous after the third and fourth injections; these reactions were not dangerous but they were troublesome and caused many patients to stop treatment. They were relieved by dexamethasone and antihistamines. In a later report, Convit (1974) states that 26,963 cases have now been treated in the field without any deaths due to treatment. The total dose was 5–6 gm during 5 to 6 weeks. Since the beginning of 1974, patients who still have microfilariae in the skin 4 weeks after finishing suramin treatment, have been given diethylcarbamazine, 200 mg daily for 3 days.

In the West Nile province of Uganda, Nelson (1955) treated 56 patients. After treatment, 8 out of 41 patients were free from microfilariae. There were many minor toxic effects especially skin eruptions after the fourth or fifth dose, and he considered that suramin treatment was not practical or acceptable unless under close medical supervision. By contrast, in the Jinja region of Uganda, Cherry (1960) treated 276 patients with apparently no ill effects. He recommended that further treatment with diethylcarbamazine should be given.

In North Cameroon, in patients heavily affected with savanna onchocerciasis, suramin (or any other effective antifilarial treatment) seems to cause many severe reactions (Anderson *et al.*, 1976). On the other hand, from their experience in Ghana, Conran and Waddy (1956) describe the partial return of sight in many blind patients (due to improvement of corneal opacities and cataracts) and the great relief from cessation of general pruritus.

Probably suramin should be given to all heavily infected patients with considerable pruritus or with danger of ocular complications, e.g., microfilariae in the skin of the head. Marked albuminuria, pregnancy, hypertension, anemia, or poor general condition would all be counterindications. The safety and acceptability would depend largely on how well the field staff were trained to select patients and to administer the injections.

3. *Wuchereria bancrofti*

It is often stated that suramin has no action on *W. bancrofti*, but this is incorrect. Thooris (1956) in Tahiti treated 20 patients who suffered from recurrent lymphangitis (average 2.9 attacks per month). At the end of treatment, the frequency of lymphangitis was reduced by 87% and 1 year later, by 74%. By the end of the year the microfilariae were gradually reduced to 5% of their original number. Because *W. bancrofti* respond so well to diethylcarbamazine, the action of suramin is not of practical importance, but these results show that suramin does act on the adult worms of other filariae besides *Onchocerca*.

C. In Treatment of Nonparasitic Diseases

In the past, suramin has been used to treat a variety of nonparasitic diseases. In these cases the action of suramin (if any) was probably due to its large polyacidic molecule rather than to its specific antiparasitic grouping.

1. *Angioneurotic Edema (Quinke's Disease)*

This is a hereditary condition due to lack of C1-esterase inhibitors that normally inhibit the first component of complement (C1). Accordingly, the complement system is too active, and pharmacologically potent substances, such as anaphylatoxin and kinin-like C2 fragments, tend to be set free, increasing the permeability of capillaries and producing the edema. Suramin is a powerful inhibitor of C1 activators and of many other components of complement so that the use of suramin is well justified scientifically (see Section IV,D). In actual practice, some patients appear to respond well; others give a poor response to suramin but respond better to other agents such as ϵ-aminocaproic acid or traxenic acid (Brackertz and Kueppers, 1973; Brackertz, 1974; Schulz, 1974; Eisen and Loveday, 1973; Fong and Good, 1972).

2. *Pemphigus and Other Conditions*

During the 1930s, suramin was used for treating pemphigus, frequently in very high doses, e.g., 10 gm in 19 days. According to Bolgert (1970), pemphigus can also be treated with quinacrine, Aureomycin, corticosteroids, or mercuric chloride. Mizonova (1969) treated 28 patients with suramin and corticosteroids and most of them improved. Senear Usher's syndrome is a special form of pemphigus (pemphigus foliaceus), and it has been treated with suramin in large doses (Samtsov, 1966; Terao, 1969). There seems, however, to be little scientific basis for the administration of suramin to pemphigus patients, and the multiplicity of other therapeutic agents suggests that it was not very effective and not specific. A modern "Textbook of Dermatology" (Rook *et al.*, 1968) recommends treatment with corticosteroids but does not mention suramin. Similarly, Moschella *et al.* (1975), in "Dermatology" do not mention suramin. It may be concluded that treatment of pemphigus with suramin is no longer justified. Dermatitis herpetiformis similarly has been treated with suramin in the past but the two recent textbooks of dermatology just cited do not mention it.

During the nineteen-thirties, even multiple sclerosis was treated with suramin—a treatment for which there was no justification except desperation because of the absence of any effective therapy.

Acknowledgements

This review of suramin, with special reference to its use for the treatment of onchocerciasis, was prepared in 1976 while I was holding a World Health Organization consultantship. Grateful acknowledgments are due many members of WHO for assistance, criticism, and advice; the WHO library staff for search of the literature and many other facilities; and Professor G. Lämmler for helpful comments. The opinions expressed here are the responsibility of the writer and do not involve WHO.

References

Anderson, J., Fuglsang, H., and Marshall, T. F. de C. (1976). *Tropenmed. Parasitol.* **27,** 279.

Apted, F. I. C. (1970). *In* "The African Trypanosomiases" (H. W. Mulligan, ed.), p. 684. Allen & Unwin, London.

Ashburn, L. L., Burch, T. A., and Brady, F. J. (1949). *Bol. Of. Sanit. Panam.* **28,** 1107.

Bacchi, C. J., Hutner, S. H., Ciaccio, E. I., and Marcus, S. M. (1968). *J. Protozool.* **15,** 576.

Bolgert, M. (1970). *Ann. Med. Interne* **121,** 399.

Boursnell, J. C., Dangerfield, W. G., and Wormall, A. (1939). *Biochem. J.* **33,** 81.

Brackertz, D (1974). *Schweiz. Med. Wochenschr.* **104,** 403.

Brackertz, D., and Kueppers, F. (1973). *Klin. Wochenschr.* **51,** 620.

Burch, T. A. (1949). *Bol. Of. Sanit. Panam.* **28,** 233.

Burch, T. A., and Ashburn, L. L. (1951). *Am. J. Trop. Med.* **31,** 617.

Buys, C. H., Elferink, M. G., Bouma, J. M., Gruber, M., and Nieuwenhuis, P. (1973). *J. Reticuloendothel. Soc.* **14,** 209.

Cherry, J.K. (1960). *East Afr. Med. J.,* **37,** 550.

Conran, O., and Waddy, B. (1956). *J. Trop. Med. Hyg.* **59,** 52.

Convit, J. (1974). *Sci. Publ., Pan Am. Health Organ.* **298,** 57.

D'Addabbo, A., Kallee, E., and Heinzel, W. (1961). *Acta Isot.* **1,** 227.

Dangerfield, W. G., Gaunt, W. E., and Wormall, A. (1938). *Biochem. J.* **32,** 59.

Davies, M., Lloyd, J. B., and Beck, F. (1971). *Biochem. J.* **121,** 21.

Desowitz, R. S. (1957). *Ann. Trop. Med. Parasitol.* **51,** 457.

Dewey, H. M., and Wormall, A. (1946). *Biochem. J.* **40,** 119.

Duke, B. O. L. (1968a). *Bull. W. H. O.* **39,** 157.

Duke, B. O. L. (1968b). *Bull. W. H. O.* **39,** 169.

Duke, B. O. L. (1968c). *Bull. W. H. O.* **39,** 179.

Duke, B. O. L. (1968d). *Bull. W. H. O.* **39,** 307.

Duke, B. O. L. (1968e). *Br. Med. J.* **4,** 301.

Duke, B. O. L. (1974). *Tropenmed. Parasitol.* **25,** 84.

Duke, B. O. L., and Anderson, J. (1972). *Trop. Doctor* **2,** 107.

Duncan, J. T., and Manson-Bahr, P. H. (1923). *Trans. R. Soc. Trop. Med.* **17,** 392.

Ehrlich, P., and Shiga, K. (1904). *Berl. Klin. Wochenschr.* **41,** 329 and 362.

Eisen, V., and Loveday, C. (1973). *Br. J. Pharmacol.* **49,** 678.

Fain, A. (1942). *Rev. Trav. Sci. Med. Congo Belge* **1,** 137.

Findlay, G. M. (1930). "Recent Advances in Chemotherapy." Churchill, London.

Findlay, G. M. (1950). "Recent Advances in Chemotherapy," 3rd ed., Vol. 1. Churchill, London.

Fong, J. S., and Good, R. A. (1972). *Clin. Exp. Immunol.* **10,** 127.

Fortes, P. A., Ellory, J. C., and Lew, V. L. (1973). *Biochim. Biophys. Acta* **318,** 262.

Fourneau, E., Tréfouel, J., Tréfouel, T. B., and Vallee, J. (1924). *Ann. Inst. Pasteur, Paris* **38,** 81.

Frisch, E., and Gardner, L. I. (1958). *Endocrinology* **63,** 500.

Fuglsang, H., and Anderson, J. (1974). *Sci. Publ., Pan. Am. Health Organ.* **298,** 54.

Gage, J. C., Rose, F. C., and Scott, M. (1948). *Biochem. J.* **42,** 574.

Gibson, D. W., Duke, B. O. L., and Connor, D. H. (1977). *Tropenmed. Parasitol.* **28,** 387.

Goldzieher, J. W. (1945). *Arch. Dermatol. Syph.* **52,** 369.

Gonzalez Guerra, L., Rasi, E., and Rivas, A. (1964). *Rev. Venez. Sanid. Asist. Soc.* **29,** 90.

Guimaraes, J. L., and Lourie, E. M. (1951). *Br. J. Pharmacol. Chemother.* **6,** 514.

Harding, R. D., and Hutchinson, M. P. (1948). *Trans. R. Soc. Trop. Med. Hyg.* **41,** 481.

Harris, A. F., Cotty, V. F., Barnett, L., and Seiman, A. (1969). *Arch. Int. Pharmacodyn. Ther.* **181,** 489.

Hart, P. D. (1968). *Science* **162,** 686.

Hart, P. D., and Young, M R. (1975). *Nature (London)* **256,** 47.

Hawking, F. (1939). *Ann. Trop. Med. Parasitol.* **33,** 13.

Hawking, F. (1940). *Trans. R. Soc. Trop. Med. Hyg.* **34,** 37.

Hawking, F.(1963a). *Exp. Chemother.* **1,** 129 and 893.

Hawking, F. (1963b). *Ann. Trop. Med. Parasitol.* **57,** 255.

Hawking, F., and Sen, A. B. (1960). *Brit. J. Pharmacol. Chemother.* **15,** 567.

Hill, G. C., and Bonilla, C. A. (1974). *J. Protozool.* **21**, 632.
Hill, G. C., and Hutner, S. H. (1968). *Exp. Parasitol.* **2**, 207.
Huethwohl. B., and Jahnchen, E. (1971). *Naunyn-Schmiedeberg's Arch. Pharmacol.* **270**, Suppl. 1, R66.
Humphreys, E. M., and Donaldson, L. (1941). *Am. J. Pathol.* **17**, 767.
Jaffe, J. J., McCormack, J. J., and Meymarian, E. (1972). *Biochem. Pharmacol.* **21**, 719.
Jirovec, O. (1943a). *Biochem. Z.* **314**, 265.
Jirovec, O. (1943b). *Biochem. Z.* **315**, 69.
Kahan, D., Zahalsky, A. C., and Hutner, S. H. (1968). *J. Protozool.* **15**, 385.
Kallee, E., and Hartenstein, H. (1960). *Nucl. Med.* **1**, 273.
Kaulla, K. N. V. (1963). *Proc. Soc. Exp. Biol. Med.* **114**, 153.
Kennedy, P., and Terry, S. (1972). *Trans. R. Soc. Trop. Med. Hyg.* **66**, 27.
Kleine, F. K., and Fischer, W. (1923). *Dtsch. Med. Wochenschr.* **49**, 1039.
Lallier, R. (1958). *Publ. Stn. Zool. Napoli* **30**, 185.
Lämmler, G., and Herzog, H. (1974). *Tropenmed. Parasitol.* **25**, 78.
Lämmler, G., and Wolf, E. (1977). *Tropenmed. Parasitol.* **28**, 205.
Lämmler, G., Herzog, H., and Schütze, H. R. (1971a). *Bull. W. H. O.* **44**, 757.
Lämmler, G., Herzog, H., and Schütze, H. R. (1971b). *Bull. W. H. O.* **44**, 765.
Lämmler, G., Grüner, D., and Zahner, H. (1975). *Z. Tropenmed. Parasitol.* **26**, 97.
Lantz, M., Kahan, D., and Zahalsy, A. C. (1968). *J. Protozool.* **15**, Suppl., 23.
Layton, D., and Azzi, A. (1974). *Biochem. Biophys. Res. Commun.* **59**, 322.
Lloyd, J. B., and Beck, F. (1969). *Biochem. J.* **115**, 32P.
Lominski, I., Cameron, J., and Wyllie, G. (1958). *Nature (London)* **181**, 1477.
Macadam, R. F., and Williamson, J. (1974). *Ann. Trop. Med. Parasitol.* **68**, 301.
Mahoney, L. J., and Barrie, H. J. (1950). *Br. Med. J.* **2**, 655.
Mayer, M., and Zeiss, H. (1922). *Arch. Schiffs- Trop.-Hyg.* **26**, 237.
Mercier-Parot, L., and Tuchmann-Duplessis, H. (1973). *C. R. Seances Soc. Biol. Ses Fil.* **167**, 1518.
Mesnil, F., and Nicolle, M. (1906). *Ann. Inst. Pasteur, Paris* **20**, 513.
Milovidov, P. (1961). *Planta* **57**, 455.
Mizonova, T. P. (1969). *Vestn. Dermatol. Venerol.* **43**, 64.
Moschella, S. L., Pillsbury, D. M., and Hurley, H. S. (1975). "Dermatology," pp. 462 and 1748. Saunders, Philadelphia, Pennsylvania.
Nelson, G. S. (1955). *East Afr. Med. J.* **32**, 413.
Nnochiri, E. (1964). *Trans. R. Soc. Trop. Med. Hyg.* **58**, 413.
Picq, S. S., Rolland, A., and Roux, J. (1974). *OCCGE Conf.* p. 192.
Riedel, H., and El-Dakhakhny, M. (1964). *Arzneim.-Forsch.* **14**, 1025.
Rivas, A., Gonzales, G., Zsogon, L., Rasi, E., and Convit, J. (1965).*Acta Med. Venez., Suppl.* p. 1.
Rodger, F. C. (1958). *Trans. R. Soc. Trop. Med. Hyg.* **52**, 462.
Rodnight, R. (1970). *Biochem. J.* **120**, 1.
Rook, A., Wilkinson, D. S., and Ebling, F. J. G. (1968). "Textbook of Dermatology," p. 1178. Blackwell, Oxford.
Samtsov, V. I. (1966). *Vestn. Dermatol. Venerol.* **40**, 74.
Sarkies, J. W. R. (1952). *Trans. R. Soc. Trop. Med. Hyg.* **46**, 435.
Satti, M. H., and Kirk, R. (1957). *Bull. W. H. O.* **16**, 531.
Schulz, K. H. (1974). *Hautarzt* **25**, 12.
Sewell, P., and Hawking, F. (1950). *Br. J. Pharmacol. Chemother.* **5**, 239.
Shaikh, M. R., and Lominski, I. (1975). *Zentralbl. Bakteriol., Parasitenkd., Infektionskr. Hyg., Abt. 1: Orig., Reihe A* **230**, 237.

Shinozawa, T., Yahara, I., and Imahori, K. (1968). *J. Mol. Biol.* **36,** 305.
Smeesters, C., and Jaques, P. J. (1968). *Proc. Int. Congr. Cell Biol., 12th, 1968* Excerpta Med. Found. Int. Congr. Ser. No. 166, Abstr. No. 143, p. 82.
Spinks, A. (1948). *Biochem. J.* **42,** 109.
Stoppani, A. O. M., and Brignone, J. A. (1957). *Arch. Biochem. Biophys.* **68,** 423.
Talbott, J. H., Lever, W. F., and Conzolazio, W. V. (1940). *J. Invest. Dermatol.* **3,** 31.
Taylor, A. E. R., and Terry, R. S. (1960). *Trans. R. Soc. Trop. Med. Hyg.* **54,** 33.
Terao, T. (1969). *Jpn. J. Dermatol.* **79,** 339.
Thoma, K., Ullmann, E., and Loos, P. (1967). *Arch. Pharm. (Weinheim, Ger.)* **300,** 577.
Thooris, G. C. (1956). *Bull. Soc. Pathol. Exot.* **49,** 311.
Tomlinson, C. C., and Cameron, O. J. (1938). *Arch. Dermatol. Syph.* **38,** 555.
Tuchmann-Duplessis, H., and Mercier-Parot, L. (1973). *C. R. Seances Soc. Biol. Ses Fil.* **167,** 1717.
Van Hoof, L., Henrard, C., Peel, E., and Wanson, M. (1947). Cited by Wanson (1950).
Vierthaler, R. W., and Boselli, A. (1939). *Arch. Schiffs- Trop.-Hyg.* **43,** 149.
von Jancso, N., and Jancso-Gabor, A. (1952). *Acta Physiol. Acad. Sci. Hung.* **3,** 537.
von Jancso, N., and von Jancso, H. (1934). *Zentralbl. Bakteriol., Parasitenkd. Infektionskr. Hyg., Abt. 1: Orig.* **132,** 257.
Wanson, M. (1950). *Ann. Soc. Belge Med. Trop.* **30,** 671.
Waring, M. J. (1965). *Mol. Pharmacol.* **1,** 1.
Wells, H. G., Humphreys, E. M., and Work, E. G. (1937). *J. Am. Med. Assoc.* **109,** 490.
Wesolowski, H., Olszewska, M., and Makowski, J. (1972). *Folia Biol. (Krakow)* **20,** 395.
Williamson, J. (1965). *Proc. Int. Congr. Protozool., 2nd, 1964* Excerpta Med. Found. Int. Congr. Ser. No. 91, Abstr. No. 77, p. 81.
Williamson, J. (1970). *In* "The African Trypanosomiases" (H. W. Mulligan, ed.), p. 125. Allen & Unwin, London.
Williamson, J., and Desowitz, R. S. (1956). *Nature (London)* **177,** 1074.
Williamson, J., Macadam, R. F., and Dixon, H. (1975). *Biochem. Pharmacol.* **24,** 147.
Wills, E. D., and Wormall, A. (1949). *Biochem. J.* **44,** xxxix.
Wilson, J., and Wormall, A. (1949). *Biochem. J.* **45,** 224.
Wolf, E. (1976). Inaug.-Dissertation d. Doktorgrades, Fachbereich, Vet. med. Justus Liebig-Universität, Giessen.
Wong, P. C., and Ma, L. (1963). *J. Trop. Med. Hyg.* **66,** 99.
Yesaiv, D. W., Wodinsky, I., Rogers, W. I., and Kensler, C. J. (1968). *Biochem. Pharmacol.* **17,** 305.

Subject Index

8 9 0 1 2 3 4 5